EATING
FOR THE
EIGHTIES

EATING
FOR THE
EIGHTIES

A COMPLETE GUIDE TO
VEGETARIAN NUTRITION

Janie Coulter Hartbarger

AND

Neil J. Hartbarger

THE SAUNDERS PRESS / SAUNDERS PAPERBACKS

W. B. Saunders Company
Philadelphia • London • Toronto

The Saunders Press/Saunders Paperbacks
W. B. Saunders Company
West Washington Square
Philadelphia, PA 19105

IN THE UNITED STATES
DISTRIBUTED TO THE TRADE BY
HOLT, RINEHART AND WINSTON
383 Madison Avenue
New York, New York 10017

IN CANADA
DISTRIBUTED BY
HOLT, RINEHART AND WINSTON
55 Horner Avenue
Toronto, Ontario
M8Z 4X6
Canada

Library of Congress Cataloging in Publication Data

Hartbarger, Janie Coulter, 1952-
  Eating for the eighties.

  Bibliography: p.
  Includes index.
  1. Vegetarianism. 2. Vegetarian cookery.
I. Hartbarger, Neil, joint author. II. Title.
TX392.H29   613.2'62   80-53187

W.B. Saunders Company ISBN: 0-7216-4549-6 paperback
                          0-7216-4550-X hardcover

Holt, Rinehart and Winston ISBN: 0-03-059076-0 paperback
                          0-03-059077-9 hardcover

Print Number 9 8 7 6 5 4 3 2 1

First Edition

For our families

Contents

PUTTING IT TOGETHER: FOUR EATING STYLES

SPECIAL CASES

Acknowledgments

Many thanks to

ALICIA CONKLIN
for being an excellent and, just as important, enthusiastic editor
DR. WILLIAM CASTELLI
for taking the time and interest to review our manuscript
JANE WILSON
for seeing us through from the beginning
WILLIAM GLADSTONE
for the initial opportunity
ALEX HERSHAFT, of Vegetarian Information Service,
for generosity and dedication to a cause
ILKA SHORE COOPER
for a patient ear and good leads
FRED COOPER (a beefo-porco-vegetarian)
for general good humor
M. C. TAYLOR
for helping to develop the weight-loss diet
PEGGY and BUDDY THORNTON, M. C. TAYLOR, and ILKA SHORE COOPER
for trying the diet
JUDITH M. COULTER
for loving support, no matter what
ELLIOTT COULTER
for general concern and office privileges
L. G. and L. B., two special friends

Capri M. Fillmore; Inez Murphy; Patricia Hausman of Center for Science in the Public Interest (CSPI); Vic Sussman; Lyn Dobrin of *Food Monitor;* Eleanor Williams of the University of Maryland; Ana L. Standard of the Cooperative Extension, White Plains, NY; Ruth N. Klippstein of Cornell University; Dr. John A. Scharffenberg; H. Jay and Freya Dinshah of the Vegan Society; Kathleen Jannaway of the Vegan Society of the United Kingdom; Marcia Pearson of the Seattle Vegetarian Society; David and Nikki Goldbeck; Dr. Basil M. Rifkind of the National Heart, Lung, and Blood Institute; Dr. Walter Troll of the New York University Medical Center; Dr. Doris Calloway of the University of California at Berkeley; Robin Hur; Dr. John H. Weisburger of the American Health Foundation; R. E. Newberry of the Food and Drug Administration; Frank Ray Rifkind of *Nutrition Health Review;* the Nutrition Department, Loma Linda University; Robert J. Avery, Jr., of the National Cancer Institute; Michael F. Jacobson of CSPI; Deborah Stapell-Schlosser of the United Fresh Fruit and Vegetable Association; Mary J. Carlson, R. D., of the National Live Stock and Meat Board; Jane Anderson of the American Meat Institute; Karen H. Brown of the Food Marketing Institute; Myrtle L. Brown of the Food and Nutrition Board; Odonna Mathews of Giant Food, Inc.; and the Nutrition Foundation

for their giving of precious time and information.

Foreword

We live, unfortunately, in a society that is in the middle of an epidemic, although most of us seem to be unaware of this fact. The disease that is sweeping our country is coronary heart disease —heart attack. In general, one in five men in the United States will develop a heart attack while he is still relatively young, in his forties or fifties, but certainly before reaching age 60. One in seventeen women will experience the same fate. The disease is not contagious like smallpox or measles; we don't leap out of the way when we pass these people at work or on the street. Yet the next time you are out walking, reflect on the fact that every time you pass five men and seventeen women, virtually anywhere in the United States, you have just brushed by one man and one woman destined to become early victims of heart attack.

Why do so many Americans develop this disease at so young an age? Finding an answer to this question is the objective of many medical investigations in this country. In the Framingham Heart Study we have followed a sampling of the population for 30 years, and have uncovered strong evidence of coronary heart disease developing in people with high blood cholesterol, high blood pressure, and a history of smoking cigarettes. By taking these measurements on people early in life, we have found it possible to predict, with great accuracy, which individuals are likely to become victims of premature heart attack.

Of course, two of these major risk factors are related to diet. If you consider that, in the vast majority of cases, a high cholesterol level is almost a necessary precondition of heart attack, it becomes increasingly important to understand what factors affect our serum cholesterols (the amount of cholesterol in the blood).

In about five percent of the population genetics plays a very important role in serum cholesterol levels. These people have inherited a tendency to manufacture blood cholesterols at an alarming rate—a tendency that is greatly aided by eating the typical, high-cholesterol American diet. This doesn't mean that the genetic factor doesn't also affect the rest of us. If I put everyone on the same standard American diet, we would all have different cholesterol values, at a rather high level, and we would all be part of the American epidemic of cardiovascular disease. Half of us would die from this disease, and another 20 percent would have some of the basic lesions in our blood vessels, even though we died of something else. However, if I put all of us on a diet with less animal fats and cholesterol, we would all still have different cholesterols, but at a much lower level, and few of us would ever have a heart attack.

A major problem we face in medicine today is that most people do not know what an ideal level of blood cholesterol should be. Many people (even doctors) feel that if your cholesterol is average you are normal. Too few people realize that an average American cholesterol level (about 210–230 mg%*) is a dangerously high level indeed. As we have discovered from studying the natural history of this disease as it occurs in America and elsewhere in the world, a safe cholesterol level is one around 150–160 mg%. Very few Americans over age 30 (fewer than five percent) have such a value. Most of the heart attacks in America develop in people whose blood cholesterols are between 230–250 mg%, levels few doctors consider serious enough to treat. Yet when we were teenagers most of us had a cholesterol around 150–160 mg%.

How can we get people in this country to lower their cholesterol in a safe and nutritious way? Well, there's certainly no lack of debate about that! Among the most recent assertions have been those of vegetarians who tell us that such levels can be attained on vegetarian diets. Many people—especially in orthodox nutrition circles—are afraid of vegetarian diets. Not enough protein, they say. Not enough vitamin B12. Besides, everyone knows that vegetarians are the nuts among the berries.

This book should serve as an introduction to many of the arguments about vegetarianism. It is specially suited to debate many of these issues. It cannot, of course, give a definitive scientific answer to the questions posed. Nutritional research in this

*milligrams per centiliter

country has lagged so far behind where it should be, that such answers will not be seen for a long time.

We are only recently beginning to question whether atherosclerosis, the basic process that blocks our blood vessels with cholesterol and elastic tissue deposits, is reversible. That someone who develops atherosclerosis can either let the process continue or try to reverse it is intriguing to many. It should be pointed out here that, in virtually all instances where reversibility occurs, the level of cholesterol attained is in the vicinity of 150–160 mg%. Such a level is attainable in humans, without the aid of drugs, practically only in people who have gone largely vegetarian.

Put this together with the fact that societies that practice vegetarianism, like the Seventh Day Adventists, outlive the rest of us and have lower cancer rates as well, and you will begin to see that very great issues are at stake.

Finally, a word of caution: We live in imperfect times; this is a book, not a bible. It should serve to enlarge your thinking in this field, but not everything printed here is gospel. It is an excellent resource to stimulate all of us about these issues—and, I hope, to separate what is true from what is untrue.

WILLIAM P. CASTELLI, M.D.
Medical Director
Framingham Heart Study
Department of Health and
    Human Services

January 9, 1981
Framingham, Massachusetts

1
Why We Eat What We Eat

*E*ating is a reflexive act for most people—it involves very little conscious decision beyond looking into the refrigerator to see what's handy. Life has changed considerably since obtaining and eating food occupied most of people's waking hours. Through the centuries our world has become much more complex, and a greater portion of our time is now devoted to other things—witness the relatively recent growth of frozen and convenience foods and fast-food restaurants.

Of course, we don't ignore food entirely. It still has important functions in our society. We share food at happy (or unhappy) occasions, and its preparation gives us an opportunity to demonstrate our artistic skills. Food gives intense sensory pleasure. We learned this as babies, and as adults we may try to recall the childhood comfort and security we derived from eating.

Modern society, however, has tended to blind us to the most important function of food—nourishing our bodies. We could live without the physical pleasure, the emotional gratification, the social bonds, and the ego-building attention food can provide us, but we can't live without the nourishment. Nevertheless, we continue to act as though this were its least important feature; the other functions have overshadowed the biological one, and hedonism seems to have become the guiding principle of our national diet. Unfortunately, our enjoyment of eating is coupled with a notable lack of good taste. Our present national culture, including our eating traditions, developed during history's period of most rapid change in agriculture, technology, transportation, and communication, so we have no long-standing tradition of good eating on which to base our national taste. If we could tell good

1

food from poor by taste alone, our pleasure-seeking might at least guide us toward a decent diet. But ask any American child to name her favorite food, and more often than not the answer will be a Milky Way bar or a McDonald's hamburger or a bag of potato chips and a Coke. These are the "treats" we have grown to love, and they have led us to a sugar-laden, fat-laden, salt-laden diet that is killing us, perhaps slowly, but ever so surely.

Some recent signs indicate that this situation may be starting to change. People seem to be developing a new awareness of their bodies and of health in general, and they are becoming more aware of food's contribution to health. Government groups study nutrition and issue weighty declarations. Popular magazines report the latest information. Self-proclaimed experts tell us how to lose weight, how to take care of our hearts, how to live to be 100.

The problem is that we don't really want to change. We cling to the foods we grew up with and learned to love. It is so hard to alter a lifetime love of ice cream, butter, and birthday cake. We resent nutrition's coming in and messing up our lives. The rules are being changed in the middle of the game, and it disturbs our sense of fairness.

Worse still, the expert recommendations rarely agree with one another, and the vast flow of information becomes instead a vast sea of confusion. Whom should we believe? How can we educate ourselves to be informed consumers of nutrition information? Much research is needed to tell the truth from wishful thinking or simple marketing ploy. It is hard to know when it is worth changing our eating habits.

One way more and more Americans are changing is by eating less meat or no meat and by cutting their intake of excess fat and protein in the process. The reasons are many: Some feel eating lower on the food chain leaves more food and a better environment for the rest of the world; some abstain as part of their religion; some are morally against the slaughter and exploitation of animals; some simply can't afford the price of meat today. Even when better health is not the major motivation (as is often the case), it is usually an inevitable bonus. Yet in no other area of nutrition is there more misinformation, confusion, silliness, and general disorder than in nutrition for vegetarians.

As a result, many people interested in becoming vegetarians are confused about the issues and afraid of the consequences. Will they have to learn a complex food-combining system to get enough protein? Will they have enough to eat in restaurants? Will they be missing essential vitamins and minerals? Some individuals, who find it necessary to cut down on meat for health or economic reasons, don't know how to fill the menu gap and have vague fears of malnutrition fostered by the Meat Board. There are even established vegetarians who still regard *Diet for a Small Planet* as their bible or insist they need no vitamin B_{12}. There are the parents and grandparents of vegetarians, as well as expectant mothers, who are concerned about growth and traditional food values. Finally, there are the doctors and other menu counselors who still consider the Four Food Groups as the last word in planning nutritious diets.

At last, in 1980, the American Dietetic Association (ADA) has condoned the well-planned (as any diet should be) vegetarian diet as ". . . consistent with good nutritional status," a diet that "meets all known nutrient needs." Furthermore, the ADA, certainly a prudent and, in fact, conservative organization, states that ". . . a growing body of scientific evidence supports a positive relationship between the consumption of a plant-based diet and the prevention of certain diseases."

This brings us to the purpose of this book. As vegetarians, we feel it is time to present a guidebook that lays out the facts of vegetarian nutrition in a manner that is presifted, easy to understand, and without hundreds of footnotes to trip over, but not superficial in its treatment of the technical realities. Our intention is to provide a primer and a reference book for new and confirmed vegetarians alike, one that describes the hows and whys of nutrition in a presentation that is admittedly opinionated but doesn't gloss over truth or controversy.

Sometimes nutrition does get complex and controversial. A good example is the recent brouhaha concerning fat and cholesterol. The Food and Nutrition Board (FNB) contradicted years of advisements from almost every health-related agency and organization when it released a report in mid-1980 stating that "normal" Americans don't have to worry about their intake of cholesterol and saturated fat. In reaching this conclusion, the FNB looked at exactly the same research findings that their own RDA (Recommended Dietary Allowances) committee had examined scarcely six months earlier when the committee recommended cutbacks in fat and cholesterol.

If the American people were confused before, this pronouncement left us with even more questions. What is a "normal"

American? Is polyunsaturated fat still better than saturated fat? Can we eat as many eggs as we want now? If America's most respected agencies can't make up their minds, how are "normal" Americans going to? What *is* the lowdown on fat and cholesterol, not to mention sugar, fiber, protein, vitamin B$_{12}$, organic vitamins, and meat? *Is* there a lowdown, or are these things just a matter of interpretation?

Good questions, ones we address ourselves to in the pages to come.

We Americans find ourselves in a unique time and place in the history of the human race. For most of us the question is no longer, "Where am I going to get enough to eat?" It has become, "What shall I choose to eat today?" The abundance of food, this most basic necessity, in our country is unprecedented, and we are poorly equipped by nature to handle it.* It is little wonder that most of our nutritional choices must now concern what to avoid rather than what to select. Again, it seems unfair. Why should we be presented with this heaven on earth, simply to be told that if we partake we'll damage our bodies? To understand it, we must understand how we came to have the bodies—and the minds—we now have.

We tend to forget that we are animals, ruled by the same general forces as our less intelligent cousins. All that separates us from them is our genes, as of course genes separate all species from one another. All living things receive their form and function from the information encoded in the genes they get from their parents. This information can change over a long period, changing the form and function of the creature. If accidental alterations give the creature an advantage in the world, he/she/it will be more likely to live and reproduce, and thus pass the improved genetic material along to future generations.

This process is known as *evolution through natural selection*. The better you are at playing by nature's rules, the more likely it is that your genes will be added to the gene pool for your species. This is how we came to be who and what we are. The process is

---

*Of course some Americans don't get enough to eat, and for them the real question is still where the food is coming from. However, poor Americans base their food choice decisions on the prevailing cultural guidelines. For example, poor people spend virtually the same amount of money per capita as do rich people on meat, even though it represents a much greater percentage of their food budget. So poor Americans act similarly to "comfortable" Americans when it comes to food choices. Thus this concept of abundance is still the national guiding principle.

incredibly slow; in fact, over the time of our recorded history, evolutionary changes in the human species are imperceptible.

Most animal and plant species have evolved to fit into specific ecological niches. Each needs a certain food and a certain climate, because it has evolved to fit into that natural "space." Humans are one of a small group of species characterized by adaptability—the ability to fit into many environments and to eat almost anything in the natural world. Our intelligence has given us the first ability, because we can create for ourselves our necessary environment almost anywhere on earth. And our digestive system has given us the second.

Very few other animals can eat as broad a diet as can humans, and this ability is one of our tremendous evolutionary advantages. It has taken us millenia to come to this point, however, and changes in the composition and nature of our food supply have, of necessity, also been slow, allowing us to adapt.

Unfortunately, the ability to alter our environment to suit our desires has begun to cause us problems in adapting to our diet. As we took control of our environment, first through agriculture and later through industry, we brought about dietary changes more rapid than our evolutionary pace could accommodate. Over the course of recorded history, change has occurred more and more quickly, so that in the past thirty years we have been faced with the most radical dietary changes in our entire history.

Our diet is no longer in any way a "natural" one. The normal environmental controls that have functioned well during the earth's history no longer apply, since humans can alter them at will. For example, instead of the natural environment's selecting which variant genetic traits will succeed and which will fail, we humans capriciously make the choices. We have altered the gene pool of thousands of species, from dogs to marigolds to oak trees, by consciously selecting which individuals will be allowed to reproduce. We have driven thousands of species to extinction—best estimates indicate that between 1980 and 2010 *one million* species of plants and animals will cease to exist on the earth as a result of human intervention in the world environment.*

We're playing the same game with our own species, but we are

*Howard Phipps, Jr., quoting Dr. Edward O. Wilson of Harvard's Department of Zoology in a speech delivered to the 84th Annual Meeting of the New York Zoological Society, February 13, 1980. Mr. Phipps is president of the New York Zoological Society.

not controlling the game. We're simply playing with variables and waiting to see what happens. We alter the air, the water, even the light that reaches us through the filter of the upper atmosphere. And we alter the food supply. We add chemicals whose long-term effects are unknown, we add to or remove nutrients from individual foods, and we choose certain food components, e.g., sugar, to play a major role in our diet with no regard for the effects of these changes on the health or the very survival of the species.

How can we know what we should be eating? The first and most obvious rule is that, as much as we can, we should eat foods close to the form in which they come from the earth. These foods have been our companions for millions of years of slow, painstaking evolution, and we know they are safe to eat. We haven't had time to adjust to altered foods, and their effects on our internal environment are unpredictable. Of course, our adaptability serves us well here, decreasing the dangers we would face if our digestive system were as specialized as that of a termite or a strict carnivore, for example. Even so, we can't predict the effects of technology on our food supply and our health.

We said earlier that technology has also given us a land of plenty—another unprecedented experience in the history of the earth. Barring war or some other unimaginable calamity, the American people as a group will probably never starve, nor even have a significant limitation in food choices. When we can get as much as we want of any particular food, how can we know when we've had too much? Again, the natural controls of limited availability or prohibitive effort no longer apply.

Our best hope for guidance is to try to determine what our pre-agricultural ancestors ate. This can give us some idea of what a "natural" diet for humans would look like.

It is popular to think of our ancestors mainly as hunters—it is in some strange way romantic, appealing to our image of Man Against Nature. The impression is supported by the presence of picked animal bones in prehistoric camps in many parts of the world. However, since the mineral content of bones makes them persist much longer than do plant remains (plus the fact that there is less to throw away from most plant foods), these fossil remnants can be misleading.

Recent study of the patterns of scratches and marks on the teeth of fossilized human jawbones—characteristic wear patterns that indicate the predominant diet—has shown that our ancestors ate flesh rarely. The basis of their diet was plant foods. This is only logical—plant food is much more abundant and less evasive or downright dangerous. Our bodies are poorly equipped to deal with dangerous or evasive prey. In this, primitive humans were much like modern apes—they'll eat meat if it falls in their laps, but by far the larger portion of their diet is plant foods.

This physical evidence should give us guidance as to what we have been naturally selected to eat (we assume that little has changed since then in our metabolism—not an unreasonable assumption, and the best we have to go on). The more vegetarian your diet looks, the closer it comes to this theoretical natural diet for humans.

In this book, we begin with this assumption—that no (or very little) meat is best for our bodies—and go on from there to look at it in depth. You will find, however, that this is not a book solely about vegetarian nutrition; it is also a guide in the many nutritional issues that face all of us at each meal.

Just to get our definitions straight, we refer to *lacto-ovo-vegetarians* as those people who eat no red meat, fowl, or fish but do eat dairy products and eggs; *vegans* as those who eat no red meat, fowl, fish, dairy, or eggs; and *meat-eaters* as those who eat red meat, fowl, or fish. Of course, we recognize that there are levels within levels (people who eat dairy but no eggs, people who eat fish but no red meat), and our definitions are simply convenient general terms.

It is important to remember, when talking about health, that it's not only what you don't eat but how you do eat that counts. A vegan can eat plenty of junk food while a meat-eater might eat a minimal amount of fish and lots of grains, fruits, and vegetables. So as you read, decide which information and advice apply to you. Here is a book in which there's no need to read around the meat to find out how to make good nutrition a natural, fuss-free part of your life.

The first section, The Nutrients, which discusses carbohydrate, fat, protein, vitamins, and minerals, provides the basis for the rest of the book, as indeed nutrients provide the basis for what we eat. It is important to make the distinction, however, between the separate nutrients and the fact that they appear together in each food. Americans tend to categorize (protein foods, carbohydrate foods) when, in fact, individual whole foods contain all these components in varying degrees. Who needs "enriched" or "fortified," when all the food you eat is rich in vitamins, minerals, carbohydrate, fiber, protein, and the essential fatty acid? And a varied diet that doesn't overemphasize a particular food or group of foods likewise tends not to overemphasize a particular nutrient to the detriment of others.

The crux of the matter is that nutrients aren't just components, like the interchangeable parts of a car. They interact to make whole, live foods, as they interact in your body when you eat them. It is no surprise that naturally rich sources of carbohydrate such as wheat and rice are also generally rich sources of thiamin and niacin, two vitamins needed to metabolize carbohydrate. Similarly, foods high in protein, such as beans or milk, generally also provide phosphorus, zinc, and many B vitamins necessary for our bodies to use protein properly.

Nature provides us with a complete diet. As long as we use it wisely, not playing with food too much, stripping it of nutritional value in our attempts to "improve" it, that abundance can feed us well and keep us healthy. As we will show, there's no need to include meat. It is variety that balances everything out.

The most dangerous foods are the extracts, the concentrated foods like butter, sugar, salt, and meat. Any food that provides high concentrations of any one thing is a food to beware of. While it may have its benefits, as high-fat nuts do, for example, too much will skew the balance. All in all, the best foods have many things to offer. In a sound, varied diet, they have everything to offer.

Still, the nutrients maintain their separate identities in your body. And it's helpful to understand ourselves from the inside out.

The Carbohydrate chapter emphasizes that complex carbohydrates should be the mainstay of your diet, while sugar and alcohol are best avoided. Fiber, incidentally, is good for you, and low-carbohydrate diets are not.

Chapter 3 tells why fat is a nutritional monster, linked to, among other things, obesity, cancer, and heart disease. Advice on how to cut down can be found there.

In Chapter 4 we finally dispense with the protein juggling act many vegetarians go through seeking perfect protein complementarity. A normal, healthy adult need only get enough calories from a variety of foods and the protein will take care of itself.

Chapter 5 describes how vitamin and mineral requirements can be met by eating a variety of fresh, whole foods, stored and cooked to preserve that freshness. We describe them, vitamin by vitamin and mineral by mineral, with a special section on how they interact. Recommendations for supplementing are included, along with a chart summarizing everything.

In Chapter 6, Putting It Together—Four Eating Styles, we outline several approaches you can take to incorporate your nutritional awareness into your eating patterns, from an instinctual approach to weekly menu planning. In this chapter you will find a list of simple ways to improve meal quality, a Daily Food Groups chart, a week's worth of menus, and a list advising which foods to choose and which to avoid.

The section on Special Cases addresses some of the people—pregnant women, babies and children, athletes, and dieters—who don't meet the description of "normal, healthy adult" that we refer to throughout the rest of the book. There are four chapters regarding their special needs.

During pregnancy (Chapter 7) all nutrient needs are higher, and we explain in detail how and why. *Of course* you can be pregnant and vegetarian, despite your parents' or doctor's fears. Included are a comparison between pregnant and normal nutritional needs and a Daily Food Guide.

In the chapter on babies and children, we look at your child's needs from birth through adolescence. We begin with a discussion of breast- and bottle-feeding. Selections from our Children's Food Group Guide can be the basis of a diet for a lifetime. Vegan children can certainly be healthy children—just be aware of their needs, as all parents should be.

Carbohydrates are the best source of energy for athletes (Chapter 9), so forget that traditional pregame steak. The myths about athletes are many. Did you know, for example, that water is the most crucial nutrient for athletes in competition?

The weight-loss diet in Chapter 10 shows that the most efficient and healthful way to lose fat is still a balanced, low-calorie diet. We provide you with one, complete with a week's recipes.

Chapter 11, Is Vegetarianism Healthier? pits the meat-eaters against the home team in a face-off that examines everything from vitamin deficiency to cholesterol to salmonella poisoning. We win.

Our last section gets down to the practicalities of food in daily life.

The shopping and storing chapter underscores the importance of reading labels (and how to do it). We also offer suggestions on where to shop (even the supermarket) and how to choose foods.

You'll find a selection-and-storage guide for fruits and vegetables and a list of kitchen timesavers.

Even though this is definitely not a cookbook, we didn't want to leave you with a lot of theory and nothing to put in your mouth. Branching Out from Your Own Recipes presents more than a dozen model recipes that include options to yield hundreds of different dishes. Sample recipes are also included. A mini-glossary of foods with which you may not be familiar is also here.

In Eating Out—and Other Matters we answer questions on subjects such as changing to vegetarianism, living with meat-eaters, traveling, and dinner invitations.

After each chapter (except this one) you'll find a list of Guidelines—handy summaries of the main points in the chapter.

Next come the Appendices, which many people routinely skip over, but which we hope you will use. Included are the 1980 Recommended Dietary Allowances (RDAs), the FAO/WHO nutrient recommendations, a summary of guidelines for vegans, a food group guide listing the many foods included in each group, addresses for mail-order sources, a bibliography of suggested reading, and a chart for converting pounds to kilograms, as well as a metric conversion table.

Finally, if you care to pursue threads that intrigue you, the chapters are separately annotated in the Bibliography.

We don't push vegetarianism as the Answer—of course it is a good diet, and it can do your health as much good as diet alone can. But many factors enter into the health of an individual: diet, to be sure, but also environment, heredity, stress, general emotional health, and everything else that makes up a life.

To your health.

THE NUTRIENTS

Carbohydrate
Fat
Protein
Vitamins and Minerals

2
Carbohydrate

Carbohydrate is the victim of possibly the biggest nutritional smear campaign in history. When in response to questions about what vegetarians eat we answer bread, pasta, beans, and vegetables, the listener's first response is, "Don't you gain weight eating all those carbohydrates?"

No, we do not gain weight from eating carbohydrates. People gain weight from eating too much food, whatever specific nutrients it may contain. Carbohydrate per se is completely innocent— although you may gain weight from it if you eat too much.

As a matter of fact, carbohydrate in general gives exactly the same number of calories per unit of weight as does protein and less than half of fat's. Try to separate the two concepts of "carbohydrate" and "fattening."

Carbohydrates—sugar, starch, and more complex carbohydrates —are not bad for you. They simply have a bad reputation that, as it turns out, is mainly undeserved. Carbohydrates are *good* for you, especially in natural combination with other nutrients. The best natural sources of carbohydrate are not only potatoes and grain products such as rice, bread, and pasta, but also fruits such as bananas, grapes, melons, and berries, vegetables like mushrooms, Brussels sprouts, onions, carrots, beets, and peppers, and the various legumes, nuts, and seeds such as pecans, garbanzos, pumpkin seeds, and pistachios. In fact, most foods that don't have a goodly dose of fat are rich in health-giving carbohydrate.

The nutritional problems associated with carbohydrate generally occur when it is separated from its natural source, as sugar is separated from cane. The sugar is no longer doing its proper dietary job of providing energy while using its significant taste appeal to

13

"sell" the other valuable nutrients the whole food has to offer. Since it is separated from its source, it sells only itself, and because refined sugar is so concentrated, we tend to eat a lot of it when available. It doesn't fill us up, since it is absorbed so quickly, and it's metabolized so fast it can leave us *hungrier*. We needn't point out just how available sugar is in today's world. By the best estimates of consumption, Americans get from 20 to 25 percent of their calories from refined sugar, either by itself or as added to processed foods.

Refined sugar is the black sheep of an otherwise upstanding and righteous nutrient family. The best, most complex forms of carbohydrate are accompanied by vitamins, minerals, protein, unsaturated fats, and food fiber (mostly another carbohydrate).

Carbohydrates—those from fruits, vegetables, whole grains, beans, and seeds (see the Food Group Guide in the Appendix for an expanded list)—should compose the largest portion of your daily calories. This will probably come as a shock to many people, whose view of carbohydrates (or "starches," as they were known in the old days) was formed sitting at the dinner table. Foods high in carbohydrates were always those tasty "fillers" you ate when you didn't really want any more meat. They weren't considered good nutrition, so our mothers discouraged our eating too much ("Don't fill up on bread or you won't have room for *dinner*"). Cultures in which the staple food was high in carbohydrate—the cornmeal of Mexico, the pasta of Italy—were looked upon pityingly for their poverty and lack of nutritional "knowledge."

But they were right all along. There is no reason to load up your diet with protein and fat and many reasons not to. Carbohydrate is the ideal fuel for our bodily processes: cheap, available, easily metabolized, very efficient. Protein can be changed into carbohydrate by the body for metabolic purposes, but the process is much less efficient and releases somewhat toxic byproducts. Most of these byproducts are usually detoxified as quickly as they are made, except in cases of metabolic screwups or poor nutrition.

When your diet depends on fat and protein for the largest part of its calories, your liver and kidneys must do a heroic job to rid your body of these byproducts. They may enlarge (*hypertrophy*) to cope with the load, a load they obviously were not evolved to handle. In some lab animals this hypertrophy is accompanied by kidney irritation.

Sometimes your housecleaning organs simply can't deal with the load, as when you go on a poorly designed reducing diet that emphasizes eliminating carbohydrate. Then the byproducts build up in your blood, making you nauseated and uncomfortable and, in some cases, triggering an underlying kidney disease of which you may be unaware.

Overconsumption of fats and protein is harmful for other reasons too. These are outlined in their respective chapters. In addition, using protein for energy needs in place of carbohydrate is hard to rationalize when people go hungry in many parts of the world, including the United States. Only the Western nations can afford this luxury, and even there only the rich practice this waste continually. Although they don't suffer from hunger and under-nutrition, they must face the diseases of overconsumption—heart disease, adult-onset diabetes, some cancers, obesity, high blood pressure. The call for drastic cutbacks in our consumption of fat and protein can best be met by replacing them with unrefined carbohydrates.

WHAT ARE CARBOHYDRATES?

The simplest carbohydrate is a simple sugar, like glucose. When you digest carbohydrates or the leftovers from protein breakdown, your liver converts these to glucose for use by other tissues. The simple sugar glucose is thus a kind of common unit of energy exchange for your body's metabolism.

Glucose, like most of the other molecules that take part in metabolism, is made of carbon, hydrogen, and oxygen. The carbon atoms make a skeleton for the molecule, and the hydrogen and oxygen atoms latch on to the sides and ends of the chain. Glucose itself has the chemical formula $C_6H_{12}O_6$. The C stands for carbon, the H for hydrogen, and the O for oxygen. The other simple sugars, fructose, mannose, and galactose, have the same chemical for-mula, but their atoms are arranged differently. After absorption, all the other simple sugars are converted into glucose.

Besides these simple sugars based on a six-carbon chain, your digestive tract may, from time to time, run across five-carbon sugars, a group known as *pentoses*. These include ribose, xylose, and arabinose, and they never appear in free form in foods. They are always in combination, either in chains known as *pentosans,* which are found in some fruit and vegetable gums, or as part of nucleic acids in cell nuclei.

Sucrose, lactose, and maltose *(disaccharides)* are made from two six-carbon sugars *(monosaccharides)* bound together. Sucrose is common table sugar, composed of a molecule of glucose and one of fructose. Lactose is milk sugar, made from glucose and galactose. Maltose is the sugar present in sprouted grain. It is composed of two glucose molecules stuck together.

Polysaccharides are made from more than two monosaccharides, fastened together to form large molecules. The most common digestible forms are starches and dextrins, found in grains and vegetables. Meat-eaters may also get very small amounts of glycogen, the starchlike chemical that animals use to store carbohydrate in their muscles and liver for emergency use.

Some polysaccharides are only partially digestible; because of their molecular structure, your body's enzymes can't break them apart completely into absorbable simple sugars. These include inulin, mannosans, raffinoses, and the pentosans mentioned above. These carbohydrates occupy a gray area in nutrition because so many variables affect their absorption. For example, Jerusalem artichokes, which contain inulin, also contain an enzyme that "digests" the polysaccharide into simpler and more absorbable carbohydrates. Since this process changes a partially absorbable carbohydrate into a fully absorbable one, it also changes the calorie content of the food! Fresh-dug Jerusalem artichokes are lower in calories than those that have been stored for a while.

Finally, some polysaccharides can't be broken down at all by our digestive apparatus. These include cellulose, hemicellulose, and pectin, the most important components of the cell walls of plants. These, along with lignin, an indigestible, almost plasticlike substance, compose what nutritionists generally refer to as *fiber.* You get fiber from plants—animals don't make it. Thus, almost all foods of plant origin except oils, refined flour, and sugar contain fiber, and no foods of animal origin, including lacto-ovo-vegetarian foods like milk, have any at all.

WHAT DO CARBOHYDRATES DO FOR US?

The most important role of carbohydrate is as a source of energy for our body processes. Every gram of pure, digestible carbohydrate you eat provides four calories to fuel your body. You use carbohydrate when you move, when your cells divide, when you synthesize hormones, when you think, when you sleep. In every case they provide the energy for the process to take place.

Of course, the other two major components of food—protein and fat—yield calories. In fact, fat provides a good deal more calories per gram than does carbohydrate or protein. But only certain organs can use fatty acids for energy; the nervous system, a notable exception, can run only on glucose.

Protein must be converted into carbohydrate before its energy can be used. And portions of the structure of fat and protein are left over when they are used. These toxic leftovers can build up in individuals whose diet is composed mainly of fat and protein. Since carbohydrate is already in a fully usable form (once it is broken down into glucose), it produces no byproducts except water and carbon dioxide when used for energy.*

A high-carbohydrate diet also tends to "spare" protein, saving it for use in building new tissues instead of for energy. People who eat a low-protein, high-carbohydrate diet are using their food protein more efficiently than those who eat more protein and little carbohydrate. Your liver uses carbohydrate to build the carbon skeletons of the nonessential amino acids, again improving your protein supply.

As we mentioned, other dietary components can be used for energy in place of dietary carbohydrate, notably protein, since it can be converted into glucose. But if you insist on getting food energy from protein and fat, be prepared to pay the price in your health. Carbohydrate is *the best* general source of energy for your body. Since the largest part of our daily food need is simply for calories, most of our diet should be composed of carbohydrate. The Senate Select Committee on Nutrition and Human Needs recommends that Americans increase the proportion of carbohydrate calories in their diet to about 58 percent. You should consider this a minimum because, as you cut your fat and protein calories to optimum levels, carbohydrate should fill the calorie gap. A good diet should probably contain about 70 percent carbohydrate calories, and as much of these as possible should come from whole, fresh foods.

WHAT HAPPENS TO CARBOHYDRATE IN YOUR BODY?

Your intestines absorb only monosaccharides, simple sugars, so all the carbohydrates you eat must be reduced to simple sugars

---

*In the exceptional case when cell oxygen is insufficient, as in violent exercise, lactic acid can build up in muscles as a result of partial glucose metabolism. This condition, known as "oxygen debt," corrects itself when enough oxygen again becomes available.

before they can cross your intestinal lining and be absorbed into your blood.

The process starts in your mouth. As you chew, the enzymes in your saliva mix with your food and begin to work on the starches and dextrins, breaking them into maltose, a disaccharide. The acid secretions in your stomach stop the enzymes but continue their job, breaking the polysaccharides and disaccharides down further and further. If the food stayed in your stomach long enough, the carbohydrates would all be broken down into monosaccharides (except for the undigestible carbohydrates).

Usually, food moves into your intestinal tract before the stomach acid has fully digested the carbohydrates. Here, intestinal secretions provide more enzymes to break up the sucrose, maltose, and lactose, and to a lesser extent inulin, mannosans, raffinose, and pentosans, into simple sugars. These can finally be transported across the borderline between the interior of your intestines and your bloodstream. They travel quickly to your liver, where all the six-carbon sugars, or hexoses, are changed into glucose.

We leave the monosaccharides for a moment to follow the residue carbohydrates—those our bodies can't digest. Since we can't use them, they have no place to go but out. They continue through the large intestine and are finally excreted. Along the way, the friendly bacteria that inhabit your intestines go to work on these carbohydrates, partially digesting them into simple sugars. Although we may be able to absorb a very small amount of these sugars, our large intestine is not really an absorptive organ. The effect is probably minimal.

Back at your liver, the simple sugars are being converted into glucose at a rapid pace. Your kidneys may also be involved in converting the simple sugar fructose into glucose. Your blood level of glucose rises, triggering a complex series of metabolic events. Your hormonal system tells your pancreas to secrete more insulin. The insulin "pumps" circulating blood glucose into fat and muscle cells, where it is converted into fat and glycogen, respectively. Your liver also converts large portions of glucose into glycogen, a starchlike carbohydrate your body uses for emergency stores of quick energy.

Altogether, most of the glucose is quickly changed into fat for storage in your adipose cells (fat cells). This stored fat is used to provide energy when glucose is no longer entering your bloodstream from your intestines. The adipose cells release fatty acids to fuel the organs, such as muscles, that can use them.

The two different storage forms for dietary carbohydrates have different functions in your body. Fat is used for fuel under normal circumstances, when the demands for energy are at a relatively low level. When your body is under an energy stress, however, as when you run hard, your muscles and heart need more energy than they can get from stored fat and the glucose circulating in blood. This is where glycogen is important. Your muscles and liver store glycogen for just such an emergency, because it can be converted into energy quickly and with a minimum of steps. In addition, some organs require a constant source of glucose. Glycogen provides this.

Different diets give your body different levels of stored glycogen. A high-fat diet produces the lowest levels of glycogen in liver tissue. Less fat and more protein does a better job, depending on how easily the particular amino acids of the protein can be converted into sugar. A high-carbohydrate diet is the best of all for stored glycogen. The exact form of the carbohydrate doesn't seem to be important (as long as it is digestible).

Because of this, athletes are finally beginning to realize the importance of carbohydrate in their diets. Today "carbohydrate loading" is all the rage before a big race or a hockey game. Athletes use this technique to pack their muscles with extra glycogen to give them the energy and stamina they need to perform in competition. As one researcher discovered, athletes can perform hard exercise nearly three times as long on a high-carbohydrate diet as they can on a high-protein diet.* Someday all coaches will know this.

DIABETES

Diabetes mellitus is a medical term for the body's inability to respond to rising blood glucose levels by storing the glucose as fat and glycogen. The result is an abnormally high blood glucose level, with glucose spilling over into your urine. This is how doctors detect diabetes—by testing for glucose in urine. Diabetes affects nerve transmission and the small blood vessels, and in severe cases

---

*Danish researchers studied the performance of nine athletes on a variety of diets, using a stationary bicycle to test endurance. After a standardized mixed diet for three days, they averaged 114 minutes of bicycling. The next three days they got a high-protein diet, centered on meat, eggs, and milk. In the next test their average performance dropped to only 57 minutes. Finally they ate a high-carbohydrate, low-protein, low-fat diet for three days. In the last test they averaged 167 minutes of cycling, and a couple of the athletes lasted more than four hours. One more athlete's myth shot full of holes.

can contribute to coronary heart disease, blindness, stroke, atherosclerosis, and gangrene of the extremities.

Nobody knows for certain what causes diabetes, although diet and heredity are both involved. There are strong indications that carbohydrate other than sugar is *not* to blame, and equally strong indications that plain old obesity is very much to blame.

Diabetes appears to spring from two separate causes, although any particular case may be based on both to a greater or lesser extent. In some cases the pancreas is unable to produce enough insulin to cope with the glucose influx from food. Insulin is the hormone that instructs fat and liver cells to store glucose as fat and glycogen, respectively, so too little insulin results in too much glucose waiting to be stored. This type of diabetes appears to be strongly linked to heredity, since the body's system is unable to cope with a normal dietary component in normal amounts.

In other cases, the blood insulin level is high enough, but the glucose-processing organs, notably the fat cells, ignore its message and fail to process the extra glucose. Meanwhile, the pancreas's insulin-producing cells crank out more insulin in an attempt to deal with the high glucose levels in the bloodstream. This resistance to insulin appears to be brought on by obesity, and it can usually be reversed or at least mitigated by returning to a normal weight. Perhaps the fat cells are complaining that they're already over-loaded and can't take any more fat.

Although both types can be controlled by insulin injections, diet and weight loss together comprise the method of choice for con-trolling diabetes related to obesity. Insulin injections coupled with weight control and an improved diet seem to have the best results overall, and many diabetics can stop medication altogether once they get their weight down and their diet straightened out. Diabet-ics who have no weight problem, whose diabetes is based mainly on insulin insufficiency, will find a dietary change less effective. However, this type of diabetes appears to be much less common than the insulin-resistance type.

Complex carbohydrates play an important role in an improved diet for diabetics. First, a high-carbohydrate diet can help in weight loss by taking the place of much of the fat the dieter must eliminate. Since carbohydrate has less than half the calories of fat by weight, it will be more difficult to eat too much. Some researchers have found that a high-carbohydrate diet can improve diabetics' re-sponse to a large influx of glucose—the standard clinical gauge of the severity of the disease. Finally, high-carbohydrate diets also tend to be high-fiber diets, and fiber also appears to help diabetics deal with blood glucose.

Sugar's role in diabetes is still unclear. Since the major symptom of the disease is too much glucose (that is, sugar) in the blood, it is tempting to blame dietary sugar for the original problem. But this connection is by no means clear. Some studies seem to show that a high sugar intake can promote the disease, while other studies show no such connection. Sugar quite clearly can have a role in promoting obesity, however, so it may have an indirect effect on diabetes even if a direct role can't be shown.

Diabetes is almost unknown in most countries outside the affluent West and our dietary imitators in the up-and-coming East. In most countries people are too poor to get fat, so diabetes is limited. In those countries (with a few exceptions) the dietary staple is some kind of high-carbohydrate food, and carbohydrates provide up to 85 percent of the total calories.

Diabetes is a disruption of the metabolism of carbohydrates, but it apparently is not caused by them. In fact, a high-carbohydrate, high-fiber diet can be helpful in controlling the disorder and returning metabolism to a healthy state.

CARBOHYDRATE AND CHOLESTEROL

In the early Sixties several reports stated that high carbohydrate diets boosted serum cholesterol and lipid levels. Indeed, the studies seemed to show that this did happen. When people were placed on a high-carbohydrate diet their blood triglyceride levels shot up, and blood cholesterol increased slightly as well. As soon as they ate a high-carbohydrate meal, however, the levels dropped back to normal, rising again slowly between meals.

It later turned out that the research project did not continue long enough to provide an accurate picture of people's response to a high-carbohydrate diet. After a period of adjustment, the triglyceride levels dropped back to normal or even lower than normal. Apparently, the elevated blood fat count was a result of the sudden dietary shift rather than a fault of a high-carbohydrate diet itself. High serum lipid count is in fact much rarer among people who eat a high-carbohydrate diet than among those who eat a lot of fat or protein. A slow dietary change avoids even the temporary elevation of blood fats for those who can little afford to raise their fat levels.

A high-carbohydrate diet is now generally accepted by researchers as a useful way to lower blood lipid and cholesterol levels, since the carbohydrate takes the place of fat in the diet.

CARBOHYDRATES AND TOOTH DECAY

Tooth decay is undeniably linked to carbohydrate consumption. In fact, this is the only harmful effect ascribed to the consumption of carbohydrates in general. Because most people think of tooth decay as a fact of life, it is not normally considered a very serious disorder, but the facts are otherwise. It is debilitating, obviously dangerous to your teeth, causes gum diseases and infection, is expensive, difficult, and stressful to correct, and can be dangerous to life in some advanced cases. Americans spend billions of dollars a year for dental care, most of it for routine maintenance work to fill all those little holes that seem to appear so regularly.

Those little holes, called *caries* (the word is both singular and plural), are eaten into the tooth enamel by metabolic byproducts from bacteria living on and between your teeth. These bacteria live on carbohydrate, and they aren't too choosy about the particular type of carbohydrate. But don't jump to the conclusion that the only way to avoid tooth decay is to avoid carbohydrate. Although the exact type of carbohydrate is not very important, the *form* in which it is eaten is very important. Foods that stay in your mouth a long time, bathing your teeth in a solution of sugar or starch, are the worst offenders because they give the bacteria the longest time to work on food and produce acid byproducts. Sticky candies and hard candy that you dissolve slowly in your mouth have become notorious among dentists as the worst of all, while other foods that contain carbohydrate, like whole fresh fruit, may have a beneficial effect because they clean your teeth as you chew them.

The plaque that builds up around the base of each tooth and in the gaps between doesn't get there by accident. Bacteria build it to be their home because it keeps them safely anchored to your tooth, where they won't get washed away or exposed to too much oxygen. When you eat something like an apple, its crunchy texture scrubs the plaque from around your teeth as you chew. Brushing your teeth has the same, if more efficient, effect.

The best way to avoid tooth decay is not to avoid carbohydrates, which is nearly impossible anyway. The best ways are (1) avoid foods that just sit in your mouth, washing your teeth with dissolved sugar; (2) eat fresh, crunchy, whole carbohydrate foods to help with cleaning, even as you eat; and (3) keep your teeth clean. That doesn't necessarily mean brush vigorously whenever you think of it—it simply means brush well once or twice a day, and in between if something is stuck in your teeth. Dental floss does a much better job between teeth than a toothbrush, but you have to learn to use it without hurting your gums. Get a dentist or dental technician to show you how if you don't know already.

Avoiding between-meal sweets is one more good way to keep your teeth healthy, since that extra dose of sugar gives the bacteria an extra opportunity to act.

WHAT GOOD IS FIBER?

Remember that fiber is the remains of the carbohydrate after your intestines have digested all they can (plus some lignin). Some researchers call this "residue," because it is left over. Even though your body throws it away, it is far from useless.

Carbohydrate is strongly attracted to water because of its chemical structure. What this means to your intestine is that a little bit of carbohydrate residue can absorb a comparatively large amount of water. This keeps the waste products soft and easy for your intestine to handle as it pushes them along toward the exit. It also makes these waste products move through your intestines more quickly. In cultures where the normal diet includes a large percentage of unrefined carbohydrate foods, and thus a good dose of fiber, the intestinal transit time is approximately half that of our culture, for example.

Since your intestines are cleaning house more often and more quickly, any toxic products of your digestion or of the bacteria who inhabit your intestines have less chance to build up. This may be the reason for the much lower incidence of bowel cancer in countries more "primitive" than ours.

A second advantage of this quicker bowel transit is that bile salts secreted by your liver have less chance of being reabsorbed by your intestinal wall. An important constituent of bile salts is cholesterol, so if you have a higher net loss of bile salts, you also have a higher net loss of cholesterol. Many doctors and heart researchers think that lowering your body's total cholesterol level is a very good idea. This may help.

Fiber is good for you in several ways. It softens and moistens your intestinal contents (plus adding bulk), so they move more quickly and easily. It also eases the passage of waste matter and thus diminishes the chances of developing hemorrhoids. A higher-bulk diet can also help you avoid diverticulosis, a painful and dangerous intestinal disorder caused by too-high pressure on small portions of your intestines. The greater bulk apparently evens out the pressure over a longer stretch of intestine, protecting the small sections from being pushed out of shape and damaged. Finally, a quicker transit time flushes dangerous digestive byproducts out of your intestines more quickly and also causes a greater intestinal cholesterol loss.

Unfortunately, different plant foods have different types of fiber, some more helpful than others. Bran, for example, though the most commercially popular "fiber food," is relatively ineffective in binding bile salts and thus reducing blood cholesterol. It does have a laxative effect, however, binding a good deal of moisture in the intestine. The fiber from foods such as carrots and legumes is much more effective in binding bile salts, and it also holds large amounts of moisture. Thus, you should try not to get all your fiber in a single form. Eat a variety of whole foods to gain the greatest benefit from your diet.

ALCOHOL

The stuff that makes you drunk is not really a carbohydrate at all. It is ethyl alcohol, made commercially by the action of yeast on carbohydrates; it is not, however, a carbohydrate or any other nutrient.

Not much good can be said for alcohol. It's a toxic, addictive drug, with almost no medical use and a tremendous potential for abuse. Ten million American alcohol addicts can attest to that abuse potential, as well as to its destructive effect on their health and the lives of themselves and their families and loved ones.

Alcohol gets you drunk by putting your brain in a state of moderate to severe asphyxiation. As the alcohol concentration of your blood increases, red blood cells start to clump together. These clumps are too big to pass through the tiniest capillaries in your brain and other organs, so they effectively block the flow of blood and thus oxygen. The more alcohol, the more clumping, the sillier you feel. Your brain is affected first because it is the organ most dependent on a continuing supply of oxygen to operate properly. You also notice the effects on your brain first, since all your perceptions are affected. Alcohol also acts directly as a sedative drug on your central nervous system.

Your movements become less coordinated, your senses less clear, your judgment less acute. If you really tie one on, your respiration reflex can be suppressed to the point that you stop breathing altogether (we all know the name for *that* phenomenon).

Beyond the immediate effects of alcohol toxicosis, we should also look at the long-term effects of alcohol consumption, especially as it relates to nutrition in general. The organ hardest hit by alcohol in the long run is the liver. The liver is the main metabolic processing center of the body, because it produces most of the enzymes used to change one chemical into another or burn nutrients for energy. We can metabolize or store fats, proteins, and carbohydrates in other tissues, but the liver is the only organ that can metabolize alcohol (and alcohol can't be stored at all). Your liver bears the brunt of a drinking bout because it must carry the load in getting rid of the alcohol.

Alcohol ties up many of the metabolic systems in the liver, forcing that organ to neglect its other duties, like fat, protein, and toxic-chemical metabolism. When you're drunk your liver can't detoxify foreign chemicals as quickly. An obvious example is the relationship between alcohol and sedatives. The sedatives last much longer in the bloodstream of an intoxicated person than in a sober person.

After chronic consumption of alcohol for as little as four or five days, structural changes begin to appear in liver cells. The neglected fat and protein start to build up in cells, leading to a further decrease in liver function. Blood flow is also restricted, and this can lead to the death of some liver cells. Finally, fibrous scar tissue begins to appear, blocking liver function still further. These scars are the classic symptoms of cirrhosis, an often fatal liver disorder common in many long-term alcoholics.

Alcohol disrupts other body systems as well. As it interferes with proper protein metabolism, the protein conversion system stops producing glucose and starts producing lactic acid, a toxic chemical. Blood glucose levels drop, cutting off essential fuel for many body processes, especially in the nervous system. The lactic acid interferes with the excretion of uric acid from the kidneys. As uric acid builds up in the bloodstream, it can trigger an attack of gout.

The liver's functions in activating various vitamins, especially vitamin A, are also interrupted, leading to moderate to severe malnutrition. This malnutrition interferes with intestinal absorption of a wide variety of nutrients, leading to worse malnutrition.

Finally, alcohol contains seven calories per gram—more than protein or carbohydrate, though less than fat. Besides all that, it's carcinogenic.

All these negative effects are balanced against studies showing that people who consume small amounts of alcohol daily—about the equivalent of a glass of wine—show a decrease in the risk of suffering a heart attack. Alcohol consumption at this low level shouldn't cause most of the ill effects outlined above (although cancer can be triggered by disappearingly small amounts of chemical carcinogens). But after the first glass, the benefit disappears and the risk increases again.

SUGAR—THE EVIL WHITE STUFF

Nowadays sugar leads a double life. Although many people pay lip service to reducing their sugar consumption, those same lips can't seem to get enough sweet stuff. Sugar represents 15 to 25 percent of our daily caloric intake. This is generally true of Americans only, however; other Western countries with different food traditions, such as Italy, get more dietary carbohydrates from starches.

Yet if carbohydrates are absorbed from our intestines as sugar, why should we not eat the sugar itself? Sugar is less desirable for several reasons. First and most important, any refined food is a food taken out of its nutritional context. Sugar is no longer accompanied by the other nutrients that "keep it honest": vitamins, minerals, fiber, protein. It is truly empty calories, and empty calories leave less room for the nutritious ones that literally enrich your life. Second is that when you eat refined sugar it slips into your bloodstream with almost no formality. Your glucose blood levels soar, triggering the Islands of Langerhans in the pancreas to secrete a big squirt of insulin. The insulin pushes your adipose cells into high gear, storing that glucose as fast as they can. Before you know it, your blood glucose has rebounded to a below-normal level, leaving you irritable, hungry, and unaccountably tired. So you thought sugar was an energy food?

Third, it is extremely hard to know when to stop eating sugar. It just doesn't make you full—after all, there's nothing to it but little crystals of very soluble, very absorbable white stuff—so it is easy to eat too many calories when a good deal of them come from sugar.

Complex carbohydrates don't cause any of these reactions. They are digested and absorbed more slowly, so you don't get a glucose high, they come with good fibrous material to fill your stomach, and they have all kinds of other good nutrients with them. Obviously, they are much better than refined sugar.

Researchers and popular writers have blamed sugar consumption for tooth decay, obesity, heart disease, diabetes, and high blood lipid levels. We have already discussed tooth decay, and it appears that sugar is no more to blame than are other carbohydrates. At least one laboratory test with animals showed an increase in the diabetes level on a diet high in refined sugar, but the conclusions don't relate clearly to humans under "normal" circumstances of consumption. Diabetes, heart disease, high blood lipid levels, and obesity are closely related in that they all can come about from an overconsumption of calories. Here sugar can clearly bear at least part of the blame. It is simply too easy to eat too much sugar. It tastes very good, and our internal metabolic controls tend to get bypassed by our appetites. At one time this sweet tooth was probably beneficial to the survival of the race. It showed our ancestors exactly which foods were good to eat—the fruits and vegetables that naturally contain sugar.

Humans are nothing if not inventive, and they found a way to remove this tasty substance from the healthful foods that contained it. In recent times manufacturers have gone one better, putting sugar into virtually every processed food on the market. We now consume about three times as much "invisible" sugar in these processed foods as we put into or on the food ourselves. The result is a basically valuable food component run amuck. We respond to the flavor and eat more and more, but in nutritionally worthless forms.

Along the way, the naturally occurring controls that limit our appetites are refined out of the foods—mainly fiber, which fills us up on its own and also holds water to increase the bulk of the food. Sugar is the most refined food of all, containing calories and nothing else. Hand a kid a bag of candy and see how long it lasts, even a big bag; but give him a bag of apples, or even cut sugar cane, and see if he eats more than is healthy. The odds are that he won't eat enough to displace other important foods in his diet *by his own inclination.*

People can easily eat thousands of calories of refined sugar, as they can refined fats and to a lesser extent refined carbohydrates other than sugar, in one sitting. The sugar itself is not so much to blame as is the *lack* of other nutrients that naturally accompany it. The finger of blame thus points straight at people, not at food components. People separate out these delicious, deadly ingredients, and people put them into made-up fantasy food. People, therefore, must be the ones to exercise control over what they eat.

It matters very little the form in which we eat the sugar—it is just too concentrated a taste for our rather primitive instincts to handle. It should be avoided as much as possible, except as it occurs naturally in foods. However, this shouldn't be construed as a license to buy a bushel of sugar cane to chew. While sugar cane is undeniably much more nutritious than the extracted sugar, it isn't sufficiently nutritious to become a dietary staple. And who knows? Your instincts may by now be so far out of joint that natural controls no longer function.

Of course, we as a nation are not going to swear off rich desserts tomorrow. We are, after all, getting exactly what we want in these high-sugar processed foods. What we must do is try to reeducate our wants so they are more in line with good nutritional practice—a slow, difficult process.

WHAT ABOUT LOW-CARBOHYDRATE DIETS?

Dr. Irwin Stillman's diet, known variously as the Water Diet, the Protein Diet, or the Stillman Diet, was only one of the most recent and best publicized salvos in the "calories don't count" campaign. Others include the Drinking Man's Diet, the Ed McMahon Diet, and the Atkins Diet. They are all very similar, so we'll use Stillman's for purposes of discussion. His claim is that if you eat only certain foods, which are high in fat and protein and low in carbohydrate, and eschew others that give reasonable amounts of carbohydrate, you can lose weight *without eating less*.

As it happens, you will indeed lose weight on Stillman's diet, but you certainly won't lose much fat—unless you cut your calories as well. If the calories come into your body, *something* must be done with them—either they are used for energy needs or stored as fat. Although your body uses its calories less efficiently on a low-carbohydrate diet, that effect is not sufficient to help you lose weight if your calorie intake is uncontrolled.

What you'll lose is body fluid, or *electrolyte*. When you cut your carbohydrate intake drastically, your body must keep its blood glucose level up some other way. It tells the liver to convert whatever is handy—that is, amino acids—into glucose and get it into the blood. Of course, your muscles can use fatty acids for fuel, so at least part of your energy needs can be met by fat.

Some of your body fat will be broken down, as will some of your body protein to make glucose. But most of your energy needs will still come from the fat and protein supplied by your food. Even under these metabolic emergency conditions, if you eat more calories than you need you will gain weight, and if you eat fewer you will lose.

When fat and protein are used for energy, their breakdown results in the release of chemicals called *ketones*. Normally, these are also used for energy or broken down more fully, but when your body is in a state of carbohydrate starvation, the ketones build up in your bloodstream faster than your body can take care of them. Your kidneys must work overtime to clear these poisonous chemicals through your urine. Kidneys require a certain amount of fluid to do their job, and they get it from your bloodstream. Thus, you run to the bathroom constantly, losing weight. Of course, this temporary dehydration will correct itself, and so will your weight loss.

Along the way, however, you do your body harm. All those high-fat foods raise your blood lipid levels. Your blood pressure may drop dramatically as a result of the fluid loss, and you may feel faint when you stand up from a sitting or prone position. You may build up toxic products of protein breakdown in your blood, sometimes even resulting in gout. Finally, you may overtax your kidneys, exacerbating any hidden kidney problems.

In his introduction to the diet, Stillman implicitly acknowledges the dangers when he limits the duration of the diet to two weeks and instructs dieters to drink *eight* glasses of water a day. Ironically, he says he designed the diet in response to his heart patients' need for quick weight loss. In this case, the cure may well worsen the disease.

CARBOHYDRATES ARE THE FOUNDATION

If we haven't made it clear so far, it's now time to make the major point of this chapter: Carbohydrates are the foundation of a healthy diet. They are the most efficient energy source for your body's needs, and they are best at building stores of muscle and liver glycogen for emergency activity needs and stamina. They produce the fewest toxic products when broken down for energy use. They spare protein, saving it for use in its primary role of building tissue instead of being burned to keep your body functioning.

Energy is the first consideration for all living things. It is the sine qua non of life itself. Carbohydrate fills this role admirably and much more healthfully than either fat or protein. You should try to get as much of your day's carbohydrate ration from unrefined sources as possible—grains, beans, fruits, and vegetables.

Food carbohydrates are perhaps the best example of the cardinal rule of good nutrition: Eat it as it grows. When you begin to separate different components from a basically healthy food to combine them again some other way, you lose much of the nutritional quality of the food. If you leave a food in one piece—not necessarily in one chunk, but with all its parts present—it has a much better chance of nourishing you adequately. "Purified" sugar is the best example of a dismembered, nutritionally empty food, as are other separated carbohydrates such as cornstarch and bleached white flour. They are nutritionally useless, but enough like food to stand in its place. You can't fool your body forever, though.

GUIDELINES

Complex carbohydrates—those from fruits, vegetables, whole grains, beans, seeds, and products made from their whole forms—are the foundation of a good diet. They should compose from 60 to 80 percent of your calories.

Get healthy amounts of fiber by eating whole grains, beans, fruits, and vegetables. It's good for you.

A high-carbohydrate diet may be helpful in managing diabetes, high blood lipid levels, and obesity.

Stay away from refined sugar and products that contain it.

Take care of your teeth, especially by keeping them clean, avoiding sugary or starchy foods that stay in your mouth, and avoiding between-meal snacks.

Alcohol is damaging to every organ in your body. We haven't evolved ways to use it without toxic effects, although very small amounts may slightly improve your statistical risk of heart disease.

Low-carbohydrate reducing diets are basically unhealthy and not terribly helpful in losing weight.

3
Fat

*F*at has gotten a lot of media attention recently, most of it confusing and, in fact, uninformed and unhelpful. Yes, high fat consumption *is* associated with a variety of ills, ranging from heart disease to maturity-onset diabetes; and saturated fat *is* more harmful than polyunsaturated fat, but only comparatively. Beyond these generally accepted points, there is quite a bit of disagreement.

WHAT IS FAT?

Fat shares some structural components with many other food and body chemicals—it's made of carbon, hydrogen, and oxygen. The carbon portion forms fat's skeleton, with hydrogen and oxygen hung on the carbon chains like ornaments on a Christmas tree. Fat differs from carbohydrate in an important respect: It has fewer oxygen molecules already attached. This means a larger part of a fat molecule's weight is made up of the "combustible" carbon and hydrogen atoms; thus, more of it is available to provide your body with energy. Since energy is calories, fat provides more calories in a smaller amount than do carbohydrate and protein. Fat yields nine calories per gram, compared with four from both protein and carbohydrate.

A fat molecule has two main components—*glycercol* and *fatty acids*. Glycerol is an alcohol with a greasy texture, also known as *glycerin*. It is metabolized much like a carbohydrate, to produce blood glucose for energy. Glycerol can have one, two, or three fatty acid molecules attached to it, forming mono-, di-, and tri-glycerides, respectively. All of these are fats.

Several different fatty acids have been identified. They differ structurally in the number of carbon atoms and in whether they are "saturated" or "unsaturated" (and to what degree). Any fatty acid can occupy any of the three attachment points on a glycerol molecule, forming a great variety of different fats.

DIETARY AND BODY FAT

Although the fat you eat and the fat in your body are constructed the same way, they are not exactly the same thing. When you eat a slice of avocado, the oil in that avocado is not deposited directly in your body as fat. It may be broken apart and reassembled to form other fats, used to make hormones or the hormonelike phospholipids, or burned to make energy. Its fatty acids can perform many roles in cell metabolism and membrane transport, brain function, and the proper function and absorption of fat-soluble vitamins. In other words, it is not simply some inert substance that goes into your mouth, through your digestive system, into your bloodstream, and straight to your hips. It does many things along the way.

Second, and equally important, your body fat does not necessarily come from food fat. Body fat deposits are storage centers for calories (as well as for fatty acids), so any extra calories you eat *from whatever source* will end up as fat, except for a comparatively small portion stored as glycogen. If you managed to eat no fat whatsoever but did eat more calories than you needed, as sugar, for example, those extra calories would be chemically converted into body fat. Since your body fat can serve quite well as a source of fatty acids for most functions listed earlier, you don't need food fat for most of those purposes. (We'll discuss fat's one essential contribution to your diet later.)

At times we will refer to body fat; at other times we will refer to dietary fat. The distinction is important, although their roles overlap somewhat, since they are both sources of fatty acids.

WHAT DOES BODY FAT DO FOR YOU?

Everybody has body fat, even the leanest or most malnourished of us. You can't live without some fat reserves. Its major role is as an energy store. Since we don't eat constantly, we store food energy for later use. The fat we have stored up is mobilized by a complex interplay of hormones when we need more energy than is available in our bloodstream and cells.

A second important job for body fat is as a source of fatty acids for a range of chemical reactions in our bodies. These fatty acids are stored as part of triglycerides, which can be broken down by enzymes when the individual fatty acids are needed. Fat deposits, especially in the liver, also act as storehouses of fat-soluble vitamins—A, D, E, and K.

Fat is stored in your body in specialized cells, known as adipose tissue cells (or fat cells). These cells resemble tiny balloons that fill with fat if you eat more calories than you need, and shrink again if you consume the fat for energy. This is how you gain and lose fat, by expanding or shrinking your fat cells.

Beyond simply storing calories for later use, adipose tissue serves in other capacities. It is very soft, so it acts as an excellent cushioning material for many internal organs. Without protective layers of fat humans would suffer many more internal injuries from comparatively minor accidents.

Fat tissue is also a good heat insulator. In the winter it cuts down on our heat loss when we go outside (and when our ancestors lived outside). In the summer it can also offer some protection when the air temperature is well above body temperature. This effect is limited, though, because we generate our own heat internally through our metabolic processes.

We are aware, of course, of what excess body fat can do *to* us as well. Overweight shortens our lifespan significantly, and the life-shortening effect seems to increase as the degree of overweight increases. "Overweight" here means having too much body fat, not simply weighing more than the average for your statistical group.

WHAT DOES FOOD FAT DO FOR YOU?

Fat is the most concentrated source of energy you can eat. We mentioned that fat provides more than twice as much energy pound for pound as does either carbohydrate or protein. A limited percentage of calories from fat can round out your daily diet nicely to provide all the calories you need. On the other hand, most of us will have no difficulty getting enough calories. The problem is the opposite—getting too many—and in this fat can be the major culprit.

Some vitamins we need dissolve poorly or not at all in water, our most common body solvent, but they do dissolve easily in fats. These are vitamins A, D, E, and K. For them to be absorbed properly they must be accompanied by a minimal amount of fat in your intestines. Again, this should not be a source of concern for most of us—we eat plenty of fat and should have no problem absorbing vitamins for that reason.

Food wouldn't taste very good with no fat in it. Many of the chemicals in foods that provide its taste are *esters,* chemicals related to fats in their structure and soluble in fats in food. Food fat tends to help blend the flavors of two or more foods you cook together, bringing out their aromas and making the entire meal more satisfying. And fat is digested very slowly, so when you eat you feel satisfied longer.

Theoretically, we need almost no fat at all in our food. We can get all the calories we need from carbohydrates and protein. We need a small amount of fat to absorb certain vitamins. But our direct need for dietary fat is limited to one fatty acid—linoleic acid. We need linoleic acid for a broad range of chemical reactions, and we can't manufacture it in our bodies. For this reason, linoleic acid is called the essential fatty acid, or EFA, as amino acids that our bodies can't manufacture are essential amino acids, or EAAs (see "Protein" chapter).

Vegetable oils are excellent sources of EFA, with safflower oil at the top of the list, followed by soy, corn, and cottonseed oils. Animal fats are poorer sources, with butter providing only a trace of EFA.

The best estimate of our EFA requirement is an amount equal to 1 or 2 percent of total calories. For most of us that is equivalent to a tablespoon of vegetable oil. Beyond that, the only dietary fat we need is a small amount to help our intestines absorb the fat-soluble vitamins. We can make the rest of the fat we may need for metabolic purposes. It is interesting to note that fat comprises about half the calories in a standard American diet. We certainly get a lot more than we need.

We should warn you at this point that "eat less fat" will be the primary refrain throughout the chapter. Since fat is such a tremendous portion of the diet for most of us, and since it without a doubt makes a major contribution to many of society's health problems, the theme bears repeating. Eat less fat.

WHAT HAPPENS TO FAT WHEN YOU EAT IT?

Not much happens to fat in your mouth or stomach, because the digestive enzymes in those parts of your digestive system are designed to work on food elements that dissolve in water, like carbohydrate. The fat is simply broken into smaller parts, so that further along the line the fat-digesting enzymes have more surface area to work on.

In your intestines, an enzyme called *lipase* goes to work on the triglycerides (fats). Lipase gets its name from "lipid," a chemist's general term for fats, and "-ase," the general ending for the names of enzymes. The lipase breaks loose two of the three fatty acids of a triglyceride molecule, leaving two fatty acids and a monoglyceride. These form compounds with intestinal chemicals so they can be absorbed by the cells of the intestinal lining. In turn, the cells reassemble the fat molecules and wrap them in a jacket of protein so they can travel through your bloodstream to storage areas or to your organs for use as energy or for chemical synthesis.

Once they pass through your intestinal wall, they may be broken up and reassembled into triglycerides many times as they pass through the lymphatic system, the liver, the bloodstream, and individual cell walls, depending on how they are to be used or how they travel.

SATURATED AND UNSATURATED

"High in Polyunsaturates" blares the label on the margarine package. "The Goodness of Corn Oil" shouts another. We are bombarded with advertising slogans that extol the virtues of fat and oil products that have a high percentage of polyunsaturated fats. "It's good for your heart and circulatory system," some say. "Lowers serum cholesterol," others brag. But what does "polyunsaturated" mean, exactly? And what does it do for you?

Fatty acids fall into three general categories—saturated, monounsaturated, and polyunsaturated. To understand these terms, we have to understand how carbon atoms link up with one another to make organic molecules.

Almost every atom has connection points where it can link to other atoms, forming molecules. Carbon has four points where it can link up with another atom. When two carbon atoms link together, they can use one, two, or three of their connection points. There will always be one, two, or three points left over on each atom to link to other atoms. For this reason, carbon is very good at forming long chains whose chemical structures look like this:

$$-C-C-C-C-C-C-C-C-C-C-C-$$

Each side of the chain has points where other atoms can link up, forming a tremendous variety of different chain molecules.

Fatty acids have this sort of chain as part of their structure, with hydrogen atoms tied on along the sides of the chain:

$$\begin{array}{ccccc} H & H & H & H & H \\ | & | & | & | & | \\ -C & -C & -C & -C & -C- \\ | & | & | & | & | \\ H & H & H & H & H \end{array}$$

Hydrogen atoms have only one tie point, so they can use up only one carbon connection point.

Sometimes carbon chains can form in which a few of the carbons hold on to one another with two bonds, instead of one:

$$-C=C-C-C=C-$$

Since carbon has only four tie points for each atom, however, these double bonds use up some of the tie points, cutting down on the number of other atoms that can attach to the sides of the chain.

When fatty acids have double carbon bonds in their chain, they lose some hydrogen atoms. Compare these two chains:

$$\begin{array}{ccccc} H & H & H & H & H \\ | & | & | & | & | \\ -C & -C & -C & -C & -C- \\ | & | & | & | & | \\ H & H & H & H & H \end{array} \qquad \begin{array}{ccccc} H & H & H \\ | & | & | \\ -C=C & -C & -C=C- \\ | & | & | \\ H & H & H \end{array}$$

Since the second chain has two double bonds, it has four fewer hydrogen atoms than does the first chain.

With fatty acids, a chain that has all the hydrogen atoms it can possibly hold is called *saturated*. If there is one double bond in the carbon chain (meaning two fewer hydrogen atoms), the fatty acid is called *monounsaturated*. Even more double bonds and the fatty acid is *polyunsaturated* ("poly-" means many).

The difference among these three forms at the molecular level is the number of double bonds in the carbon chain. At a larger level, where our senses operate, the difference is in texture.

Saturated fats, such as butter or lard, are solid at room temperature, while polyunsaturated fats, like corn oil, are liquid. Fats with a lot of monounsaturated fatty acids, like olive oil, are thick, but more liquid than solid.

Generally, the fats found in animal products are composed mostly of saturated fatty acids (hard fats), while fats that come from vegetable sources are mostly unsaturated (oils). There are some exceptions. Some fish oils are just that—oils—and are much higher in polyunsaturated fatty acids than are other animal fats. On the other hand, cocoa butter and coconut and palm oils are hard fats, or close to it, and they are even higher in saturated fatty acids than most animal fats.

Because vegetable oils are cheap and popular among consumers, food manufacturers like to use them in their products. But vegetable oils don't always have the characteristics required for every single product a food manufacturer may make. In particular, oils may not be stiff enough to give a bread dough, for example, the proper "body." Vegetable oil isn't really the right texture for consumers to use as a spread on bread or over vegetables.

The answer is to take the unsaturated, liquid oil and make it into hard fat. But how? By hydrogenating it—adding hydrogen to the carbon chains to fill them up with hydrogen atoms. And what do we end up with? A more saturated fat. Liquid oils can be hydrogenated by being heated and exposed to hydrogen gas in the presence of nickel. The result is a product, such as margarine or Crisco, that sounds like highly unsaturated fat (which it used to be), but tastes and looks like more saturated fat (which it has become). In many cases, if you start out using vegetable oil products to avoid saturated fat, you end up eating just what you wanted to avoid.

Of course, there are margarines and then there are margarines. Some remain high in polyunsaturated fats, even though they have a more acceptable texture because of their chemical treatment. Others are disasters, using cheap byproduct oils like coconut and cottonseed, hydrogenating them beyond recognition, dyeing them to look like stale butter, and then flavoring them with (ready for this?) butter. The lesson here is: If you want to use margarine to cut your saturated fat, READ THE LABEL. Using a bad margarine in place of butter is worse than not using one at all. Of course, people with heart disease should not use even a little butter or other saturated fat, so for them margarine can help cut saturated fat and balance it with polyunsaturated. The best margarines are only about 20 percent saturated and as much as 50 percent polyunsaturated, with the rest monounsaturated.

Hydrogenation also partially or completely destroys the only nutritionally necessary component of fat—linoleic acid. The more completely hardened the fat, the more the linoleic has been converted to oleic and stearic acids, both useless for the reactions that require linoleic.

In most foods, the benefit of hydrogenation is to the processor, not the consumer. The majority of products with hydrogenated oil use it in place of more expensive alternatives or because it has a longer shelf life than does polyunsaturated, or simply as a marketing ploy. An example of this is its role in peanut butter. Its only function is to keep the peanut oil from separating. Some people don't want to be reminded that peanut butter has a goodly helping of oil in it, so they'd rather not see it floating on top when they open the jar. Or they may not want to stir the oil back in before they use it. So processors have given them peanut butter that stays stirred, by making the oil too thick to flow out of the peanut meal. However, the integrity of this noble-in-its-simplicity food is violated. If you don't want to stir peanut butter, refrigerate it. It will stay fresher, too.

We've indicated that the best sources for unsaturated oils are vegetable products, particularly grains, nuts, seeds, and the oils extracted from them. Avocado and olive oils are also mainly unsaturated, although most of this is from monounsaturated oleic acid. Coconut oil and cocoa butter are more than half saturated, and palm oil is nearly half saturated.

The only animal fats in a lacto-ovo-vegetarian diet are butterfat and the fat present in egg yolk. Butter is, of course, butterfat, as is the fat component of cream, whole milk, yogurt, and cheese. It is well over half saturated fat, and it gives only a trace of linoleic acid. Egg fat is slightly better, much lower in saturated and higher in monounsaturated fatty acids. Still, it provides little EFA (linoleic acid).

CHOLESTEROL

We include cholesterol in this chapter because it is related to dietary fat in some important ways. However, it is not itself a fat, but a greasy alcohol, like glycerol, but thicker.

"Cholesterol" is a word known to most of us because of the publicity it has received, mostly about its relationship to coronary heart disease. High levels of cholesterol in the blood are related to an increased risk of heart attack, and indeed, cholesterol itself is a major component of the artery-blocking plaques that cause many heart attacks.

We can get cholesterol from food, and different foods have widely different amounts of cholesterol. Thus, different diets can provide widely differing levels of dietary cholesterol. Dietary cholesterol and blood plasma cholesterol are two separate things, however, just as dietary fat and body fat are two different things.

Most of the cholesterol in your body is manufactured by your own organs, notably your liver and intestines. A portion comes from food, but food cholesterol is only partially absorbed in your intestine. Moreover, the higher your blood cholesterol, the less your organs manufacture and the less your intestine absorbs from your food. This is known as a *negative feedback system,* because the results of an action—synthesizing or absorbing cholesterol—inhibit the continuation of that action. Your body systems, particularly those regulating your blood chemistry, provide many examples of this kind of feedback.

The system's efficiency varies widely from one person to another. Some people can eat tremendous amounts of cholesterol-laden foods and still maintain relatively constant blood levels. Others have little control at all, and their blood levels may soar after a high-cholesterol meal. These are the minorities at each extreme; most people fall somewhere between in blood-cholesterol-regulating efficiency. Therefore, different people will show different effects from an attempt to limit blood cholesterol by limiting food cholesterol.

Other factors complicate the picture. When your diet contains less than 300 to 400 milligrams of cholesterol a day, any change made in your cholesterol intake has a proportional effect on your blood cholesterol (depending on how efficiently your internal regulators work). Once your intake goes above 400 milligrams, however, changing your intake has a lessened effect on your blood level.

The average American gets about 450 milligrams a day, and it's easy to see how—a single egg yolk contains 250 milligrams. For a dietary cholesterol cutback to have a significant effect, many of us would have to make drastic changes, because we would have to cut our intake in half.

Exactly what effect would this change have? According to most researchers, a drastic cutback in food cholesterol intake will make at most a 10 to 15 percent change in blood cholesterol levels.

Other factors complicate the issue even more, because they have an even greater effect on blood cholesterol than does dietary cholesterol. The most significant is your weight; that is, your fatness. The fatter you are, the higher your blood cholesterol level, and the more weight you lose the lower you can force it. This functions independent of dietary cholesterol; in fact, you can conceivably eat *more* cholesterol and still lower your blood level by losing weight (but don't try it to see if it works). This one factor has the strongest influence of all on blood cholesterol.

Another very important factor is the amount of saturated fat you eat. The more saturated fat in your diet, the higher your plasma cholesterol level. This factor is also relatively independent of your food cholesterol intake, although many foods that contain saturated fat also contain cholesterol.

Finally, the saturated fat in your diet can be balanced to a limited extent by polyunsaturated fat (monounsaturated fat apparently has no effect at all). Eating polyunsaturated fat in place of saturated fat can lead to a significant lowering of blood cholesterol level. The strongest effect on blood cholesterol occurs when you eat half as much saturated as polyunsaturated fat. This is known as the P/S ratio (polyunsaturated/saturated ratio) of your diet. When your P/S ratio is about 2 (twice as much P as S), you've reached the theoretical ideal. In contrast, the average P/S ratio in this country is about 0.4 or 0.5 (half as much P as S). Vegetarians certainly have an easier time maintaining a good ratio, since most fats of vegetable origin are high in polyunsaturated fatty acids, and since the fat in meat is very high in saturated fatty acids.

Consumption of food fiber also has an effect on blood cholesterol. Cholesterol is a necessary constituent of bile salts, substances secreted by your liver into your intestines to help in fat digestion. The food fiber in fruits, vegetables, nuts, legumes, and some grains (but not wheat bran) ties up some of these bile salts so they are excreted instead of being recycled as normally would happen. You lose whatever cholesterol you would have reabsorbed.

Evidence also indicates that your primary protein source may have a profound effect on your blood cholesterol level. Researchers fed subjects with elevated blood cholesterol a diet that substituted soy protein for meat. Even when the intake of dietary cholesterol remained high, average blood cholesterol fell dramatically. Other research indicates that casein—milk protein—works to elevate blood cholesterol. In fact, animal protein in general seems to have this effect.

One other factor affects the level of cholesterol in your bloodstream. We mentioned earlier that fats travel through your blood in combination with protein. These aggregations of triglycerides and protein molecules are called *lipoproteins,* and they also function to transport cholesterol, since it is insoluble in water, as is fat. Chemists can differentiate among several different types of lipoproteins; the two most common forms are *high-density lipoprotein* and *low-density lipoprotein* (HDL and LDL).

HDL and LDL are two of several factors that carry cholesterol in your blood, but they have opposite effects on your potential for heart disease. LDL is bad for you and HDL appears to be good. The most important factor in the risk of heart disease is the proportion of your total blood cholesterol represented by LDL and HDL. If a relatively high proportion of total blood cholesterol is LDL, you've got a problem. If a high proportion is HDL, your risk is significantly reduced.

An important point here is that your absolute levels of HDL and LDL are less important than are the proportions of the total they represent. If your total blood cholesterol decreases but the HDL decreases *less,* the ratio—and your risk of heart disease—has improved. It's the reverse for LDL. If LDL levels decrease less than total blood cholesterol, you could be in worse shape than before.

Irrespective of your diet, you can improve your HDL ratio and cut the odds of heart disease by making hard exercise a part of your daily life. Researchers have found that people who exercise hard, with mountainclimbing, long-distance running, etc., have elevated HDL ratios. Of course, this vigorous exercise has other health benefits, including lowering your weight and sometimes your blood pressure (both of which affect your risk of heart attack).

In a way, high blood cholesterol is a warning signal. It tells you that you are probably not treating your body as well as you should if you want to live a long, vigorous life. You're not eating well, you're probably overweight, and you don't exercise enough. Of course, this is all too common today, even with the recent growth in interest in active sports participation and a growing awareness of the importance of nutrition. Our average energy expenditure is continuing to drop, while our consumption of fat and sugar continues at an excessive level.

This is a matter of opinion, of course. Others disagree with this indictment of the popular diet, saying we don't yet know enough to make recommendations for dietary change for the whole country. The Food and Nutrition Board (FNB), an organization under the general leadership of the National Research Council, released a report in mid-1980 that stated in part that normal Americans need not reduce their consumption of fats and cholesterol.

Both the content of the FNB's report, *Toward Healthful Diets,* and the manner in which it was released to the public were attacked immediately by professionals and by lay people. Most organizations that have reviewed the evidence connecting diet and coronary artery disease, including the American Heart Association, the Food and Agriculture Organization of the World Health Organization, the office of the Surgeon General, the Inter-society Commission for Heart Disease Resources, and even the RDA Committee (formed under the FNB), have recommended diet changes to cut the risks of heart disease.

Suddenly, a government-sponsored organization had contradicted the recommendations of a score of scientific bodies, few of whom had any particular ax to grind. The FNB was assailed with charges ranging from conflict of interest (many of the Board members were consultants to industry organizations and companies that stood to gain or lose from the Board's statement) to ignorance to sloppy scientific work.

The FNB's major reservation against making recommendations for dietary changes to reduce the risk of heart disease in the entire population is reasonable. The causative link between blood cholesterol level and the incidence of heart disease has not been unequivocally demonstrated. No one has actually *proved* that high blood cholesterol causes heart attacks, and more to the point, nobody has proved that lowering blood cholesterol will necessarily protect an individual from a heart attack.

The FNB acknowledged that dietary changes might be appropriate for people "at risk" of developing heart disease, but the implication was that these individuals are a minority. According to the FNB, normal Americans need not alter fat or cholesterol eating habits.

However.

The group of "at-risk" individuals is much larger than the document implies. Dr. William Castelli, director of the Framingham Heart Study, a 32-year study of the people of Framingham, Massachusetts, responded to the report: "The report says that only people at risk should worry about their fat and cholesterol intake. But who is at risk? One-half of all Americans have a family history of heart disease, one-third are overweight, and the majority have high blood cholesterol levels. In fact, nearly all Americans are at risk to get a heart attack." Dr. Castelli's point of view is borne out by the fact that heart disease is the nation's number one killer.

In addition, there are many strong indications that cholesterol does, indeed, have a causative role in heart disease. Several animal feeding studies have shown that the single addition of cholesterol to the diet can lead to atherosclerotic lesions—the plaque deposits that build up to block blood vessels and cause heart attacks. Other feeding studies have shown that these lesions can be decreased by lowering the animal's blood cholesterol level. This is a very strong indicator that lowering blood cholesterol through diet can protect individuals from heart disease.

We feel that the questions have been answered sufficiently to recommend a diet that would produce lowered blood cholesterol. Of course, this issue, like most others in nutrition, may never finally be answered. We look forward to the results of the many research projects either under way or planned in this crucial area.

Even if the evidence finally proves that lowering blood cholesterol has no significant effect on your risk of a heart attack, the dietary changes required generally fit in with a more healthful life style anyway. They eliminate unnecessary fat and concentrated protein; so they can't be harmful and may be very good for your total health. Cholesterol-lowering changes, in order of effectiveness, are as follows:

Lose weight. If you are overweight, getting closer to some kind of "ideal" weight can cause a dramatic drop in your blood cholesterol level.

Cut back on saturated fat. This is obviously much easier for a vegetarian than for a meat-eater, since meat (especially red meat) is high in saturated fat.

Moderately increase your consumption of polyunsaturated fats. This is best done by eating whole foods that contain polyunsaturated fatty acids as natural components, such as beans, nuts, and seeds. Don't overdo, and certainly don't end up eating more total fat than you did before you cut down on saturated forms.

These three actions are known to be effective in lowering blood cholesterol levels. In addition, there are two other steps you can take, both of which have variable effects, depending on how your body reacts.

Cut your consumption of food cholesterol significantly. The richest sources are dairy products (particularly eggs and butterfat), shellfish, liver, and other organ meats.

Let high-fiber foods—fruits, vegetables, grains, seeds, legumes, bread—*play a larger role in your diet.* These drain off part of your blood cholesterol by binding with intestinal bile salts made from blood cholesterol and taking them along to be excreted.

Cut down on animal protein, whether you are nonvegetarian or lacto-ovo-vegetarian. Although the exact causative relationship is unclear, changing to vegetable protein sources, especially soy, appears to lower serum cholesterol level significantly in people with a cholesterol problem.

You will have the most worthwhile results by following the first three steps on this list. Losing weight and cutting down on saturated fat, especially, will help your health in other ways and are good for you in general, whether their cholesterol-lowering effect proves helpful or not.

CALORIES

"Fat" and "calories" are nearly synonymous to many people, and fat is actually the most concentrated calorie source you can eat. One gram of fat—less than a quarter-teaspoon of butter, for example—gives you nine calories. Both protein and carbohydrates pale in comparison, with their measly contribution of four calories per gram.

The average American gets more than half of his or her day's calories from fat. In contrast, most authorities, including the U. S. Senate's Select Committee on Nutrition and Human Needs, recommend that Americans cut their fat intake considerably, a minimum of 25 percent. The caloric slack would then be taken up by carbohydrates and, to a lesser extent, protein.

In fact, many Americans would do well to cut out 25 percent of their daily fat intake and not replace it with anything at all. Life expectancy appears to be directly linked to body weight—the more you weigh above the national average, the shorter your life expectancy compared to the average. A less publicized but potentially much more important aspect of weight loss is that if you weigh *less* than average, your life expectancy is *longer* than average (up to a point, naturally). Remember, too, that the national average is significantly above ideal weight. Cutting 12 or 13 percent of your daily calorie intake by cutting out a quarter of your daily fat intake is an excellent way to lose weight. And losing weight is, as we've shown, a great way to climb up that Great Actuarial Table of Life.

Fat is an especially handy place to cut calories, because it is such a concentrated calorie package. Cutting out a given amount of fat from your diet will have twice the calorie effect of cutting down on protein or carbohydrate by an equal amount. The result is that you have more to eat if you cut down on fat than if you cut down on the other two—a lesser change in your eating pattern. Many low-fat foods, such as vegetables, grains, and legumes, have an appreciable amount of fiber to help fill your stomach and give you a satisfied feeling.

This is all well and good until you consider what you will be losing by eliminating this fat. Unfortunately, most of us *like* fat—a lot. Fat provides quite a bit of sensory gratification when we eat, because it carries most of the "taste chemicals" contained in food (except sugar and salt). Because fat lingers in your digestive tract longer after eating, since it's digested slowly, you feel satisfied longer after a high-fat meal, even if you are no longer feeling full. Therefore, decreasing fat intake will probably make you hungry faster than usual. This is usually all right, though, because the food you eat will be less fattening, so you can eat more and still get fewer calories. Of course, since you don't eliminate fat from your diet completely, you get the benefits of both.

It becomes clear why food fat and obesity are related. We like fat—it tastes good and satisfies our hunger pangs longer. Unfortunately, it carries a disproportionately high load of calories, so when we indulge our tastes (as we affluent Westerners are famous for doing), we load our diets with highly caloric food that not surprisingly makes us fat. Of course, it is simplistic to say that fat is fattening, any more than anything else is when eaten to excess. The point is that it's much easier to eat fat to excess because (1) it yields more calories than does protein or carbohydrate and (2) it gratifies the senses completely out of proportion to the nutrition it brings with it. We should probably add this to the list of reasons: habit. We eat a diet with 50 percent of its calories from fat because we're used to it. This is excessive fat consumption by any measure, especially considering the other health risks we describe later.

More conservative nutritionists, that is, those who would make the smallest changes in the traditional diet, advocate a decrease in fat to 35 percent of total calories. The more radical, however, advocate cutting back to as little as 10 percent of calories from fat. This is impossible without radically restructuring the way you eat and live. For your diet to average 10 percent of calories from fat, most of what you eat must be well below that level to make up for the few things you'll probably eat that are much higher. Your diet could include most grains (but not oats), most beans (but not soybeans or chickpeas), and all fruits and vegetables except olives and avocados. Nonfat milk products would, of course, also be included, as would defatted soy and wheat germ products. Nuts and seeds average about 75 percent of calories from fat, so you'd have to all but cut them out of your diet to keep down to 10 percent fat. Whole-milk dairy products get from half to three-quarters of their calories from fat, so you would have to minimize them as well.

A tough diet, all in all, but probably a very healthy one. In our culture very few people could structure their lives this way, and it seems reasonable to set a goal that more people could rationally aspire to. Twenty percent of calories from fat would give most of the health benefits, and would be much easier for the average person to accomplish. But don't be misled—it's still very difficult to achieve. Vegetarians have it much easier than do meat-eaters, of course, since red meat gets about half its calories from fat, pushing the proportion to the high side immediately (prepared meats, like cold cuts, are much higher in fat, while poultry and fish are significantly lower). On the other hand, vegetarians who eat chunks of hard cheese and handfuls of nuts as a snack will be getting even higher levels of fat from these foods. Fat is a problem for almost all of us.

FAT AND CANCER

At this point you may be so tired of cancer warnings that you're tempted to skip this section. "What doesn't cause cancer?" you say.

Actually, the number of chemicals that cause cancer is rather limited. Unfortunately, the few that do act as carcinogens or as tumor promoters are widespread. The food you eat, the air you breathe, the work you do, the sun that shines, the water you drink and bathe with, and the other organisms around you, both microscopic, and visible, may all have some factor or another that can increase your cancer risk. A major challenge of the coming years will be to identify these factors and eliminate them from the environment.

Luckily, many are avoidable. Ten years ago a deep suntan was looked upon as a sign of good health. Today many people are aware of the unhappy consequences of all that solar ultraviolet light pouring into defenseless skin cells, and many people now avoid overexposure to the sun.

Food carcinogen warnings, on the other hand, have been coming so quickly lately you may be bewildered—what's the latest on what I can and can't eat? Sometimes the warnings tell you to stay away from the very things you thought were good for you. The saccharin you used to avoid sugar was possibly giving you cancer, for example. (Of course, it was later given a conditionally clean bill of health, until the next round of experiments condemns it again.)

Such is the case for fats. Although the evidence is far from complete, it now appears from tests with laboratory animals that polyunsaturated fatty acids may promote cancer, and they may be worse in this respect than monounsaturated or saturated fatty acids. Understand, we aren't saying they *cause* cancer; rather, they may cause accelerated growth in tumors caused by other carcinogens. Remember that the other types of fatty acids didn't get good marks; their effects are simply less pronounced than those of polyunsaturates.

These fatty acids are implicated as promoters of skin and breast cancers in rats, but they may affect other types of tumors in other animal species. Thus if you tried to increase your consumption of polyunsaturates to protect your heart from circulatory disease, you may have been furthering damage to other parts of your body.

Unfortunately, it is unclear how this research relates to humans. Population studies of widely divergent groups indicate that, in people at least, saturated fat and especially animal fat are more closely associated with a variety of cancers. These studies that compare whole population groups statistically are called *epidemiological studies,* from the same Greek roots as the word *epidemic.* They can't prove causative links, but they can show strong associations between two or more factors in the life style of an entire country's population, for example. Over and over, such studies have connected increased cancer incidence with increased consumption of animal fat, as well as sugar, alcohol, and total calories. Until the exact mechanism is worked out, we are left somewhat in the dark.

The situation is a double bind, and the best solution is to avoid most fats as completely as you can. A reasonable goal for lowering fat consumption is to get 20 percent of calories from fat. Getting even that fat through food—rather than as separated fat—may be beneficial. An interesting side note, for those who are worried about eating foods naturally high in polyunsaturates, is that some of these foods contain a substance that may *inhibit* tumor development. Soybeans, in particular, have an enzyme described as a *protease inhibitor* that several researchers are investigating to determine its tumor-inhibiting properties. It may well offset the tumor-promoting effects of polyunsaturated fatty acids contained in the same foods. Again we see the benefit of eating foods in their natural state as much as possible.

This factor may also explain the differences in the conclusions reached by the epidemiological studies on the one hand and the laboratory research into polyunsaturated fatty acids and cancer on the other. Since the animals in the experiments were fed purified fatty acids, they did not have the benefit of the whole natural food that populations of humans—in the wild, so to speak—would get. Of course, animal foods containing fat afford no such protection, since they contain none of these tumor inhibitors.

CALCIUM AND FAT

In some cases fat can have a negative effect on the absorption of calcium in your intestine. The calcium is present as a dissolved salt, and thus as a free ion. Fatty acids can bond with this free calcium ion, making an unabsorbable soap.

This process, called *saponification,* becomes significant only when the concentration of fatty acids is relatively high, so if your intake of fats is moderate to low, the effect is unimportant. If you eat a lot of fats and if you are marginal in your calcium intake to begin with, however, it may have some effect on your health. Calcium from your bones may be drained to maintain the necessary blood levels. Since calcium blood levels are crucial to your metabolism, your body will sacrifice bone strength.

Very few of us need worry about this, however. We only mention it here to indicate another aspect of fat's negative influence on health.

GOALS TO AIM FOR

It should be clear by now that, of the three main nutrients, fat is the major nutritional bad guy. Whether saturated fat or unsaturated fat is worse is still not clear. What is clear, however, is that we should all try to cut fat from our diets as much as we can. Fat is implicated in heart disease and in promoting cancer of the colon and breast in humans and other cancers in research animals. It contributes to obesity, a disease on its own and a primary cause of diabetes. It can even interfere with absorption of the essential mineral calcium. And it displaces other important nutrients in your total diet.

Balanced with these negative points are a few rather limited pluses. First, we need a small amount of fat in our intestines to absorb the fat-soluble vitamins. Second, we need a small amount of polyunsaturated fat to provide the essential linoleic acid. The only reported cases of EFA deficiency to date have been in newborns, and in no way should it be a problem for adults. Children may sometimes need a certain amount of fat in their diets simply because they need the concentrated calories it provides to cover their disproportionately high energy output. Athletes who put out tremendous effort over extended periods may need a certain amount of fat for the same reason—they may not be able to eat enough otherwise to get the required calories.

A reasonable goal for dietary fat is 20 percent of calories. This is within the reach (barely) of most Americans. Going below this level is apparently harmless, as long as you can get enough calories to keep yourself healthy. (We assume you won't eliminate fat totally, of course.)

The debate over polyunsaturated fat versus saturated fat still rages, and conclusive evidence linking saturated fat to heart disease may never be obtained. Even so, it seems prudent to keep your intake of these fat types in an approximate 2 to 1 ratio: half as much saturated as polyunsaturated fat.

As far as cholesterol is concerned, the evidence is also not yet in, but most vegetarian sources of cholesterol are also sources of abundant fat, which should be avoided on its own. Eggs do indeed provide large amounts of protein, but you don't need that much protein anyway (see Chapter 4). If you eat great numbers of eggs, you miss the vitamins, minerals, carbohydrate, and fiber that would take their place if you ate a healthy, more varied diet.

HOW TO CUT DOWN

You may be convinced by now that it is important to decrease your fat consumption as much as possible. There is no such thing as a good fat, beyond our limited need for EFA in polyunsaturated oils.

There is a great difference between realizing something must be done and determining *how* to do it. When you go to a restaurant and eat three pieces of bread and butter before you are served, which do you regret, the bread or the butter? Most people immediately think of the bread the next day when the grim reality stares up from the bathroom scale. They don't remember the butter, because spreading butter on bread is a childhood reflex, not something you even notice, let alone scrutinize.

When you pass up a baked potato at dinner because it's "too fattening," do you think about the butter or sour cream spread liberally on it? The unadorned baked potato is certainly not fattening—it has only about 100 calories—but we've been schooled into thinking of it that way. The way we eat it makes the potato fattening.

Unfortunately, many of us have a difficult time facing a slice of bread or a potato without their customary accompaniments of butter and other fatty flavoring ingredients. Parents used to think fat was good for children, so many of us grew up with plenty of it on our plates.

We mention this only to show that we realize how difficult it will be for many people to eliminate even a little fat from their diets. They would rather pass up the bread completely than try it plain. This would be a mistake, because foods like bread and other grain products, potatoes, and vegetables, plus other foods to which we don't add fat such as fruits, beans, and seeds, are the best choices to fill the calorie and volume gap left by the fats you are going to avoid. They have protein, vitamins, minerals, and, most important, lots of health-giving carbohydrates.

Specific places to eliminate fat include changing from whole milk to part skim and then skim, eating much less cheese (except low-fat cheeses like ricotta, farmer, and cottage cheese), eating fewer nuts and eating them raw rather than roasted in oil, and finding things to use in place of butter or other fats as spreads on bread and vegetables. For example, unsweetened applesauce is delicious on bread, muffins, or baked potatoes, and lemon juice is an excellent flavoring for vegetables. In addition, there are usually low-fat alternatives to almost every dairy product (except, of course, butter and cream).

In a restaurant order baked potato or spaghetti instead of french fries, have vegetables plain instead of in cream sauce, eat pasta with tomato sauce instead of sauce Alfredo. In general, avoid fried foods and pay attention to the foods you know have added oil, such as salad (in the dressing). Steamed vegetables are better than vegetable tempura, and strawberries in wine are better than chocolate cake with buttercream icing. Remember that huge amounts of fat can be hidden in foods; in fact, a restaurant may make its tomato sauce with a lot more oil than you do at home.

Many cookbook recipes were formulated before the most recent research about diet management was published. Don't be shy about experimenting—for example, in making a cheese sauce, you needn't mix the flour thickener with butter to get it to blend with the milk or stock base. Simply blend it well with the finely grated cheese, and pour the mixture into the hot liquid. Simmer the entire mixture together until it thickens. Remember to think before you add. Try the recipe with half the oil called for; you might even like it better, and it probably won't hurt the result, whatever the outcome.

If, in addition, you want to alter the ratio of saturated to polyunsaturated fat in your diet, you can use polyunsaturated oils in almost every case when you fry or saute food. Save butter for spreading on bread, and even then use it only rarely and in very small amounts. Pretend that it's very, very expensive and you have to conserve it. If you have a great deal of trouble cutting down on your use of spreading fats, consider using a high-polyunsaturate margarine. Even though it is chemically processed and often preserved, colored, and flavored with other lab products, it will probably be better for you in the long run than saturated fat. Read the cautions in Chapter 12, Shopping and Storing, before buying margarine. And remember, there's no such thing as a good fat.

It's not a good idea to increase your intake of polyunsaturated fats to somehow compensate for a high saturated fat intake. Your total fat intake should never increase, no matter what dietary changes you make. Although polyunsaturates do help lower serum cholesterol, they give you very little nutrition for their calories and they may promote cancer, just like other fats. Take your pick—neither heart disease nor cancer is a great choice. The safest course is to cut your fat intake at least to 20 percent, and make your largest cuts in animal fat.

But you may have a passion for something that has far too much fat. You know there's no way you'll stop eating it. But you do have to remember it does matter, no matter what you'd like to think. Make up for the transgressions against your body somewhere else—make a low-fat main dish and don't butter your bread and baked potato to offset the dietary "problem" you feel you can't pass up. This is only the mature thing to do—no make-believe about how it's just this once. Your body keeps track, even if your head doesn't.

GUIDELINES

Your body fat acts as a cushion, thermal insulation, and a reservoir for energy and fatty acids.

Food fat provides the EFA linoleic acid, aids in the absorption of fat-soluble vitamins, and gives eating enjoyment and calories.

Beyond these relative pluses, fat is a nutritional disaster. It can crowd out more nutritious food or aid and abet us in growing obese. It has been linked to a variety of ills, especially cancer and heart disease.

A reasonable dietary goal for most Americans is to cut fat intake to 20 percent of calories.

We should try to eat half as much saturated as polyunsaturated fat.

Fat yields nine calories per gram. Carbohydrate and protein yield four.

Avoid whole milk, cream, butter, fried foods, and ice cream. Cut down on cheese and nuts.

4
Protein

We Americans as a nation bow down to the altar of the pagan god Protein, sacrificing fatted calves and all manner of other unfortunates at a mind-boggling rate. Of course, our national overemphasis on protein intake can be blamed partially on the public relations efforts of the meat and dairy industries and the Department of Agriculture. But protein's mystique has, until recently, been furthered by scientists as well as flacks.

In 1838 Jan Mulder, a Dutch chemist and doctor, coined the word "protein." Scientists in his day found that certain nitrogen-containing chemicals were necessary to life, and research took off at a great pace. Professor Liebig, a respected physiologist, stated that energy expenditure required protein, and although this was quickly disproved, the idea has persisted even 'til today.

Carl von Voit of Germany determined that adult males required about 118 grams of protein a day, although he made this determination by simply measuring protein intake of a group of men, without attempting to manipulate experimentally their intake. Around the turn of the century, W. O. Atwater, an American follower of von Voit's protein "research," declared that laborers needed 145 grams of protein and sedentary people needed only 125.

During World War II, the United States government formulated a set of Recommended Dietary Allowances (RDAs) for most nutrients, including protein. Although the recommended amount was still quite high, it was, at least, based on some sketchy research. The RDA for protein has been lowered at every revision, until today it is significantly below the amount consumed by the average American. Perhaps we can now begin to think of protein in a

54

realistic context, as a necessary nutrient just like carbohydrate, vitamins, minerals, and fat, and no more or less important than other nutrients.

One question immediately arises. If protein is no more important than fat and carbohydrate to full nutrition, why is it the only energy-providing nutrient* that has an RDA?

The answer is twofold. First, more research has been done concerning the need for protein than on the other two major nutrients. Thus, the National Research Council has more information to use in determining a minimum need and in making their recommendations. Second, although there are literally millions of different proteins, a general structure is common to all, and they are all relatively interchangeable as far as nutrition is concerned. Fat and carbohydrate have many forms, some good and some bad, some more absorbable or more necessary than others. This complicates the issue so much that a simple recommendation for intake is almost impossible to make. But certain forms of carbohydrate and fat are needed just as much as protein is in your diet.

WHAT PROTEIN DOES

If carbohydrate and fat are the fuel of life, protein is the structure of life. All living things, from humans on down the evolutionary scale to viruses, are built of protein, and various proteins take part in our every life process. Cells build proteins called *enzymes* to control chemical changes inside the cells and in the rest of the body. The growing portion of bones is first protein, and is later filled in with minerals to harden it. Any part of your body that grows requires new protein to create its structure. Hair, nails, and skin have a protein called *keratin* as one main component. Most hormones are mainly protein. The structure of muscles, connective tissue, and the various glands and other organs is also protein.

Protein is ubiquitous because it is so useful. The number of different forms it can take is almost unlimited, each form with a different possible biological function.

Plants and certain protozoa are the only living things that can

---

*Carbohydrate, fat, and protein are energy-providing nutrients because they all provide calories—this is the major role of fat and carbohydrate, but only a secondary role for protein. Nutrients such as vitamins and minerals don't yield any calories.

create protein from water, air, soil, and sunlight. The rest of us must get it, either directly or indirectly, from plants. If you eat meat you are still eating plant protein, because the animals got their protein from plants or from other animals who ate plants. At each stage of the process the animal takes the protein from the food, uses what is needed, and discards the rest.

WHY PEOPLE NEED PROTEIN

The need for protein is universal in humans, although it varies from one person to another, and in any person from season to season, day to day, even hour to hour. Although most of us are well aware of our protein need, since it has been drummed into us since early childhood, we probably haven't stopped to question why we need it. This article of faith should be examined so we can make some sense of it.

Because they are growing and increasing the physical mass of their bodies, children's need for protein is obvious. Likewise, adults recuperating from surgery, injury, or debilitating disease obviously need protein to heal, as do athletes in training who are building more muscle mass (although this need has been greatly overemphasized for athletes).

However, why should normally healthy adults need food protein? After all, the organs, muscles, skin, skeletal structure, and blood are already *there*. They don't need to be created anew.

This question sounds reasonable on the surface, but it assumes that the human body is a static system, that once built, it no longer changes. Actually, every organ and part of your body is in a continual state of turnover. Cells are constantly dying and being replaced, proteins are broken down and built up again, blood and skin are continually lost (although generally in quite small amounts).

Your body is a little like a large city in this respect. A city is in a constant state of flux, as buildings are torn down and rebuilt, facades are changed, streets are realigned. Even if your body isn't destroying entire city blocks and rebuilding them from the ground up, it is still in a constant process of interior remodeling and housecleaning.

Unlike a city in the throes of rebuilding itself, however, your body discards very little old building material. There is little waste, because the broken-down proteins are recycled into new body proteins. This explains why we refer to your body's use of protein as a process of turnover. In a healthy person under normal circumstances, the body proteins are in a state of dynamic equilibrium—constantly changing, but staying more or less the same over time.

The protein-recycling system is normally relatively efficient, but it can't be perfect. Protein is still lost from your body because of the changes it is constantly undergoing. This lost protein travels two main paths. First, your body loses protein directly, through losses of small amounts of skin, hair, nail trimmings, and body secretions such as sweat.

Second, small amounts of protein are broken down and converted into blood glucose to be burned for energy. This is the major path for protein loss, and it becomes even more significant in people who eat a poor diet, especially one low in carbohydrates.

Your daily need is simply for enough protein to replace these losses. Excess food protein is either burned for energy or changed into fat and stored for future use as an energy source. You can't store it as protein, as carbohydrate is stored as glycogen or food fat as body fat.

HOW MUCH DO YOU NEED?

Any protein you eat over your basic daily need is wasted, at least as protein per se. It would be helpful to know, therefore, how much protein you need daily.

Most authorities agree that an adult's protein need equals the day's body protein loss, plus a factor to account for any food protein your body doesn't use. Put more simply, "in" equals "out." This is the normal state for healthy adults—equilibrium.

If you lose more than you take in, you are in negative balance. This means your body proteins are breaking down faster than you are replacing them, an unhealthy situation. This can occur when you're sick and some of your body tissues are being rapidly destroyed, or if you get too little protein or too few calories in your diet. Too little dietary protein or calories is very unusual in the United States.

On the other hand, if you are retaining protein for new tissue growth, as does a child, a pregnant woman, or a convalescent patient, "in" is greater than "out." This is called *positive balance,* and these people need comparatively more protein than do adults in normal health.

Since the turn of the century, researchers have watched human protein metabolism in carefully controlled studies to find the minimum adult protein need. To determine the protein requirement for experimental subjects, the researchers needed to measure their protein intake and loss.

Proteins are very complex chemical compounds composed of thousands of atoms connected together into a unique pattern for each different protein molecule. When our bodies lose protein, what we excrete is often just a remnant of the protein molecule. That remnant, however, contains the one chemical element that sets protein apart from the other nutrient chemicals. Although protein contains carbon, hydrogen, and oxygen, just like fat and carbohydrate, it also contains nitrogen. This nitrogen is lost when protein is lost, either through direct loss, as in bleeding or nail trimmings, or through energy use. Thus, researchers could measure nitrogen intake and loss, and from these they could infer protein intake and loss. The studies came to be known as *nitrogen-balance studies,* because nitrogen was the indicator that showed protein balance.

Nitrogen is relatively easy to detect, so researchers had a useful tool for measuring the presence of protein. However, measuring minimum protein need is more complicated than simply comparing protein intake to protein loss. Recall that any protein you eat over your minimum need is simply burned or stored as calories. When it is converted into calories, the nitrogen portion is broken off and discarded. It is excreted in your urine, and thus appears as part of your nitrogen loss. Under normal circumstances, then, *any* protein intake over the minimum looks like simple protein equilibrium, like filling a glass to overflowing.

To find the *minimum* level, negative balance (losing more protein than taking in) was created in subjects through fasting or some other protein-depleting regimen. Once they were losing more than they were taking in, researchers could give them increasing protein rations until they were again in equilibrium. This was the true minimum protein requirement. Of course, the volunteers were fed enough calories in carbohydrates to keep them from burning protein for energy and increasing their nitrogen loss.

This minimum level varied from one person to another. The researchers calculated an average minimum from all their experimental data.

WHAT IS YOUR RDA?

The average figure for a number of experimental subjects in several different studies was 0.32 grams of protein for every kilogram (2.2 pounds) of lean body weight (obese people need less proportionately). This is the amount of easily digested protein they needed every day.

Since the Forties, the U. S. Food and Nutrition Board has formulated and revised its Recommended Dietary Allowances (RDAs) for a number of essential nutrients, including protein. They used the results of these nitrogen-balance experiments as a basis for their figures.

Because the data were arrived at in the rather idealized environment of a metabolic lab experiment, the FNB decided that not enough leeway was included. The experimental average minimum was not enough for all people eating a variety of diets—life is not a laboratory, and nobody is average.

The FNB decided to add two separate safety margins. They first added about 45 percent, bringing the total to 0.47 grams per kilogram, because people eat foods of tremendous variety, some of which yield less of their protein to be used than did the easily metabolized proteins in the research trials. This safety margin assumes we can use only 68 percent of the protein present in the mixed diet common in America, compared with 100 percent for the egg protein used in the test.

As the first safety margin accounts for variations in diet, the second, raising the total by another 70 percent to 0.80 grams per kilogram, accounts for variations in individual need. This estimate of an ideal protein intake is very generous by almost any measure. If the experimentally determined minimum of 0.32 grams per kilogram body weight was enough for at least half the group of subjects to be in nitrogen balance (since it was an average for a whole group of experiment subjects), we can reasonably assume that half the adult population can get along on this level of protein intake, as long as it is in a very available form.* The RDA is a total of 150 percent higher than this minimum average level.

This figure should guarantee virtually all of us sufficient protein in our diets, so in this book we'll use the RDA as the standard. Keep in mind, though, that for most of us the RDA is more than our actual need. It's interesting to note that every time the protein RDA has been changed, it has been set at a lower figure. Getting the protein RDA covers our minimum need and gives enough extra to cover temporary increases in our need.

To figure your own protein need according to the RDA, take your body weight in pounds and divide it by 2.2 to get kilograms. A 170-pound person weighs 77 kilograms. Next take that weight and multiply it by 0.80 grams per kilogram. Our 77-kilogram subject thus needs 61.6 grams of protein a day.

$$\frac{170}{2.2} = 77 \text{ kilograms} \qquad \begin{array}{r} 77 \\ \times 0.80 \\ \hline 61.6 \text{ grams} \end{array}$$

Individual RDAs can range quite a bit. A 100-pound person has an RDA of only 36.4 grams; for a 190-pound person it climbs to 69 grams.

It you are overweight—that is, too fat—the calculation becomes more complicated. Fat tissue requires much less protein than do other organs and tissues because it is only a storehouse for a relatively inert material: fat. This is why the RDA is based on relatively lean body mass. Thus, fat people require less protein than do lean people of the same weight. The fatter you are, the less

---

*An average has the effect of evening out the highs and lows of a sample group, while taking these variations into consideration. Thus one or two very high or very low need levels can throw off the average by a few points, even over a relatively large sample group. In the individuals studied in the nitrogen balance research, we can expect that there may have been some with protein need much greater than that of the rest of the group, either because of heredity or some other factor. On the other hand, it is unlikely that there would be even a few people whose need was significantly lower than that of the group as a whole, because this would imply a protein-use system *more advanced* than that of the others in the sample. This is much less likely.

The upshot of this discussion is that it seems more likely that the average was pushed higher by individual variations rather than lower, and consequently, it should cover the need of more than half the "average" population.

you require compared to your actual weight. A doctor can help you calculate your actual protein need, based on your lean body weight.

If 90 percent or more of your daily protein comes from plant sources (this obviously includes all vegans), you must figure your need higher. Plant proteins are somewhat less digestible than animal proteins (which include dairy products), so less of their total protein actually enters your bloodstream. Common vegan diets provide protein at about 80 percent of the efficiency of lacto-ovo or mixed diets.

The math is somewhat complicated, but to get the same yield from a diet of 80 percent efficiency, simply add 25 percent to the total. You get the same result by figuring your weight in kilograms and using that figure for grams of protein. Our 170-pound vegan would need 77 grams of protein to fulfill his RDA, instead of the 61.6 a lacto-ovo or omnivore would need.

If you eat a good, varied diet and get enough food, you'll still get quite enough protein, even with lowered digestibility.

WHO IS COVERED

The RDA is not guaranteed to cover 100 percent of the adults in our society, only 98 percent. Before you begin to wonder whether the figures are right for you, understand what the 98 percent figure means. It is a result of the size of the experimental sample—the researchers did not have a large enough group to test so that they could guarantee that all adults would fall within the experimental range. Dr. Doris Calloway, a researcher at the University of California at Berkeley and a member of the 1974 RDA committee, said, "There is no way to know if you are an individual who is not within the statistical group covered by the RDA. However, in our research we have never found anyone whose protein need exceeded the RDA."

In other words, the 98 percent figure is a measure of the scientists' uncertainty, not an absolute measure of the portion of the adult population covered by the RDA. It is quite possible that *every* adult is already given ample insurance by the protein RDA. As more research is carried out, the RDA's formulators will either become more certain of their figures or they will revise them to reflect the results of experiments.

Of course, the figure is also limited to adults who are in normal health. Children, pregnant women, and women who are breast-feeding all have RDAs different from normal adults, and they are quite a bit higher. People recovering from disease or trauma, such as surgery or severe burns, similarly need significantly more protein to replace the tissue that has been lost. These individuals are (or should be) aware of their greater protein need as a part of their broader need to regain their health.

DOES OUR DIET LIVE UP TO THE RDA?

The RDA is a recommendation for gross protein intake, and as such it contains certain assumptions about the usability of dietary protein to our bodies. We'll discuss that issue later in the chapter. But how does our gross dietary intake of protein compare to the RDA?

The popular American (nonvegetarian) diet provides 100 grams or more of protein each day. Using the RDA of 0.80 grams of protein per kilogram of body weight, that's enough for a 275-pound person. Since it refers to a lean 275-pound person, we are talking about a *large* individual.

Looked at another way, 100 grams of protein is 62 percent more than a 170-pound person needs for a day. Note that 170 pounds is a good weight for a 6-foot tall man of medium build. Few adults will need more protein than he.

What about vegetarians? After all, we don't eat the most popular sources of protein in the nonvegetarian American's diet—red meat, fish, and poultry. Doesn't that make us lose a major share of our protein need?

No.

In fact, lacto-ovo-vegetarians have nearly the same protein intake as do their meat-eating counterparts. The vast majority of vegans also eat well over the RDA for protein. In addition, neither group does it by cramming their meals with concentrated protein foods such as soybeans.

The notion that vegetarians do not get enough protein is based on a misconception of the nature of food. Certain foods are not "protein" foods or "carbohydrate" foods, even though different foods are rich sources of different nutrients. *Most* foods provide *most* nutrients, including protein, to a greater or lesser degree.

Even green vegetables provide protein at a remarkably high level. If a 170-pound man got his entire caloric need of about 2650 calories from broccoli, he'd be getting 272 grams of protein! Of course, he'd have to eat about 17 pounds of broccoli to accomplish this feat, and he might experience a variety of unpleasant side effects. All in all, it would be rather stupid, but it does prove our point—protein is almost everywhere in the food we eat. Only refined carbohydrates, such as sugar and cornstarch, and refined fats, such as oil and butter, give no protein at all.

The one thing that may interfere with getting enough protein on almost any vegetarian regimen is receiving a large portion of your calories from highly refined junk food—such as candy, desserts, or soft drinks—and refined fats. If you get a quarter of your calories from these non-nutritive sources, you must depend on the other three quarters for *all* your nutrients.

When we assure you that you get enough protein we assume, of course, that you get enough calories to support your energy needs. This may seem like a strange point to raise. After all, who in our affluent society lacks for *calories?* Besides the obvious group— those too poor to afford enough food—people who eat a very coarse, bulky diet, centered around raw vegetables, may have some difficulty eating enough food at a sitting to keep up with their caloric needs. Our somewhat ridiculous example of the broccoli shows how difficult it can be to get enough calories from fresh raw vegetables. This would be accompanied by a surfeit of protein, which would only be burned for energy.

If you eat insufficient calories to support your body weight, your body will begin to draw upon its energy stores—glycogen stored in the muscles and liver, fatty acids, and, finally, tissue protein. The less stored glycogen and body fat you have to depend on, the more quickly your body will have to consume its protein to keep the fires of life burning. Protein is the only energy source that can stand in the place of carbohydrate when your glucose and glycogen supplies run low. Although fat breakdown releases glycerol, which can be converted to glucose, the amount equals only about 4 percent of the calories in the fat. Because certain organs, notably your brain and nervous system, require glucose as their fuel, fat can't supply all the energy you need to function.

If, for some unexplainable reason, a person decided to live only on broccoli and vegetable oil, he could function on 4 or 5 pounds of broccoli and 7 or 8 ounces of oil a day. It would be a boring and nutritionally inadequate—in fact, decidedly unhealthy—diet, but since the calories are sufficient from this diet he probably wouldn't lose weight or tissue protein.

It is crazy for anyone to eat so limited a diet, however. Every instinct we have points toward a more varied, and consequently more healthy, way of eating. The average vegetarian, if there is such a person, has no trouble obtaining enough calories and protein.

Below is one day's typical eating for our 170-pound man. His protein need is 61.6 grams according to the RDA; he needs about 2650 calories a day to maintain his weight.

BREAKFAST
Oatmeal with milk and fruit
Orange juice
2 slices of whole wheat toast with apple butter

LUNCH
Peanut butter and jam sandwich on whole wheat bread
Vegetable-barley soup

DINNER
Pasta with broccoli, mushrooms, and pignolis
Large salad with dressing

This sample should put the entire question into perspective. This one day's food gives him enough calories and plenty of protein. A vegan could eat the same foods, substituting soy milk (or even fruit juice—the protein content of the rest of the diet is high enough) for the cow's milk at breakfast.

CONCENTRATED PROTEIN SOURCES

We hope it is now clear that vegetarians can get ample protein without overeating, that is, staying within their calorie needs. It may still seem that a lot of bulk is required just to obtain those calories. This is a borderline possibility only in the case of raw-foods vegans with light appetites and people with elevated protein needs such as children and pregnant women. They should take extra care that their calories are sufficient and that all the food they eat contributes to their nutritional requirements.

Many nonflesh foods provide a concentrated source of protein without prohibitively high caloric levels or amounts of water or sheer bulk. Below is a list of a few foods at the top of the scale. These may well already be in your diet, whether you are vegetarian or not. Don't take this as a guideline for what you should be eating. Instead, realize that these foods make a significant contribution to your diet in the form of concentrated protein. Don't overdo, since you don't *need* much concentrated protein.

Legumes:
　Soybeans
　Lentils
　Garbanzos
　Peas
　Pinto beans, etc.

Most Cheeses:
　Swiss
　Cheddar
　Parmesan
　Cottage cheese
　Ricotta

Other Foods:
　Eggs
　Wheat germ
　Wheat bran

Less familiar foods:
　Soy grits or flour
　torula or brewer's yeast
　Gluten flour

Many other foods contribute significant amounts of protein to your diet, including most dairy products (but not butter, for example), whole grains and whole grain products, and vegetables. Even the much-maligned potato is a good source of protein in the context of your entire diet.

WHAT YOUR BODY DOES WITH PROTEIN

Protein is surrounded by mysticism. When it was discovered in the middle of the last century it was touted as the stuff of life. Even its name builds up its importance, derived from *prōteios,* a Greek word meaning *chief* or *foremost.*

Even now, protein is approached with great reverence. Coaches direct their athletes to tank up on it so they'll be strong. The meat industry publishes pamphlets hinting darkly about protein deficiency. Adelle Davis and Carlton Fredericks, the twin oracles of the health foods movement, advocate double or *triple* the RDA for protein. People view protein as a panacea, protecting them from the flu and old age, and giving them an energy boost.

The only reason for such mysticism is ignorance. Few people know exactly what food protein is needed *for* and exactly how it is converted into body protein.

We keep referring to *body protein* and *food protein*. This is an important distinction, because your metabolic system does not use food protein directly. Instead, the protein is broken into smaller component parts, then reassembled into body protein.

This is the secret of the incredible usefulness of protein in nature. Remember that we referred earlier to the multitudes of forms protein can take. It is so changeable because it is composed of a series of small standardized parts that can be strung together to make a large protein molecule.

These small pieces are called amino acids. At one end of every amino acid is an atom of nitrogen, locked in a combination called an *amino group*. This characterizes an amino acid and is also what allows different amino acids to link together—the amino group on the end of one links up with the acid group on the end of the next.

The amino acid nitrogen is the very same nitrogen that the researchers used to measure the presence of protein. Besides nitrogen, amino acids contain carbon, hydrogen, oxygen, and a couple of other optional chemical elements.

To make protein, a cell's machinery links various amino acids together to form a long, chainlike structure. If the chain has fewer than 100 amino acids, it is called a *polypeptide;* more than 100 make it a protein. The differences among proteins are (1) the lengths of their chains, (2) the different amino acids occupying places in the chains, and (3) the twists and kinks they may have. The structure is basically the same for all.

Given the variety of forms proteins can take, it is amazing that there are only two dozen or so known amino acids. These few "beads" string together to construct every single life form we know. Certain amino acids are known to exist in only a few species of plants or animals. Others are virtually everywhere.

When you eat lunch, you generally crush it mechanically (chew it), mix it with a few digestive enzymes to help break down some of the carbohydrates, and swallow it. Nothing happens to the protein until it reaches the stomach and then the intestines. Stomach acid and digestive enzymes attack the junctions between amino acids, breaking the chains into smaller and smaller parts, and finally leaving individual amino acids to be absorbed by your intestinal wall. Sometimes the cells of your intestine absorb two or three linked amino acids, but the cells break them apart before they deliver them to the bloodstream.

Note that your body can't absorb protein as a whole molecule; only the individual amino acids are absorbable. Once those amino acids enter your bloodstream, your body has no notion about what kind of protein they came from, so it is pointless to argue the relative merits of different proteins, as long as they supply you with the amino acids you need.

Once the amino acids are in your bloodstream, your cells absorb them to replenish their supplies. The cells draw from these supplies when they construct new proteins, and all the needed amino acids must be available in the cell to make a specific protein. If one amino acid is unavailable, the cell can't substitute another, for that would mean it would be making a completely different protein, with completely different properties.

Your liver can build up many of the amino acids by building the framework and the acid group from glucose or from remnants of amino acid molecules. It then steals the amino group from another amino acid and attaches this where needed. This "stealing" of the amino group is called *transamination,* and it allows your body to have a complete supply of almost all the amino acids, as long as there are enough amino groups to go around (i.e., enough gross protein in the diet).

ESSENTIAL AMINO ACIDS

The liver can't construct all the amino acids. Some specific amino acids must come from your food, because your body is incapable of making them from scratch. Because these amino acids are essential in your diet, they are called *essential amino acids,* or EAAs. This term causes a certain amount of confusion because it implies that the EAAs are somehow more important in your body than all the other amino acids. "Essential" in this case refers to their importance *in your diet,* not in your body. You can't get them anywhere else, so it is essential that you get them in your food.

Although exactly which proteins your body is synthesizing varies widely from moment to moment, and thus your need for individual amino acids varies from moment to moment, that need is remarkably constant over a period of time. The largest portion of your protein requirement is nonspecific. Since your body can make most of the amino acids, it simply requires the nitrogen portion of most of the amino acids. About 20 percent of your total protein need is for the essential amino acids.

Thus your daily protein need has two distinct components: dietary nitrogen and essential amino acids. If you fulfill these two protein requirements, you are getting enough protein. You could, of course, receive all your dietary nitrogen from EAAs, but 80 percent would simply be stripped of their amino group so your liver could manufacture other needed amino acids.

In some foods—carrots or cassava, for example—the EAAs make up less than 20 percent of the total amino acid complement. These foods don't provide enough EAAs as a proportion of their total protein, so you would have to eat disproportionately large amounts of them to get enough EAAs. Coincidentally, these foods also contain little total protein compared with their calories, so they can't be a basis for your protein nourishment. This is not to say that they shouldn't have a place in your total diet; they simply don't contribute much to your protein need. If you live where a variety of food is available, this needn't concern you. Most other whole foods supply at least 20 percent of their protein as EAAs.

"COMPLETE" VERSUS "INCOMPLETE" PROTEIN

Your body is composed of a variety of differentiated tissues, all of them made up of characteristic proteins. Each of these proteins has a characteristic pattern of amino acids. Your liver may be particularly rich in one or two specific amino acids, and consequently will need proportionately more of them for routine repair and synthesis than will some other organ. This is true of every organ of your body, but because most bodies are made up of about the same proportions of each specific tissue, the proportion of the total requirements of each essential amino acid is remarkably constant from one person to another. A certain fraction of food amino acids must be lysine, another fraction should be tryptophan, another methionine, and so on.*

Over the past generations nutritionists have spoken in terms of some ideal protein food that provides all the essential amino acids in their ideal proportions so that the protein contributes precisely

---

*There are nine EAAs: lysine, tryptophan, methionine, histidine, leucine, isoleucine, threonine, valine, and phenylalanine. As a practical matter, the most critical are the first three because as the amino acids occur in nature, when lysine, methionine, and tryptophan are sufficient the others are also.

the amino acids our body systems need for best utilization. Foods were compared against this theoretical ideal and were thus broken down into two categories, "complete" and "incomplete" proteins.

Because animal proteins are more similar to our own body proteins than are those from plants, they provide amino acids in a ratio more similar to our needs. The natural proteins closest to this ideal are found in milk and egg. Vegetable sources of protein may be proportionately higher or lower in individual EAAs than the theoretical ideal.

Thus animal proteins were generally classed as "complete," while plant proteins were "incomplete." The implication of these classifications was that plant proteins were not suitable for supporting life for humans.

For rich humans, that is. This theory did not explain how most of the world, those too poor to afford animal protein, could get enough protein to live. According to the "completeness" theory, they should be suffering from protein malnutrition, yet much of the world's population get enough protein for their needs, even though they don't eat meat or get much milk. How do they get the amino acids they need while eating mainly vegetable protein sources?

Very few proteins, no matter how "incomplete," are completely devoid of a particular EAA. Even if one or more EAAs are supplied at less than perfect proportions, a shortage of that EAA will exist only if there simply isn't enough of it in the entire diet. In marginal economies, where perhaps only one or two different foodstuffs are available, people can still obtain enough usable protein by eating enough of those one or two foods. As long as the requirement for the least-available EAA has been fulfilled, the individual has eaten enough protein to live and to remain in nitrogen equilibrium. This is a wasteful way to eat, however, because all the other amino acids you must consume will simply be stripped of their nitrogen and burned for energy. Still, it is a sufficient diet, and you needn't overeat calories to achieve it with most staple foods.*

---

*Even if your protein intake drops suddenly (if you go on a poorly designed weight loss diet, for example), your body has some reserve capacity to keep you going. When you eat normally and maintain nitrogen equilibrium, you are using your protein intake at about 70 percent efficiency. If your protein intake suddenly drops, your body compensates by increasing its protein-processing efficiency. It can't take up all the slack, but it can minimize the ill effects.

Your body is remarkably flexible in dealing with variations in your food supply. It will keep you reasonably healthy and functioning over a wide range of protein intake. This is not a license to abuse your metabolism, but it should reassure you.

Some foods are unsuitable bases for this kind of protein "monodiet," either because they have too many calories compared with grams of protein or because they are simply far too deficient in an EAA. Foods too high in calories include high-fat foods like nuts, many processed foods, and most fruits, whose low protein content is compounded by their high sugar content. The best example of a "food" extremely low in a particular EAA is gelatin, an animal protein extracted from bones, horns, hooves, and other slaughterhouse leftovers. It is nearly devoid of the EAA tryptophan. Some other foods, such as cassava and yams, are also deficient in one or more EAAs.

The whole idea that even desperately limited diets can provide adequate protein may seem radical—we've been taught that humans can't live by bread alone. Interestingly, it has been known for 60 years that we *can*. Sixty years ago a researcher fed a group of men a diet of bread made from wheat flour. This was their only source of protein. He found that wheat bread alone, though low in the EAA lysine, was enough to keep his subjects in nitrogen equilibrium. Nitrogen balance is the final authority on the protein sufficiency of any diet, for it measures whether we are replacing our body protein loss with sufficient food protein. If we don't get enough of any EAA we can't stay in equilibrium, because we can't synthesize any proteins that need that EAA. Even on a monotonous wheat-based diet this was not a problem.

Most grains, legumes, and vegetables are sufficient protein sources for adults (dairy products are, too, of course). You should not try to live on one of them solely. You need other nutrients besides protein, and a monotonous diet can't supply them. Other nutrients will run short long before protein does. A varied diet rich in whole grains, legumes, fruits, and vegetables (and dairy products) will insure not only enough protein but also a good supply of all the other essential nutrients as well.

Once you eat a variety of foods, you will likely need a more efficient protein source than that offered by a monodiet. As soon as you eat nuts or oil or fruit or dessert, you lose some caloric leeway and need a smaller amount of food that supplies the same amino acids. Likewise, people in positive nitrogen balance need more concentrated sources. That is why many people insist on eating "complete proteins." Such foods are still not necessary, however. A varied diet has its own built-in protection.

COMPLEMENTARITY

Plant foods divide into broad families that share EAA strengths and weaknesses. Foods from one group can fill the gaps in the EAA complement of foods from other groups, thus making the protein use of the entire diet more efficient. Although wheat and other grains are comparatively low in lysine, legumes and vegetables have an abundance of that EAA and they can bring the lysine level of the entire diet up to a suitably high level. Likewise, the grain products compensate for the EAA weaknesses of the other foods.

This is known as the complementary effect of varying protein sources. The concept first gained wide recognition after the publication of Frances Moore Lappé's groundbreaking book, *Diet for a Small Planet,* in which she publicized the then-revolutionary notion that vegetarians could be well nourished.

The original concept was based on animal-feeding studies performed with rats, which indicated that two different plant foods caused better growth when fed in combination than they did when fed singly. Lappé limited her discussion to only the foods used in the experiments, but more recent authorities have generalized the findings to whole families of foods. The complementing families are (1) whole grains; (2) legumes, nuts, and seeds; (3) dairy products; and (4) vegetables. Vegetables and the legume group generally compensate for the EAAs underrepresented in the grain group; dairy products can improve the protein efficiency of any of the other foods. Even within groups, the proteins often complement each other to a certain extent, since all foods have a slightly different collection of EAAs. For example, legumes complement the protein of nuts or seeds. For your daily eating, the best approach is simply to eat from all four groups (or three, if you eat no dairy products) each day.

Lappé also indicated that these foods must be eaten at the same meal for effective protein complementarity. Research had shown that infant rats fed purified amino acids could not make efficient use of them if one or two EAAs were left out of the mixture. Even a difference of two hours in completing the rats' full complement of amino acids slowed their growth.

More recent data and a reexamination of the older experimental data, however, indicate that in-a-meal complementing is not necessary. First, research carried out by Edmund S. Nasset showed that at least one organ—the intestine itself—provides large amounts of high-quality protein within the digestive tract to act as a complement to food protein. In effect, your own body acts to complement the amino acids you eat. The source of the amino acids is the sloughed-off lining of the intestine.

Second, the rat-feeding studies can't directly parallel the protein needs of adult humans. Infant rats are in positive nitrogen balance because they are growing, so their need for a full complement of EAAs is immediate and crucial. In addition, feeding laboratory animals isolated amino acids does not parallel what happens when humans eat real food. Naturally available foods are generally not completely devoid of a particular EAA. This takes the pressure off your body to provide the full amount of any EAA to complement the total of the others.

Of these two points, the first is much more important. Nasset showed that the intestinal lining (plus the protein of intestinal enzymes) provides up to 90 grams of protein a day, and since this is your own body protein, it is of a quality nearly equal to milk protein. Since dairy protein can complement that of all the other groups, it follows that your own intestinal protein can do the same.

This can be extended logically, if not experimentally, to include the entire breakdown and resynthesis process of all your body proteins. This process of protein turnover supplies your metabolism with a continuous source of a perfect complement of amino acids for the synthesis of new body proteins. The protein from the foods you eat merely contributes to this turnover pool of amino acids. It represents far less than the total free amino acids from body sources. These intrinsic amino acids are more than enough to even out temporary imbalances in the dietary amino acid supply. In addition, every cell has a small supply of various amino acids tucked away in its interior. When a cell constructs a protein, it takes amino acids from these supplies, and then restocks from bloodstream amino acids. This also serves to overcome temporary imbalances in the EAA proportions.

Thus you needn't become an accountant when complementing your protein sources if you don't eat many (or any) animal proteins. Instead make sure your diet includes foods from all the protein families each day. Your body is able to cope temporarily with variations in the EAA supply and still use your food protein at close to peak efficiency, as long as the imbalances equalize over a short period of time. More long-term imbalances may decrease your body's efficiency of protein use. This doesn't mean you won't get enough protein—as we've seen already, adults can live healthfully on a diet of proteins low in a particular EAA. But it does cut your margin for error if you eat a less than ideal diet (i.e., if you eat processed foods, fats, or sugar), since you may not be able to eat enough of your main protein source and still stay within your normal calorie range.

The best diet to insure that you get plenty of all the nutrients you need, including protein, is a varied diet of whole foods, with as few calories as possible from non-nutritive sources. We explain this diet in greater detail in Chapter 6, Putting It Together.

SPECIAL PROTEIN NEEDS

Thus far in our discussion of protein we have concentrated on the needs of adults, who are normally in nitrogen equilibrium. Negative nitrogen balance—losing more protein than you take in—is a pathological state that can result from a number of circumstances, including starvation, injury, and illness. The cause must be corrected before you can reestablish equilibrium. Luckily, you'll probably never be in negative nitrogen balance without realizing it, since it is usually just one part of a traumatic state with a number of obvious symptoms. The exceptions are crash dieting and fasting, which can both cause protein loss.

Often those in negative balance caused by injury or disease begin to retain protein as they heal. They must build new tissue to replace what was destroyed, so their total body protein increases from morning to night—i.e., they are in positive balance. Similarly, children and pregnant women retain protein, because they are building new tissues. Lactating women can't really be said to be in positive balance, since they still lose as much protein as they take in, but they are creating new, high-quality protein every day for their breast milk, so their bodies act as though they were in positive balance. Athletes at the beginning of a training cycle also go into positive balance because they are building up new muscle tissue. As they become more conditioned, they come closer to equilibrium as muscle development slows and conditioning increases.

The protein need of all these individuals is somewhat more critical than that of normal adults. They are making more withdrawals than deposits to their amino acid pool, so there may be slightly less leeway to absorb variations in the food amino acid supply. Children, for example, require 30 to 40 percent of their day's amino acids in the form of EAAs. It is even more important that their diet be varied and healthy. The best basis for their diet is fresh whole foods in wide variety. Of course, it is often difficult to get children to eat a varied diet. Parents and other adults can only do their best (see Chapter 8, Babies and Children).

Although a concentrated protein source such as milk or various soy foods can serve to assure a full complement of EAAs, other nutrients must also be included. A varied diet is again the best insurance.

YOU DON'T HAVE TO WORRY ABOUT PROTEIN

Almost any vegetarian diet that provides enough calories for your body weight contains enough protein. The exceptions are diets based on foods that are extremely low in protein compared to calories (like high-fat diets or monodiets based on plantains or nuts or refined foods) or very low in a particular EAA (like cassava or yams). In this respect other nutrients are probably more critical than protein and would run out sooner in a poor diet.

Some people have a more critical need for protein because they are in positive nitrogen balance. We look at the special nutritional needs of children, athletes, and pregnant women in other chapters.

IF SOME IS GOOD, IS MORE BETTER?

Protein is unquestionably good for you. It is a requirement for your continued good health. You must get it in your daily diet.

But if the RDA for protein is good for you, shouldn't more be even better? What about twice the RDA, as most Americans eat? Or triple, as some authors recommend?

If you eat a lot of protein, you'll have more amino acids temporarily in your bloodstream. After cells use molecules of the various amino acids, their supplies are replaced from the "unattached" amino acids in the bloodstream. The excess EAAs are quickly broken down into carbohydrate and waste nitrogen. If you don't happen to need the carbohydrate at the moment, most of it is converted into body fat and stored in your fat cells.

High blood levels of amino acids do seem to have an effect on cell metabolism, however. There is some indication that the higher your blood amino acid level, the faster your cell proteins turn over. This higher metabolic rate may cause your cells to age faster and die sooner. As your cells age, so does your body.

We know what happens to the carbohydrate portion of the extra protein, but what happens to the nitrogen part? The process of removing the amino group from an amino acid is called *deamination*. The amino group becomes ammonia, a soluble, poisonous gas.

This unfortunate state of affairs is immediately corrected by changing the ammonia into a less toxic chemical: urea. In some people it is converted into another related chemical, uric acid, which is more toxic and which produces the discomfort and swelling known as *gout*. These chemicals must be removed from the blood before they can cause any harm.

This is a job for the kidneys. They continually sweep your blood clean of impurities. Urea-type compounds make up the bulk of their housecleaning job. Under normal circumstances the kidneys do the job efficiently, keeping dissolved nitrogen concentrations below a dangerous level. In some cases, such as kidney disease or shutdown from trauma, the products of protein deamination can build up to toxic levels and cause real harm. In these cases doctors often recommend a low-protein diet.

What about the rest of us, with normal kidney function? Can we safely eat as much protein as taste and custom dictate? There are some indications that overconsumption of protein (at levels equal to that in the standard American diet) may have a negative effect on health. Your liver may hypertrophy (enlarge) in response to the need to deaminize extra amino acids. Likewise, your kidneys may enlarge to accommodate housecleaning duties they weren't designed to handle. In some animals inflammation of the kidneys accompanies a high-protein diet.

In addition to the direct effects of excess protein on your excretory system, it also appears that high protein consumption causes increased calcium loss, weakening your bones through osteoporosis (next time somebody repeats the old myth that lots of protein builds strong bones, bring this up). There are also indications that vegetarians have denser bones than do omnivores, especially after the age of fifty or so. This would tend to be a protection against the slow-healing bone breakage that is so common among older people.

Finally, there are some even less direct effects of a diet high in protein. Many high-protein foods, especially nonvegetarian ones, also carry a large dose of fat. Meat is a particular offender, since all its calories are either protein or fat. Very lean sirloin gets about 30 percent of its calories from fat, even after cooking. (The negative effects of fat on your health are outlined in greater detail in Chapter 3. They include increased risk of heart disease and the other diseases associated with obesity and increased risk of some types of cancer.)

A high-protein diet also tends to be low in dietary fiber. Besides being good for your digestive comfort, fiber may be protection against colon cancer, the most common cancer in the United States and the second worst cancer killer.

All in all, a high-protein diet is far from the panacea pushed by industry spokespeople and diet-book authors. It can be downright harmful, in fact. Babies and athletes are particularly vulnerable to the ill effects of too much protein, but all of us can be harmed by this nutritional excess, and the other dietary excesses and deficiencies that go along with it.

CONCLUSIONS

Worries about obtaining enough protein are completely unfounded in a society as affluent as ours; in fact, we normally get far in excess of our daily need. Nearly every food provides protein, although some give much more than do others.

As long as you eat a varied diet that doesn't depend on refined carbohydrates or fats for a large chunk of caloric need, you will get enough protein. In fact, other nutrients are more dependent on your getting a varied diet than is protein, so this need for dietary variation extends to meat-eaters as well as vegetarians.

People in positive nitrogen balance—children, pregnant women, convalescents, athletes at the beginning of training—are taking in more protein than they lose. They have a somewhat more critical protein need, which can still be met with a varied diet of good whole foods.

Diets mainly composed of vegetables and leafy greens may be too bulky to provide enough calories and thus enough protein. These diets will be adequate if they include enough legumes, nuts, seeds, and whole grain products.

Getting too much protein may well be as much a cause for

concern as getting too little. Several diseases and disorders of our metabolic system are associated with either high protein intake itself or with the high fat and low vegetable fiber intake that comes with a high-protein diet.

If you are getting enough calories from a decent diet, you are getting enough protein, so *don't worry*.

GUIDELINES

Normal adults need protein to replace losses that occur during protein turnover.

Any diet that keeps you in nitrogen equilibrium provides all the protein you need (as long as the proper state for your body is equilibrium).

The RDA is for dietary nitrogen (which you get in the form of protein). About 20 percent of this protein requirement must be in the form of the essential amino acids, since they can't be manufactured in the body.

To calculate your protein RDA, take your lean body weight in pounds, divided by 2.2 to get kilograms, then multiply the result by 0.80 to find the grams of protein you should eat each day. Vegans need slightly more than nonvegans—their RDA in grams equals their body weight in kilograms.

Nearly any vegetarian diet with adequate calories should provide quite sufficient protein for an adult in normal health.

A varied diet based on whole foods is your best insurance against getting too little protein. Eat whole grains, legumes, nuts, and seeds for the bulk of your protein, supplemented with dark green, leafy vegetables and (if lacto-ovo) dairy products.

Don't overdose on high-protein foods. Too much protein may cause as many problems as too little.

5
Vitamins and Minerals

"Eat your greens."
"Why?"
"They're good for you."
"Why?"
"They've got vitamins and minerals and stuff."
"But I hate greens."
"Shut up and eat your greens."

Green vegetables aren't the only source of vitamins and minerals in a good diet, but many of us grew up going through this dialogue at every dinner. No wonder becoming vegetarian seems like such a radical step, particularly considering what those greens often looked like. They might more appropriately have been called "grays."

Things have changed a little since we grew up. Now vegetables are often prepared with a little more respect for their flavor and eye appeal and for their nutrient content, including (but not limited to) essential minerals and vitamins. We dedicate this chapter to the fresh, green, health-giving soul cooked out of all those soggy plates of limp spinach and stewed stringbeans. They deserved better and so did you.

WHAT ARE VITAMINS AND MINERALS?

Everyone knows you need vitamins and minerals (although there is little agreement on how much of which), but many people have a fuzzy idea at best as to exactly what they are. They are vital nutrients, just like protein, carbohydrates, and fats. You can't live long without them. But they differ from the other nutrients in two important ways. You need them in much smaller amounts, typically less than a gram a day of any one. And they don't contribute food energy (calories).

Vitamins and minerals differ from each other, too. Minerals are very simple in structure. They may be as simple as an atom or two with an electric charge (known as an *ion*). Vitamins are much more complex. They are long chain molecules, resembling fats, proteins, DNA, and complex carbohydrates. Some minerals can be part of vitamins, as cobalt is a part of vitamin B_{12}, but vitamins are not part of minerals.

An entire book, even several volumes, could be written about the many functions vitamins and minerals play in your body. Minerals can be structural, as in the case of calcium or phosphorus in bones. They can play a part in the fluid balance of your body, as do sodium, magnesium, potassium, and several others. They can form complex compounds to carry oxygen to your cells or do other metabolic jobs, as iron does.

Vitamins generally perform metabolic roles. They form parts of enzymes or hormones, which can variously break down carbohydrates, regulate body functions, or convert one amino acid to another. They are also necessary parts of protein complexes; an example is vitamin A, which forms a part of visual pigments so you can see.

Vitamins and minerals take part in thousands of reactions crucial to the healthy functioning of your body every day. Taking care that you get enough of each of them is a sensible idea. Luckily, it's not terribly difficult to get all you need, as long as you get a good diet. Vegetarians, despite the scare stories, have no greater difficulty than omnivores, although special needs differ. We explain in greater detail below. We include the RDA when one has been set. In some cases not enough research has been done to warrant an RDA; however, a range of estimated safe intakes for these nutrients is included in the Appendix. Note that when we describe sources, we are ignoring flesh foods and concentrating on vegetarian sources.

THE VITAMINS

A vitamin is a relatively complex chemical; its absence from the diet causes a deficiency disorder that can be corrected simply by supplying the vitamin. As the vitamins were discovered they were designated by letters (vitamin A, vitamin C). As their structures were accurately determined, they came to be called by chemical names (niacin, biotin). All the vitamins now known are A, C, D, E, K, B₆, B₁₂, riboflavin, thiamin, niacin, folic acid, pantothenic acid, and biotin.

They divide into two general categories, water soluble and fat soluble. A, D, E, and K are fat soluble; the remainder are water soluble. Generally, fat-soluble vitamins are stored in your fat deposits, while water-soluble vitamins can't be stored and must be replaced daily (with some exceptions noted here).

The Fat-soluble Vitamins

VITAMIN A

The chemical name for vitamin A is *retinol*. Since retinol is a product of animal metabolism, it is present only in animal tissue and dairy products. Most animals, humans included, get their vitamin A by converting certain plant chemicals into retinol. These chemicals, mainly carotene, are the pigments of plant cells and are known as *vitamin A precursors* or *provitamin A*. Carotene gives plants a characteristic yellow or orange color, but it can be masked by the intense green of chlorophyll in many green plants. Generally, the stronger the color of a vegetable, the more provitamin A it provides.

Humans convert carotene to retinol in the intestines and liver. Once in your body, vitamin A is stored in fat deposits, mainly in your liver. Carotene doesn't build up your body's vitamin A stores as efficiently as does retinol, but newer nutrient tables should take this into account when they describe the vitamin A content of foods, expressing it in terms of retinol equivalency.

The only biochemically proven need for vitamin A is as a raw material for visual pigment—the protein complex in your eye's retina that reacts to light. In fact, night blindness is the earliest sign of a deficiency, and it can often be corrected immediately with a supplement or a diet change. Vitamin A also takes part in many metabolic functions that aren't fully understood, including glycogen and glycoprotein syntheses, building bones and teeth in children, some enzyme reactions, and regulating cell membrane stability (working with vitamin E).

Acute deficiency causes blindness from eye tissue breakdown in tens of thousands of children each year, mainly in Southeast Asia and the Mideast, where several factors limit the vitamin in the diet. This terrible situation is completely avoidable and could be eliminated by a concerted effort of governments and relief organizations to get the easily synthesized vitamin to the children when they need it. Although such acute deficiency is rare in this country, many poor adults and children still fail to meet the RDA.

The RDA for vitamin A is 800 retinol equivalents (RE) for women and 1000 for men. Infants need 420 RE, and lactating women 1200. This should be incredibly easy for everyone to get—one carrot yields 800 RE, and a slice of pumpkin pie provides more than 500. Spinach and broccoli contain tremendous quantities, and various wild greens, like dandelion and lambsquarters, have enough in a small serving for several days' RDA.

The fact that many children and adults have low serum vitamin A measurements is some indication of how far our national diet is from ideal. While vitamin A–related blindness is all but unknown in this country, lesser deficiency symptoms, including night blindness, are not at all uncommon. An improved diet that includes sources of vitamin A precursors could all but eliminate the problem.

Good sources of provitamin A or preformed retinol include:

Beet greens	Tomato juice
Carrot	Mango
Collard Greens	Peach
Lambs quarters	Butter
Kale	Whole milk
Parsley	Egg yolk
Spinach	Swiss chard
Tomato	Dandelion greens
Sour cherries	Escarole
Pumpkin	New Zealand spinach
Papaya	Sorrel
Watermelon	Sweet potato
Asparagus	Apricots
Broccoli	Nectarine
Curly endive	Prunes
Mustard greens	Margarine
Red pepper	Fortified skim milk
Winter squash	Ovaltine

Vitamin A is stored in fatty tissue, so a large amount consumed one day can carry you through several days with none at all. In fact, if you have excellent stores you could probably go for months with no additional vitamin A, so wide variations in diet aren't particularly harmful as long as your intake balances out over the long term.

Your body's ability to store this vitamin can be harmful as well as helpful, however, especially for children. Vitamin A is toxic in high concentrations, and people who take large doses of the prepared vitamin (retinol) at levels 20 to 30 times the RDA may be poisoning themselves. Infants have been poisoned with a single large dose administered by overzealous mothers. Although individual needs may vary, it seems sensible to stay close to the RDA if you choose to supplement this vitamin. Simply making sure you eat foods that contain carotene is the best way to insure that you get enough. Neither carotene nor retinol is lost to an appreciable degree during storage or cooking of food.

Overdosing is less likely from carotene in vegetables, although cases have been recorded of people eating enough carrots or squash to turn their skin yellow. The carotene isn't converted to retinol fast enough to cause a toxic reaction, and the yellowing disappears after the carotene consumption drops.

The only thing that may interfere with absorption of vitamin A is an extreme lack of fat in the diet (since the vitamin dissolves in fat). This condition is understandably rare, since almost any diet is more than adequate in fat.

VITAMIN D

The chemical name for vitamin D is *cholecalciferol*. It functions as part of a system of hormones that regulates blood levels of calcium and phosphorus and their absorption in the intestines. It also controls the mineralization of bones to form a strong skeleton.

Lack of vitamin D causes bones to lose calcium because the calcium transfer in the intestines can't keep up with loss through the urine. Blood levels of calcium must remain stable, so calcium is extracted from bones if the level starts to drop. When this condition occurs in adults, it is known as osteomalacia. If children have too little vitamin D, calcium fails to deposit in their growing bones, leaving them soft and cartilaginous. As these children start to walk, the bones deform from the weight. This disorder, known as rickets, was very common among European city dwellers in the last century.

There are few good food sources of vitamin D, mainly butter, milk, and egg yolk. Apparently, nature has designed our bodies to get our vitamin D needs a different way. Sunlight falling on skin causes a form of cholesterol to change into a vitamin D precursor, which the body metabolizes into active vitamin D. In Northern cities with smoggy skies, however, you may not be able to get enough D from sunlight in the winter to cover your needs. Whole-body exposure to the noonday sun can provide a day's ration in 15 minutes or so, so if you sunbathe in the summer, you may be able to store up enough to cover your wintertime needs. This is a good way for vegans to cover their need for vitamin D without supplements.

Milk is fortified with vitamin D, and it seems the obvious food to fortify, since it is a good source of the calcium and phosphorus that vitamin D works on. The vitamin is not lost to any appreciable degree through cooking.

The RDA for children is 400 IU. For adults it is only 200 IU, but the National Research Council assumes adults will fill their needs with sunlight. It is *not* a good idea to supplement vitamin D beyond the RDA, for either children or adults, since the vitamin builds up and can cause calcium deposits in many organs. Calcium deposits can interfere with kidney function, a very dangerous condition.

You can't overdose from sunlight-made vitamin D, because the level of the vitamin in your blood controls the skin's synthesis of D precursor.

Sources for vitamin D include:

Butter
Egg yolk
Milk
Sun

VITAMIN E

Vitamin E is nature's own preservative for unsaturated fatty acids. Because the double bonds in the carbon chains of unsaturated fatty acids are less stable than single bonds, reactive chemicals such as peroxides can attack the chains at these points, causing the fat to become rancid. Vitamin E is even more vulnerable to this attack, so it uses up the force of the reactive chemicals by sacrificing itself, thus protecting the fat from attack.

Obviously the best sources of vitamin E should be those foods highest in unsaturated fatty acids, such as grains, nuts, vegetables, and seeds, and the oils derived from them. This has been borne out in laboratory analyses of a variety of foods. The best sources of vitamin E are:

Wheat germ oil	Brazil nuts
Walnut oil	Wheat germ
Sunflower oil	Whole rye
Cottonseed oil	Whole wheat
Safflower oil	Whole cornmeal
Palm oil	Asparagus
Rapeseed oil	Spinach
Corn oil	Sweet potato
Sesame oil	Beet greens
Soy oil	Turnip greens
Peanut oil	Leeks
Almonds	Brussels sprouts
Filberts	Broccoli
Walnuts	Wild blackberries
Sunflower seeds	Apples
Peanuts	Pears

The role of vitamin E when eaten is similar to its role in the plants that produce it. Once it enters our system, it protects the unsaturated fat in our cell membranes, and it also protects the reactive vitamins C and A. Vitamin E may also play a role in our enzyme system, but this hasn't been demonstrated conclusively.

The vitamin's effects and the results of a deficiency are multiple and baffling, from infertility to brain degeneration to anemia. Beyond the functions noted, no other benefits have been proved. This doesn't mean others don't exist, but they haven't been experimentally verified. Since its function is unclear, a minimum need has not yet been set. However, the RDA for vitamin E ranges from 4.5 IU for infants up to 15 for adult men. This is an average need—it is tied directly to the amount of unsaturated fats in your diet, since its presence preserves these fats from reactive chemicals. If you consume foods in their natural state you should get enough E to cover known needs.

There are several different forms of vitamin E, whose chemical name is *tocopherol,* and they vary in biological activity. The most active form is alpha tocopherol, which seems to be most concentrated in foods whose oils have the largest proportion of unsaturated fatty acids, like safflower. There are some exceptions, however. Corn oil is high in unsaturated fatty acids, but most of its vitamin E is in the gamma form, which is only about 7 percent as active as alpha tocopherol.

Processing strips large amounts of vitamin E from its natural sources. Most of the vitamin E in grains is lost when they are turned into refined flour. The remainder is destroyed by bleaching. Solvent extraction processes common in the production of most vegetable oils remove most of the vitamin from these important sources. The vitamin can also be destroyed by freezing. This points up dramatically the importance of eating foods in forms as close to nature as possible.

VITAMIN K

Vitamin K is necessary to insure proper blood clotting. A deficiency can cause hemorrhaging leading to anemia and continuous bleeding from even small cuts. Deficiency is rare, however, because vitamin K is easy to get in most any diet. Only newborn infants and adults who can't absorb the vitamin in their intestines have shown deficiency.

We get about 50 percent of our vitamin K from food. Its distribution is similar to that of provitamin A—green and yellow vegetables and dairy products. Green tea provides tremendous amounts, but regular black tea has none.

The other 50 percent of our intake is a product of bacterial activity in our intestines. This is a heartening example of interspecies cooperation—we give the bacteria a home and food, and they give us a necessary vitamin. The reason, in fact, that newborn infants may have a deficiency is that their intestinal bacterial cultures may not be well established (coupled with low tissue stores). In many hospitals newborns get an injection soon after birth.

You need not worry about getting enough of this vitamin unless you have been on a regimen of powerful antibiotics (which kill the intestinal bacteria) or you have been taking anticoagulants (for example, if you are receiving treatment for a recent stroke). You may need supplementation until your body and its intestinal guests get back on an even keel.

The Water-soluble Vitamins

VITAMIN C

We hesitate to leap into the vitamin C controversy. It seems that vitamins cause more arguments among researchers, nutritionists, talk-show hosts, and supplement salespeople than any other nutritional component. We should start at the beginning.

Vitamin C, whose chemical name is *ascorbic acid,* is a water-soluble, heat- and oxygen-unstable vitamin present mainly in fruits and vegetables. Humans are one of three or four known species that can't synthesize the vitamin in their bodies. We therefore need to receive it from food. The still-unanswered question, and the main source of controversy, is "How much?" The RDA is set at 60 milligrams for normally healthy adults, 35 milligrams for infants, 80 milligrams for pregnant women, and 100 milligrams for lactating women. Its major function is as a chemical reducing agent in numerous enzyme reactions. It seems to be crucial to the metabolism of copper and iron into certain enzymes, and it is required for the proper metabolism of some of the amino acids. One of its most crucial roles is in maintaining *collagen,* the protein of connective and scar tissue. A lack of vitamin C causes collagen in bones, capillaries, and gums to break down, and blocks the healing of cuts, bruises, and bone breaks. Stress depletes vitamin C, because it is used to produce the stress-response hormones.

Deficiency affects nearly every tissue and process in the body, which is some indication of how useful and important the vitamin is. The traditional name for the symptoms of deficiency is *scurvy,* characterized by ruptured capillaries, bleeding gums, rough skin, loosened teeth, poor healing and resistance to infection, and muscle degeneration. Scurvy is very rare today because people have learned its cause and the importance of eating fresh fruits and vegetables for the vitamin.

Other more subtle effects have been claimed for vitamin C besides preventing scurvy. These include mobilizing our bodies' defenses against infection (for example, a cold virus), increasing the absorption of iron, and detoxifying various poisons. People under stress seem to need more of the vitamin to maintain tissue and blood levels, as do dieters and smokers.

Although many undocumented claims have been made for vitamin C as a cancer preventer, at least one is true. Relatively small amounts of vitamin C can block the formation of carcinogenic nitrosamines, both in your body and in foods. Nitrosamines are compounds made from nitrite combined with secondary and tertiary amines, chemicals naturally present in meats and in our intestines. Nitrite is present in some vegetables after unrefrigerated storage and in some processed meats, particularly bacon. Vitamin C keeps the two from combining. Although nitrosamines can be formed in bacon during cooking (since it contains no vitamin C), the vitamin C naturally present in fruits and vegetables should keep food nitrites from combining with intestinal amines. The only nitrites you need worry about—at least as far as cancer is concerned—are those added to meat.

It is safe to say that we haven't heard the last word on vitamin C, as researchers continue working on a variety of projects to confirm or disprove the many claims. It seems sensible to hold off on a final judgment until more evidence is available.

You may decide you want to take vitamin C in doses larger than the RDA. If you intend to take vitamin C in the gram doses advocated by some (a gram is a thousand milligrams), however, be advised that it may have some unhealthy side effects. The product of vitamin C metabolism is oxalic acid, which combines with various minerals to form insoluble compounds. These may build up in your kidneys to form kidney stones. In addition, people seem to develop a tolerance for high levels of vitamin C, so that if the dosage is lowered to normal or even higher than normal levels, signs of deficiency appear. High blood levels of vitamin C may even cause calcium loss from bones, eventually resulting in osteoporosis. So use caution if you supplement, or even if you eat a lot of high vitamin C foods.

Fresh vegetables and fruits are the best sources of vitamin C. Of these, the best sources are:

Broccoli greens	Spinach
Black currants	Asparagus
Kale	Gooseberries
Sweet peppers	Loganberries
Chives	Potatoes
Lemon pulp	Tangerines
Papaya	Collards
Watercress	Horseradish
Swiss chard	Parsley
Limes	Cauliflower
Okra	Orange pulp
Brussels sprouts	Beet greens
Guava	Strawberries
Turnip greens	Lima beans
Cabbage	Grapefruit
Kohlrabi	Melons
Mustard greens	Turnips

Vitamin C is lost in tremendous amounts in cooking water, so you should cook vitamin C–rich foods in little water, or steam or stir-fry them (or, of course, eat them raw). Heat itself destroys the vitamin as do oxygen and alkali (like baking soda). Fresh foods lose the vitamin rapidly during storage, especially if they are cut or bruised, so keep them cold and well wrapped to preserve as much as possible. Frozen foods may retain much of their vitamin C, depending on how they are processed.

Vegetarians have a significant advantage over flesh-eaters when it comes to vitamin C, since foods that contain it typically make up a larger portion of our diet.

THE B VITAMINS

The B vitamins have more in common than their generic name. They are often found together in foods, and their role in the body is similar. They all take part in one or more enzyme systems as a *coenzyme*. As a lock is useless without a key, the protein portion of some enzymes is useless without its coenzyme—it just can't do its job. The B vitamins, and possibly vitamin C as well, perform this function in enzymes relating mainly to energy release. Different enzymes catalyze the release of energy from glucose, amino acids, and fatty acids, and different B vitamins take part in all these reactions. Their specific roles, sources, and other details are described here.

Riboflavin (B₂)

Riboflavin is one of the B vitamins, also known as vitamin B_2. Like the other B vitamins, it takes part in a number of enzyme reactions that break down carbohydrates and fats and metabolize proteins. The full extent of its participation in various enzyme systems in humans and in other animals is still being determined, and it appears that its usefulness is very broad. Generally, it seems that it is most important in energy release and protein synthesis.

The RDA for riboflavin ranges from 0.4 milligrams for infants up to 1.7 milligrams for young men. The best sources are:

Milk	Butternut squash
Ricotta	Asparagus
Collards	Beet greens
Brewer's yeast	Brussels sprouts
Various cheeses	Chard

Peas (dried)   Almonds
Cottage cheese   Sorrel
Yogurt   Spinach
Broccoli   Avocado
Mushrooms   Millet
Okra   Pinto beans

This is not the easiest vitamin for a vegan to obtain, and those who eat no animal products should take care to get enough. Riboflavin is relatively heat stable, so little is destroyed in cooking. It is very sensitive to light, however, especially in solution, as in milk, so foods containing riboflavin should be protected from light. Since it is water soluble, riboflavin can be lost in cooking water, so foods containing it should be cooked in as little water as possible (or steamed, sautéed, or baked), and the water saved for other purposes and not thrown out.

Thiamin (B₁)

Thiamin, another B vitamin, appears to have two distinct roles in the body. It forms a part of several enzyme systems that regulate metabolism of carbohydrates and the deaminated remnants of several amino acids. It also participates directly in the nervous system as a part of the signal-transmission chemistry of nerve fibers.

Since thiamin is essential to the energy-release system in your body, the amount you need depends on the calories you consume (calories equal energy). The current RDA is 0.5 milligrams per 1000 calories of food intake. Thus, if you eat 2500 calories a day, you'll need 1.25 milligrams of thiamin a day. Even if you go on a diet and cut your calories, keep your thiamin intake above 1.0 milligram. If you eat a diet rich in whole foods, you'll probably get enough thiamin to keep up with your calorie intake, *provided* you don't get a large proportion of your calories from alcohol or sugar. These and other empty-calorie foods supply virtually no thiamin, while requiring it to be metabolized.

Thiamin is spread rather thin in foods. The best source is yeast. Beans, peas, and nuts provide significant amounts, beyond requirements for their own metabolism. Grains provide enough thiamin to account for the calories they contain, but only if they are eaten in unrefined forms. Beriberi, the thiamin deficiency disease, was common in countries where polished or "white" grains were consumed. The World Health Organization reports that beriberi has declined in most parts of the world, although the reasons are far from clear. Apparently beriberi, like many other deficiency diseases, is brought on by a general lack of health due to malnutrition. The particular form of the malnutrition is determined by the nutrient that runs low first—scurvy in the case of vitamin C, megaloblastic anemia in the case of vitamin B_{12} and folic acid, beriberi in the case of thiamin. A general improvement in the diet may ward off symptoms of beriberi, even if thiamin intake is marginal.

In the United States beriberi is virtually unknown because of our better diet and, even more, mandatory thiamin fortification of most refined grain products. This is needed to replace the nutritive value removed from the grain when it is refined.

One group, alcoholics, has higher thiamin needs than the general population. Alcohol products provide no thiamin (except home-brewed beers), so an alcoholic has a net deficit of thiamin proportional to whatever part of his daily calories he receives from alcohol. This lowered thiamin intake is apparently made worse by a folic acid deficiency or perhaps the diminished activity of folic acid. Lack of folic acid seems to decrease absorption of thiamin in the intestines. The total effect leads to a condition known as "alcoholic neuritis," with symptoms indistinguishable from "dry" beriberi.

Thiamin is water soluble, so it is easily lost in cooking water. Like most of the other B vitamins, it is attacked by oxygen and destroyed by heat. Baking soda added to cooking vegetables hastens the oxidation of thiamin, so that old-time method of keeping vegetables bright green in cooking should be discouraged.

Your body can't store much thiamin, since it is water soluble. Therefore sufficient amounts must be supplied in your daily diet. Good sources include:

Yeast	Nuts
Beans	Grains
Peas	Spinach
Oranges	Asparagus
Yams	Broccoli

Niacin

Niacin, another B vitamin, is necessary for the formation of two enzymes crucial to the energy metabolism of fats, carbohydrates, and protein, which take part in the energy release system of every cell in our bodies. One enzyme allows the body to metabolize alcohol and lactic acid, two toxic food chemicals that might otherwise build up if niacin weren't present in sufficient amounts.

Niacin is present in reasonable amounts in most adequate diets. Your body can make it from the amino acid tryptophan, so foods that have a lot of tryptophan provide niacin, even if they have little of the vitamin itself (such as milk products). The process is somewhat inefficient—it requires 60 milligrams of tryptophan to make a single milligram of niacin. Even so, a quart of milk yields 8 milligrams from tryptophan only—about half the RDA for most people.

Other foods, particularly grains, may have some of their niacin bound up in unusable forms (known as niacytin), so it is sometimes difficult to determine exactly how much niacin a food yields. Niacytin can be broken down into usable forms by alkalis, such as the lime water used in grinding corn to make *masa harina,* the staple of most poor Mexicans. Enough niacin is thus released from this rather low-niacin food to protect them from a deficiency.

The best sources of niacin are:

Dairy products	Peanuts
Beans	Kale and collard greens
Peas	Mushrooms
Nuts	Spinach
Grains	Broccoli
Yeasts	Asparagus
Avocado	Various seeds

Although niacin is water soluble, it is more heat stable than the rest of the B vitamins.

The RDA for niacin is also tied to calorie intake because it takes part in energy release. You should get 6.6 milligrams for every 1000 calories, but never less than 13 milligrams, no matter how low your calorie consumption goes (as on a diet).

Folic Acid

Folic acid is the acid form of a group of nutrients known as *folates.* They get their name from "foliage," leafy greens, one of the best sources of the vitamin. Because folates take such a tremendous range of forms, scientists have had a difficult time determining exactly how they work, how much humans need, and which forms are the most usable. We'll use "folic acid" to describe the whole group of chemicals.

Folic acid is needed for every cell to produce DNA, the chemical that encodes all the genetic information that must be passed on in cell reproduction. If folic acid is missing from the diet, the effects show up most quickly in the cells that divide most quickly—the bone marrow cells that produce red blood cells and the epithelial cells that line the intestines and the uterine cervix, for example. As folic acid deficiency sets in, the nuclei of these cells change and become enlarged. Cell division is interrupted. This can lead to a number of unfortunate consequences, the most immediate of which is anemia, as the bone marrow cells slow down their production of red blood cells.

Exactly the same anemia can be produced by a shortage of vitamin B_{12}; in fact, the only way the two deficiency anemias can be distinguished is by finding the vitamin to which they respond. This indicates that B_{12} and folic acid may be interdependent in their function, or perhaps lack of one may inhibit the function of the other.

Lack of folic acid also blocks the full absorption of thiamin, especially in alcoholics, who appear to have some impairment of folic acid metabolism.

Folic acid is required to build several of the amino acids, so it stands at an important point in cell metabolism. A cell must have at hand all the needed amino acids if it is to make a protein. If folic acid is deficient, some amino acids may also be deficient, interrupting the protein synthesis.

The best sources of folic acid are:

Leafy green vegetables	Avocados
Yeasts	Oranges
Grains	Bananas
Legumes	Cantaloupe

The RDA for folic acid ranges from 30 micrograms for infants to 400 micrograms for adults. Pregnant women need double the RDA, because a growing fetus has a great need for the vitamin. Lactating women need 500 micrograms. These amounts should not be difficult to obtain from a good whole-foods diet, provided the food is fresh and not overcooked. A good portion of the folic acid in food is lost through cooking or through a few days' unrefrigerated storage.

Again, the standard American diet is chronically low in all the foods that provide folic acid (as well as many of the other B vitamins): green vegetables, whole grains, and legumes. Some of these are the same sources for vitamin A, which is marginal in the diets of many Americans. It is no surprise, therefore, that most Americans barely squeak by with enough folic acid in their everyday diets, and as many as one third of all pregnant women have a deficiency.

Pregnant women should use caution before they take a folic acid supplement, however. Deficiency causes anemia, exactly the same as a deficiency of vitamin B_{12}. If your real deficiency is for B_{12}, a folic acid supplement can erase the anemia, but not the other damaging effects of B_{12} deficiency, such as nervous system damage. For this reason, any pregnant woman with anemia should have her blood levels of folic acid *and* vitamin B_{12} checked to be sure which deficiency is causing the anemia, before supplementing either.

Since folic acid in tablet form is about four times as available as the folic acid in food, a supplement of only 100 micrograms may cover the RDA. In fact, supplement tablets are limited by law to 100 micrograms in an attempt to limit its effectiveness in masking vitamin B_{12} deficiency.

Vitamin B_{12} appears to help folic acid in its role in bone marrow cell metabolism, so a shortage of vitamin B_{12} would seem to interfere with folic acid's job to a certain extent and trigger the same megaloblastic anemia.

Vegans, whose consumption of folic acid is unusually high and of vitamin B_{12} is unusually low, should be especially wary of this effect. As with most nutrients, folic acid can cause problems as well as solve them, and it is important to be aware of the effects of various styles of eating on the interactions of various nutrients.

Vitamin B_{12}

People who want to challenge your vegetarianism, especially if you eat no animal products at all, may bring up vitamin B_{12}. "It only comes from animal sources," they say, "so an all-plant diet can't be natural for humans." This is yet another proof of the old axiom that a little knowledge is a dangerous thing. It is completely true that plants don't make B_{12}. However, it is equally true that animals don't synthesize it either, a fact that may have escaped the notice of your argumentative friends. We all get vitamin B_{12} from the same source—the small bacteria and fungi that decompose organic material in the soil and in our intestinal tracts. Some animals can absorb it as it is produced, directly from their intestines, as we do biotin and vitamin K. Humans apparently can't; we must get it preformed in our food.

Meat-eaters and lacto-ovos have it easy when it comes to vitamin B_{12}, because the vitamin is common in flesh foods and dairy products. It is more difficult for vegans to get, though, because very few plant foods provide it. The best known are tempeh and kombu, two oriental fermented foods, one made from soy and the other from seaweed. These are not commonly found on supermarket shelves in this country, as are meat and milk.

The whole question is disturbing on another level. Vegetarians are tired of defending themselves and their diet, and rightfully so. A vegan diet is eminently healthy; in fact, vitamin B_{12} is the only nutrient for which vegans must search out special sources.

However we would caution any vegetarians, vegan or not, against getting into arguments over what constitutes a "natural" diet. We simply don't know what our forebears ate for breakfast one million years ago, although there are some indications that it was predominantly vegetarian. At any rate, man is not a "natural" animal. We reshape our environment, both internal and external, to suit our whims. We analyze our motivations, and plan for the future. We wish to dominate nature, and we will suffer no bonds on our ambition. This sets us apart from other animals and from a state of naturalness.

A more appropriate argument concerns the relative health merits of various diets. In this respect, both vegans and lacto-ovos come out very nicely.

To return to vitamin B_{12}, however, vegans should pay attention to their intake, because vegan sources are uncommon and not always easy to get. *All vegans should make sure they get the RDA for this vitamin.* Those who claim they don't need to get vitamin B_{12} from their food are playing a dangerous game with their health.

Commercial vitamin B_{12} tablets are made from bacteria cultures, so they aren't animal products. The plant foods we mentioned earlier are excellent sources, but they are hard to find outside of oriental markets.

Your body stores vitamin B_{12}, apparently enough to last several years if the vitamin becomes unavailable. This is at least a partial explanation for the ability of many people to go for years with no

B_{12} intake and no apparent ill effects. It appears that the body uses the vitamin very efficiently, and this efficiency may increase if the supply declines. Some individuals may also be able to absorb the vitamin through the large intestine, although this has not been verified. If they can, they should be able to get along on the B_{12} synthesized by intestinal bacteria; however, this is unlikely since the large intestine, where B_{12}–secreting bacteria live, is not an absorbing organ.

Human needs for the vitamin are truly miniscule—the RDA of 3 micrograms is considered quite generous by almost all researchers, and healthy individuals have been able to get along on as little as 0.1 microgram for long periods. The RDA for pregnant women is 4 micrograms, to account for the needs of the growing fetus.

Sources include:

Dairy products
Egg products
Tempeh
Kombu
Fortified yeast
Fortified soy milk

Nutritional yeasts sold in health food stores may be supplemented with vitamin B_{12}, although yeasts do not produce it naturally.

The function of vitamin B_{12} in our bodies is multifaceted and only partially understood. It participates, with folic acid, in the processes leading to cellular replication of the genetic code (DNA and RNA). It also acts to protect the sheath of nerve fibers, known as myelin. In vitamin B_{12} deficiency, the same megaloblastic anemia may develop as is caused by folic acid deficiency. This may be hidden in vegetarians, though, because their greater intake of folic acid overcomes and masks the B_{12} deficiency. However, vitamin B_{12} deficiency also causes the myelin sheath around nerve fibers to break down, resulting in generalized damage to the nervous system. The physical symptoms include loss of feeling in hands and feet, loss of positional sense ("which way is up?"), poor memory, confusion, and finally death. The earliest warning sign of vitamin B_{12} deficiency is the anemia, and the neurological symptoms may not become apparent until damage is severe. This is nothing to fool around with. Anyone with a low intake of vitamin B_{12} who develops anemia should have a serum B_{12} test to see if he or she is low in tissue stores. It is usually simple to correct, but terrible to neglect.

Vitamin B_{12} can't cross our intestinal barrier on its own; it needs a companion chemical, known as *intrinsic factor*, which is secreted by our intestines, to bond with so it can be absorbed. In some people this intrinsic factor is lacking, and they must get monthly injections of the vitamin throughout their lives to avoid deficiency. Absorption is also affected by some other factors. Iron and vitamin B_6 both increase vitamin B_{12} absorption, and absorption increases during pregnancy and decreases with age.

Vitamin B_6

Vitamin B_6 is yet another vitamin involved in many different metabolic processes, ranging from constructing amino acids to the conversion of tryptophan to niacin, as described earlier. In fact, the role of vitamin B_6 in tryptophan metabolism may be one of its most important functions, since poisonous or carcinogenic metabolites of the amino acid may build up during B_6 deficiency.

Vitamin B_6 is also part of the enzyme that converts stored muscle glycogen to glucose, which the muscles can then use for energy. It takes part in a long chain of chemical processes that creates hemoglobin, the oxygen-carrying protein of red blood cells. It may also be involved in some as yet unknown way in the body's system of hormones. Its role in the synthesis of nervous system proteins is indicated, but also unproved.

All in all, vitamin B_6 seems to be a jack-of-all-trades vitamin. There is even some indication that vitamin B_6 therapy can help people with atherosclerosis (hardening of the arteries).

The RDA for vitamin B_6 ranges from 0.3 milligrams for infants to 2.2 milligrams for adults (2.6 for pregnant and 2.5 for lactating women). Good sources are the same as for many of the other B vitamins:

Leafy vegetables
Whole grains
Beans
Peas
Lentils

And for the same reasons as the other B vitamins, vitamin B_6 may be low in many people's diets—overconsumption of refined foods like white flour that haven't been refortified with the vitamin (as most have not). High protein intake tends to increase the need for vitamin B6, as does use of steroid contraceptive pills. Alcoholics may have a B6 deficiency as part of a general vitamin deficiency brought on by malnutrition. Two antituberculosis drugs, isoniazid and cycloserine, as well as the antiarthritis drug penicillamine, interfere with vitamin B6 and increase the body's need for it.

Vitamin B6 is destroyed by light and heat, and it is lost in cooking water, so foods containing it should be appropriately protected and cooked to preserve as much as possible.

PANTOTHENIC ACID

Pantothenic acid gets its name from the Greek word for "everywhere," and indeed it is present in every living cell. As a practical matter, it is almost impossible not to receive any of the vitamin, and pure pantothenic acid deficiency has yet to be observed.

Pantothenic acid forms a part of coenzyme A, an enzyme that takes part in reactions of fatty acids, proteins, and carbohydrates. Several writers refer to it as "standing at the metabolic crossroads," and this is an appropriate description.

The RDA committee did not set an exact RDA for pantothenic acid in its 1980 recommendations, but indicated that 4 to 7 milligrams should cover everyone's needs well. Good quantities are present in the by-now familiar foods, plus a few others:

Green vegetables	Milk
Whole grains	Sweet potato
Seeds	Cantaloupe
Legumes	Dates
Egg yolk	Strawberries

Freezing destroys some pantothenic acid, and milling of grain removes most of it.

BIOTIN

Biotin is part of an enzyme system that synthesizes various fatty acids and fats. These fatty acids form part of all cell membranes, as well as being crucial to the functioning of our nervous system.

We need biotin in very small amounts, and our daily need is

easily taken care of by food intake and synthesis by intestinal bacteria. Researchers have been able to produce biotin deficiency only by feeding a biotin antagonist that blocks its function by binding to it and making it unavailable. This is the protein *avidin*, present in raw egg white. You needn't worry about eating raw eggs, however, unless you plan to eat a dozen or so—they contain little of this protein, and it would require at least this many to use up your stores of biotin. Only one minute's cooking is enough to inactivate the protein, so you needn't worry about eating cooked eggs at all, from the standpoint of biotin deficiency.

Other Vitamins and Vitaminlike Substances

Several chemicals are known to be necessary for health, or at least they may be necessary under certain circumstances. *Choline,* although necessary for several metabolic processes, apparently can be manufactured by humans in their own bodies, so it is not needed in the diet.

Another vitaminlike substance is a complex of ionized chromium, a mineral, plus niacin and water. It seems to act like a hormone, in conjunction with insulin, in regulating blood sugar levels. Some adults may not be able to manufacture this complex as fast as they need it, and they can profit by consuming it directly from food. The best sources are nutritional yeasts that have been grown on chromium-rich nutrients. We also obtain chromium from a variety of foods, and most of us can manufacture this complex in amounts sufficient for our needs from the mineral forms of chromium in our diet.

Claims have been raised about the nutritional value and need in human nutrition, of a variety of other chemicals, including para-aminobenzoic acid, inositol, pangamic acid ("vitamin B_{15}"), and many others. These have not been experimentally verified as vitamins. In the case of some, there is still a possibility that a nutritional need can be demonstrated. In addition, other chemicals may be discovered that are necessary in our diets. The issue is by no means closed, but be wary of claims for any chemicals as miraculous substances. These have been raised time after time, only to be disproved. Laboratory research may have faults, but its plodding, methodical, systematic approach provides the most reliable answers to difficult nutrition questions.

THE MINERALS

The distinction we and other writers make between minerals and vitamins may still be confusing. They are both substances that are required in the diet in small amounts to complete our nutrition.

Minerals are simple substances, not built up on a carbon-chain skeleton, as are the vitamins. Once in your body, they may become part of enzymes or other chemicals that do have this skeleton, but we don't need to consume them in this form as we do with vitamins.

Minerals are divided, rather arbitrarily, into two groups: macrominerals and trace minerals. The distinction is based on the amounts present in the body. The cutoff point varies, so different charts will show minerals in different categories. It is not too important a distinction, but it helps in visualizing the relative amounts of the different minerals we need.

The Macrominerals

CALCIUM

Most of the calcium in our bodies is in bone, in fact, about 99 percent. Calcium represents between 1.5 and 2 percent of our total body weight, so its contribution to our skeletons is obvious. It has other metabolic functions besides allowing us to stand upright in a breeze without bending. It takes part in several enzyme systems, as do the other minerals; it is necessary for blood coagulation and proper muscle contraction. Our heart muscles can't work without it, nor could our nervous system interact properly with our muscles. On the cellular level, calcium is part of some cell membranes and of the "glue" that holds cells together.

Our bodies regulate the calcium level in the bloodstream so that it stays remarkably constant because of its importance to all these metabolic and cellular systems. If the blood level drops, the parathyroid gland secretes a hormone that triggers a greater absorption of calcium through the intestines. The hormone also triggers the removal of part of the calcium in bones. In fact, our bones form an essential storehouse for this mineral to equalize variations in our dietary supplies. When calcium levels later increase, intestinal absorption decreases, and calcium is redeposited in the skeleton.

We need to consume between one and two times as much calcium as phosphorus daily to keep this calcium-regulating system in balance. Diets with an overabundance of phosphorus tend to make us lose calcium, softening our skeletal bones. Likewise, diets high in protein tend to promote calcium loss at anything less than high calcium intake.

Estimates of calcium intake vary widely. The RDA is 800 milligrams for adults, 1200 for adolescents and pregnant or lactating women. The World Health Organization's recommendation is only half the RDA for normal adults, however. Why the divergence? It seems that the National Research Council studies the United States, while the WHO is concerned with the whole world. Our very high protein intake leads to greater calcium loss and consequently to a higher dietary need. You can conclude that if your protein intake is lower than that of your neighbors, you'll probably need less calcium than they do. Your body grows accustomed to your usual intake, so if you suddenly shift to a low-calcium diet, you'll lose quite a bit of calcium before your intestinal absorption becomes more efficient and stabilizes your calcium balance.

The best sources of calcium include:

Milk

Cheese

Sesame (crushed or ground)

Tortillas

Ground limestone

Eggshell

Yogurt

Blackstrap molasses

Leafy green vegetables

Masa harina

Hard water

Chalk

Seashells

Those of us who eat a lot of whole grains and legumes also receive a sizable amount of a chemical called *phytic acid* from the outer coating of the seeds. Phytic acid has the unfortunate tendency of binding to certain minerals (mainly calcium, iron, and zinc), making them relatively unavailable. These bound forms, known as *phytates,* go right through the intestines without being absorbed. In older nutrition textbooks this was often blamed for deficiency of these minerals.

Recently, however, researchers have found an enzyme called *phytase* in human intestinal secretions. Phytase inactivates phytic acid and releases its bound minerals, including calcium, for absorption. The enzyme is also produced by yeast in breadmaking and by grains themselves when they are allowed to sprout. Phytic acid should cause no problems for anyone who is accustomed to whole grain products.

Earlier experiments that showed mineral loss from phytic acid did not allow the bodies of research subjects enough time to get used to the dietary change of introducing phytic acid. It takes a short while for our intestines to start producing the enzyme if we haven't needed it before, so for that period we do indeed lose some minerals. The effect is minimal over the long term, however. Vitamin D seems to be important to the adjustment to a high-phytate diet.

Other natural foods, mainly green leafy vegetables such as spinach, rhubarb, dandelion, lambsquarters, chard, beet greens, sorrel, pigweed, and parsley, contain *oxalic acid,* another chemical that binds minerals into unusable compounds. These greens would be excellent sources of calcium and iron if it weren't for the oxalic acid they also contain, which we have no way of digesting. As it is, some greens can provide a portion of these minerals, but the largest part is locked up out of our reach.

Calcium is absorbed best in an acid medium, such as fruit juice. Little is lost from food in storage, although it is soluble in cooking water and can be washed away if you throw out the "pot likker."

PHOSPHORUS

Phosphorus is usually absorbed as the phosphate ion, a combination of phosphorus and oxygen. Phosphate combines with calcium to mineralize bones, and it takes part in cells' energy release cycle in the form of ATP and ADP, the chemicals cells use in storing energy from "burned" glucose and fatty acids. Your phosphorus requirement is tied to both calcium and protein intake. To mineralize bones we need about 1 milligram of phosphorus for every 2 milligrams of calcium. For tissue construction we need about 1 milligram for every 2 or 3 grams of protein we eat. The RDA ties phosphorus intake to calcium intake milligram for milligram, except for babies, who need more calcium than phosphorus. But this may be a concession to our national high-phosphorus diet. We should get *at least* as much calcium as phosphorus, ideally.

No one should have a problem obtaining enough phosphorus (as long as calcium and protein are sufficient for their roles), since most foods containing calcium have approximately equivalent levels of phosphorus, and all cell-protein foods—vegetables, grains, nuts, seeds—contain plenty of phosphorus already incorporated in the cells you are eating. Milk protein, although not accompanying any tissue cells, is also accompanied by phosphorus in sufficient levels.

Overusing antacids containing aluminum hydroxide or calcium carbonate can cause phosphorus deficiency. These chemicals bind with phosphate and make insoluble, indigestible compounds. Chronic antacid taking can lead to severe muscle weakness as cell phosphate stores are depleted and red blood cells refuse to give up their load of oxygen to tissues.

Fooling with your digestive chemistry is a bad idea anyway, because you have no way of knowing the cause of your discomfort or indigestion. It may well be caused by too *little* digestive acidity, and taking antacids only makes the problem worse.

In our culture generally we are more likely to get too much phosphorus rather than too little. Two factors—eating a lot of meat and drinking a lot of carbonated soft drinks containing phosphoric acid—push our dietary phosphorus intake to 1500 milligrams a day or more. This disproportionately high level compared with that of calcium can lead to our bones' being leached of calcium to balance blood serum levels of phosphorus. At its extreme, this leaching can lead to brittle bones in adults and soft bones and easily decayed teeth in children. Calcium and phosphorus must remain in some sort of balance, whatever their intake levels may be, to avoid this problem.

The best sources of phosphorus are:

Various beans	Masa harina
Rice bran and polishings	Wheat bran and germ
Milk	Yogurt
Cheese	Pumpkin seed
Sesame seed	Nuts
Peas	Broccoli
Yeast	Tofu
Various grains	

In addition, soft drinks and meat push Americans' consumption of phosphorus far too high. Although a necessary nutrient, phosphorus should not be consumed in amounts greater than that of calcium.

MAGNESIUM

More than half the magnesium in our bodies is deposited in bones. The rest is in soft tissues and in body fluids. Magnesium participates in innumerable metabolic reactions and processes, including breaking down fatty acids, activating amino acids, transmitting messages from nerves to muscles, releasing energy for very heavy work, protein synthesis, and synthesis and breakdown of DNA.

Foods with a significant magnesium content include:

Green vegetables
Legumes
Whole grains

In addition, it is present in measurable amounts in most foods. It is also present in some drinking water. Magnesium can be lost in cooking water, and most of that found in grains is lost when the bran and germ are removed in refining. The RDA ranges from 50 milligrams for infants to 400 for adolescent boys and 450 for pregnant or lactating women. The normal-adult RDA is 300 to 350 milligrams, which gives a respectable safety margin, since magnesium deficiency is almost unknown in otherwise healthy people. Disorders that can block magnesium absorption or increase loss include kidney malfunction or shutdown, severe vomiting or diarrhea, and chronic alcoholism with malnutrition (magnesium deficiency may cause alcoholic hallucinations).

Magnesium deficiency locks calcium in your bones, throwing your blood calcium level off. This can have profound effects on a variety of body functions. Luckily, few of us need worry about it.

SODIUM AND POTASSIUM

Sodium and potassium act together to stabilize the water balance of your body, insuring that enough water is stored in cells and in circulation in body fluids. Potassium stays mainly inside cells, while sodium stays mainly outside in the extracellular fluid. Both act to hold water where it is, and a higher relative concentration of either ion will draw water to that side of the cell membrane. This effectively dilutes the more concentrated ion, reestablishing equilibrium on both sides of the cell membrane, but it also causes a net change in the water content of the extracellular and intracellular pools. Because cells can "pump" ions in or out, they can control the water content. In addition, nerve cells use sodium and potassium ions to transmit signals.

We lose sodium and potassium through similar circumstances, but different routes. When we work hard we sweat, losing water and sodium. At the same time, our muscles heat up. Their natural response is to release potassium, which stimulates blood vessels to dilate and increase the local blood flow. The heat is carried away, but so is the potassium, to be lost in the urine.

Our kidneys generally keep blood levels of sodium and potassium very stable, excreting when there is excess and retaining when there is a shortage. Our love of salt and salty food generally keeps them busy excreting sodium, while our limited consumption of potassium-rich foods, like fruits and vegetables, keeps them equally busy retaining potassium. Some, perhaps many, of us have a problem with this regulatory system, and suffer from the effects of unstable fluid balance.

When potassium is in short supply and sodium is overabundant, fluid builds up in the extracellular pool, mainly in the blood. This results in *hypertension,* or increased blood pressure. Many researchers view the hypertension rampant in our society as a nutritional disorder, stemming from our culture's distortion of the sodium/potassium balance in our bodies through excessive consumption of salt and other sodium-containing chemicals (MSG, baking soda, sodium citrate, sodium nitrite and nitrate, and others). Hypertension results in a shortened lifespan—shortened through a variety of mechanisms mainly related to circulatory breakdown.

We can improve our health and our chances by changing our diet: less sodium and more potassium. The best way to achieve this is to eat fresh fruits and vegetables, on the one hand, and to avoid processed foods and added salt on the other. Processed food has huge amounts of added salt and other sodium-containing additives, in fact, so much that you can think of sodium as a dangerous additive in these foods. Even canned vegetables have added salt, and the potassium is depleted through canning methods, as well. Fresh peas, for example, have less than 1 milligram of sodium per 100 grams and about 380 milligrams of potassium. By the time they make it into the can, they've lost 200 milligrams of their potassium and picked up *230 milligrams* of sodium, all from added salt. No wonder hypertension is a problem for Americans, if such a relatively innocuous food as canned peas shows these numbers. Imagine what truly salty food does for you!

The only reason salt is added to prepared foods is to respond to the demands of popular taste. You want it, you get it. Unfortunately, even if you don't want it, you still get it because everybody else wants it. The best solution is to use as much fresh food as you can, and don't use salt. If you eat a variety of foods you'll get all the sodium you need from those that contain it naturally. Granted, it is a strong preference to fight, but the pangs you suffer from salt "deprivation" will fade in a month or so, and food will taste good again, perhaps even better. Be vigilant about your children's diets, as well. Better to keep the salt habit from being established at all than to have to break it later.

You may need additional sodium and potassium if you perspire heavily. "Heavily" means a water loss of about eight pounds. Replacing this water, *which should occur before you replace lost minerals,* will require about a gallon of water. Any fluids beyond this should be accompanied by around 1 gram of salt for every liter (a bit more than a quart) of fluid. The salt in food should account for most of this. Get your potassium by drinking fruit juice. If you take diuretics you may need to replace both sodium and potassium. *Never* take diuretics except by order of your doctor to treat a specific medical problem. They promote water loss by accelerating mineral loss, and they can leave you mineral deficient and dehydrated.

Foods that supply sodium and potassium include:

Potassium sources

Winter squash	Orange juice
Various beans	Chard
Spinach	Bananas
Papaya	Peas (fresh)
Cantaloupe	Brussels sprouts
Raisins	Nectarines
Molasses	Other fruits and vegetables
Prune juice	

Sodium sources

Salt	Canned vegetables
Most processed foods	Canned soups
MSG	Cured olives
Baking soda and powder	Cheese
Sodium nitrite and nitrate	

IRON

Iron is one of the most familiar of the minerals. Who can forget Popeye and his magical can of spinach (which later turned out to be a very poor source of iron)? Most of us know that iron gives blood its red color as the oxygen holder of the blood protein *hemoglobin*. In hemoglobin, iron serves to hold oxygen in a relatively loose grasp, so the red blood cells can make oxygen deliveries to cells that need it. Iron is also present in myoglobin, an oxygen-storage protein in muscle tissue. About 2.5 grams of iron is present in adult men in this form. Another gram is in storage in other proteins, waiting to be released if needed for emergency hemoglobin synthesis in the bone marrow cells that build red blood cells.

Iron is one of the most difficult minerals for humans to obtain in sufficient amounts. Pound for pound, infants and pregnant women need six times the iron that adult men need. In fact, men may be the only population group worldwide not in danger of some degree of iron deficiency.

The best vegetarian sources of iron are:

Prune juice	Dates
Legumes	Kale
Millet	Wheat
Rice polishings	Acorn squash
Molasses	Torula yeast
Dried fruits	Strawberries
Chard	Potato
Beet greens	Oatmeal
Raisins	

Cooking food in iron pots increases the iron content tremendously, especially if the food is somewhat acid (tomato sauce, for example). Some people still may not receive enough iron, even incorporating these foods in their diets. The RDA for iron ranges from 10 milligrams for infants and adult men up to more than 18 milligrams for pregnant women. These levels are perhaps possible for people eating excellent diets specifically emphasizing the iron-containing foods on the list.

Vegetarians who get less than 10 percent of their protein from animal sources have much higher iron needs, according to the WHO, because the iron in vegetarian foods is much less absorbable. The WHO puts the needs of adolescent and adult women vegetarians at 24 and 28 milligrams a day, respectively. These amounts are difficult to find in the diet, if not impossible.

Why should vegetarians' iron needs be so much greater than those of nonvegetarians? First, dietary iron comes in two forms, ferrous and ferric iron. These are two different ion states of the iron atom. The ferrous ion is more reactive and, hence, more easily absorbed than the ferric ion. But much of the iron present in fruits, legumes, and vegetables is in the ferric form. Eating these foods with vitamin C, citric acid (the acid in citrus fruits), calcium, or the sulfur amino acids (such as methionine) helps absorption because it tends to reduce ferric iron to the ferrous state. The sulfur amino acids, which are especially prevalent in animal-source proteins, are especially helpful in increasing iron absorption.

Second, iron is a marginal nutrient for the majority of the world's population, even among people of the affluent Western countries. Any small variations in availability can have a large effect on the health of individuals whose needs are great anyway.

Iron deficiency causes *anemia,* which literally means bloodlessness. Bone marrow is unable to make red blood cells because iron-containing hemoglobin can't be formed. The blood, in turn, has few red blood cells, and can carry much less oxygen to the cells, resulting in exhuastion, lowered resistance to infection, and slower healing. In addition, muscle cells become depleted of myoglobin, the protein used to store oxygen for later use. This contributes to the feeling of tiredness.

Anemia may or may not be common in the United States, depending on the source quoted. Many people have blood iron levels below the normal range, but the issue is very complex—iron may be stored in tissues so that blood tests can't detect it, and different people may have different appropriate blood levels. Even so, the mineral seems to be short in many people's diets.

For these reasons, it seems a good idea for women (until menopause) and children to keep a close eye on iron intake and consider supplementing iron. On the other hand, don't be too lavish with your iron supplements. Your body doesn't have an effective means of disposing of excess iron, and it can build to toxic levels.

ZINC

Zinc takes part in several enzyme reactions controlling DNA and RNA metabolism, protein metabolism, and connective tissue formation. The most obvious sign of zinc deficiency in children is that their growth stops immediately, although this can also be caused by a number of problems. In adults, an early warning sign of zinc deficiency is small white spots on the fingernails. This is even more indicative of zinc deficiency if the spots appear in the same position on more than one nail. Zinc deficiency slows wound healing, decreases the sense of taste, and may impair the cell-mediated immune system.

Human zinc needs are similar to iron needs. Zinc appears to be more easily absorbed from animal source foods. Zinc can also be bound by phytic acid (see the section on calcium), and in certain susceptible people this can decrease zinc absorption. In one study, a group of Iranian children showed severe zinc deficiency. The researchers blamed this on phytic acid in the staple unleavened bread coupled with low zinc intake. However, the children were also generally malnourished. Malnutrition can interrupt the synthesis of many enzymes, presumably including phytase, the phytic acid–degrading digestive enzyme. This may have been a factor in their zinc deficiency. In areas of the world where people get enough to eat, zinc deficiency is uncommon.

The best sources of zinc include:

Legumes	Wheat germ
Green peas	Various grains
Spinach	Other vegetables
Cocoa	Milk
Bran	Egg yolk

None of these is an excellent source, however, so vegans especially should take care and perhaps consider supplementing (since animal food sources are the most easily absorbed). Using galvanized (zinc-coated steel) containers for cooking and storing food may contribute a certain amount of zinc to the diet; on the other hand, zinc coatings may contain traces of dangerous heavy metals, such as cadmium and lead, and you may actually overdose on zinc.

Trace Minerals

Several chemical elements are needed in the diet in very small amounts, much smaller than for the minerals already discussed. They include copper, iodine, selenium, cobalt, manganese, nickel, and perhaps fluoride, silicon, molybdenum, vanadium, and tin. Chromium's function as an essential trace mineral is described earlier, in the Vitamins section.

Many of these come from soil or water, and dietary levels obviously vary widely from one area to another. Only a few have firm RDAs, since they are needed in such miniscule amounts and since research on them has not yet progressed far. In the United States, local variations in the trace-mineral content of crops is usually overcome by our food distribution system: Our food comes from so many different places that lacks and overabundances tend to overcome each other and cancel out, at least in theory.

Recently, however, questions have been raised about the quality of our food *production* system in relation to trace minerals. When fields are farmed over many years, the soil elements removed by the crops must be replaced. The vast majority of farmers replace nutrients with artificial fertilizers compounded from relatively pure chemicals. The most common minerals returned to the soil are nitrogen, phosphorus, and potassium, since plants remove these in largest amounts from soil as they grow. But chemical fertilizers don't replace many of the trace minerals, which are just as surely removed by the roots of billions of plants each growing season. These must become depleted, since plants can't create most of them from thin air.

After an unknown period, then, the deficiencies and overabundances of trace minerals can no longer compensate for one another through the mechanism of modern food distribution. The deficiencies must become too great and the abundances too rare.

This is the strongest argument in favor of organic farming methods, with their emphasis on using wastes and "leftovers" as fertilizer to replace that which has been removed from soil. This haphazard approach to soil enrichment is neither as old-fashioned nor as radical as its detractors would like to think, since the widespread use of chemical fertilizers has occurred only since the Thirties. While it may be true that chemical fertilizers, coupled with pesticides, synthetic plant hormones, and weed killers, produce a greater yield per acre than do the older farming methods, we must still question the quality of the food, especially as the soil becomes depleted of essential minerals. Furthermore, how long can these high yields continue? There is already some indication that long-term chemically farmed fields are showing a decreasing yield that no longer responds to technologists' attempts to overstimulate growth.

Add to this the fact that organic farming uses less energy and requires more labor than modern factory farming, and we begin to see its attraction in these times of shrinking energy supplies and growing unemployment.

Perhaps this is a little too visionary to be appropriate in a discussion of essential trace elements in food. On the other hand, it is appropriate to illustrate the relationship between the demands of economics and the quality of our lives. In this case, the economics benefit a few—the owners of the factory farms—and eventually hurt many—the consumers of their high-tech produce. Adding a less centralized food production system based on local talent and local fertilizer to our existing nationwide food distribution system could go a long way toward readjusting the balance and giving us better food and better health.

The essential and possibly essential trace elements are described below.

Copper functions as part of several enzymes. The most important of these promotes iron absorption; in fact, copper deficiency can cause anemia that doesn't respond to iron supplements, but does respond to copper. It is also essential to maintain proper levels of norepinephrine and dopamine (two of the brain's messenger chemicals), maintain blood vessel tissue, and protect animals from oxygen intoxication, a poisonous state brought on by too much oxygen in the blood and tissues.

It is also very toxic in large amounts, so supplementing without medical supervision can be extremely dangerous. The best dietary sources include the same foods that provide iron:

Legumes
Potatoes
Raisins
Nuts
Grains

Iodine is part of the thyroid hormone system that regulates growth and development, protein synthesis, energy metabolism, and the creation of specialized tissues. The RDA ranges from 40 micrograms for infants up to 150 for adolescent boys and 200 for lactating women.

The iodine content of your diet is dependent on the amount of iodine in the soil on which your food is raised. Iodine deficiency used to be common in areas with low soil iodine before salt packers began to add small amounts of it to their product. Iodized salt is now a reliable source for adequate levels of this essential mineral. If you don't use iodized salt there is still little danger, at least right now, of developing iodine deficiency, because for most of us food comes from all parts of the country, depending on the vagaries of the food distribution system. Thus foods from iodine-deficient areas are balanced by foods from iodine-rich areas. But even this nutrient may become depleted in commercially farmed soil eventually, and if you raise all your own food, it might be a good idea to have your soil tested to be sure it provides this essential element.

It is possible that we now get *too much* iodine in our national diet, mainly due to the wide use of iodized salt in processed foods. Some doctors have treated cases of intractable acne as an allergy, and they report a few cases that seem to be responsive to a decrease in iodine intake. Of course, there is no reason to assume you're hypersensitive to dietary iodine just because you have bad skin. On the other hand, it might be worthwhile for your doctor to test you for iodine sensitivity, especially if processed foods are a big part of your diet.

Rich sources of iodine besides iodized salt include kelp (seaweed) and sometimes milk and eggs, depending on what the animals were fed.

Selenium forms part of an enzyme that protects lipids from oxidation that turns them into toxic chemicals. Statistical studies link low selenium intake to a higher cancer incidence, but no direct biochemical link has been found. Selenium has often been likened to vitamin E in its functions because both act as antioxidants. Selenium is very toxic in large doses. Good food sources are:

Milk
Wheat
Other grains
Seaweed
Brewer's yeast

Cobalt forms part of cobalamin, vitamin B_{12}. In fact, this is its only known metabolic use. Cobalt differs from all other necessary minerals in that it is the only mineral that must be absorbed as a part of the vitamin to have any effect on metabolism. All other minerals can be absorbed and used *as minerals,* whether they function structurally or as part of enzymes or other metabolic chemical systems. We discuss vitamin B_{12} in the Vitamins section.

Cobalt is toxic in large amounts because it competes with iron in intestinal absorption, leading to anemia.

Manganese is, again, part of enzymes in the body. The primary role of these enzymes is in synthesizing protein-sugar complexes, which are important constituents of connective tissue and the growing portions of bones. Manganese also appears to have a function in carbohydrate and fat metabolism, as well as in the metabolism of the brain. Rich sources are blueberries and bran. Lesser sources include roots, grains, tea, legumes, fruits, and vegetables.

Nickel appears to be important in human nutrition, although its functions and metabolic role are not known. Deficiencies in experimental animals have produced a range of symptoms, from impaired reproduction to increased plasma cholesterol levels.

Fluoride is the ion of the chemical element fluorine. Present evidence is insufficient to classify it as essential for humans, although many researchers feel that this will be demonstrated. Fluoridation of water in many communities is the primary source for this mineral for most people. It is also a source of controversy. Many individuals don't like the idea of having their drinking water treated with chemicals, whether or not it is "for their own good." There is no indication that fluoridated water is harmful, and it definitely protects against tooth decay. There is some evidence that it may protect older people against osteoporosis, although the intake must be higher than normal for this effect to appear. Newborns may need supplemental fluoride to help their primary teeth resist decay. Rich dietary sources are seaweed and tea.

Fluoride is toxic in large amounts, as are all nutrients. Intakes of less than 20 milligrams a day for a long period have produced some x-ray evidence of bone damage, although 20 milligrams a day over the long term seems to be the minimum for obvious bone deformities. Single doses of 2 to 10 grams are fatal, but rare; they have been recorded mainly as accidental overdoses in hospitals or dentists' offices.

Silicon is the second most prevalent element on earth. It is present in many plant tissues, so it's logical that silicon would show up in animal tissues as well. Silicon seems to have a role in the proper calcification of growing bone, similar to that of vitamin D. There are indications that silicon may have a role in connective tissue formation and in aging.

Molybdenum may be necessary for humans because it forms a part of two oxidation enzymes. Molybdenum deficiency has never been described in humans, however, so its status as essential is only conjecture. Even if it is needed, the need amounts to only a few micrograms a day per kilogram of body weight, which we can get from legumes and some grains. Molybdenum content of foods depends on soil concentration.

Vanadium and *tin* may be needed for humans; they have been demonstrated essential for some other animal species. Vanadium may have some influence over reproductive health and growth rate. Tin also affects growth rate.

Of course, the last word is not yet in concerning essential minerals, for either humans or other species. Nutritional research moves slowly because it depends on repetition of carefully controlled experiments to yield a reliable result. These experiments may require several generations of animal or human subjects before they bear fruit in the form of information. Thus, many discoveries remain to be made.

This research influences our health because we, among all the animals, consciously influence our own environment, both external and internal. Understanding our internal environment can lead us to dietary changes that may improve our health immeasureably. And, of course, we must also understand the dietary changes we've already made, and their effects on our health as individuals and as a group. When we began to mill grain and separate it into white flour and "leftovers," we didn't know the negative effects it would have on our health by removing important nutrients from our diet. Researchers discovered the link, and the results of their research showed that we had to do something about the deficiencies of this food, which had formerly been so nutritious. Fortification with some of the stripped nutrients has been the answer for industry. A better answer is eating foods more in their natural state—whole, fresh, untreated.

Of course, other dietary changes have improved our health as a nation. Food-borne diseases are now under control, if not eliminated, because we have learned their causes and keep an eye on food production to limit their spread. We have learned that eating too much fat, too much sugar, too much protein, *too much food,* is unhealthy, and we are trying to learn to change this eating pattern. More answers to important questions lie ahead, and probably more questions, as well.

INTERRELATIONSHIPS

In some ways it is a fallacy to view food as a composition of separate nutrients, as we have done. Human nutrition and human metabolism are characterized by a constant ebb and flow of these separate chemicals that make up our food and our bodies, and they interact with each other as well as with our metabolic systems.

Some may limit or increase our absorption of others, some may require the presence of others to function, and all are required in varying amounts to nourish us well. Some of the better documented interactions are outlined here.

Vitamin B6 is needed in increasing amounts as protein intake increases. The need may also increase tremendously for women on the Pill.

Folic acid may require the presence of vitamin B12 to function in the cell synthesis of DNA and RNA. Vitamin B12 deficiency can result in anemia that a much greater intake of folic acid can offset (although folic acid can't correct the destructive effects of vitamin B12 deficiency on nerve tissues). Chronic alcoholism appears to block folic acid metabolism, resulting in deficiency symptoms even when enough is available in the diet.

When *vitamin B12* is in short supply, abundant folic acid can block some of the symptoms of B12 deficiency. Large doses of vitamin C may block full absorption of vitamin B12. Supplemental vitamin B12 may not correct the problem. In some people, lack of a digestive system chemical called "intrinsic factor" can block B12 absorption.

Niacin is needed in amounts based on caloric intake, since it is crucial to energy release. In a diet short on niacin, your body may make up its need by converting tryptophan, an essential amino acid, into niacin. Vitamin B6 is required for this conversion.

Thiamin's need is also based on caloric intake, for the same reason niacin's is. Thiamin is dependent on folic acid for proper intestinal absorption.

Your need for *vitamin E* is tied to dietary levels of unsaturated fatty acids. Vitamin E supplies appear to be protected against oxidation by vitamin C. Vitamin E and vitamin A work together in maintaining the fatty acid portion of cell membranes. Selenium seems to act similarly to vitamin E, but it is unknown whether they interact with one another.

Vitamin A is protected from oxidation by vitamins E and C. A diet extremely low in fat decreases vitamin A absorption in the intestines. The activity of vitamin A may be decreased by a zinc deficiency, since zinc is required for the liver to secrete RBP, the vitamin A bloodstream-transport protein.

Phosphorus and *calcium* unite to mineralize our bones, and they are both dependent on vitamin D to be absorbed in the intestines.

Calcium should be present in amounts at least equal to those of phosphorus, since an overabundance of phosphorus can result in the leaching of calcium from bones. Too much protein can also result in bone-calcium loss, and too much dietary fat can bind food calcium into indigestible soaplike compounds. Magnesium deficiency can throw off blood levels of calcium by locking the bone calcium up so it can't be used for metabolic purposes.

The intestinal absorption of *iron* can be increased by dietary vitamin C, calcium, and the sulfur amino acids, as well as citric acid in citrus fruits. Too much dietary cobalt can result in anemia, since cobalt competes with iron in intestinal absorption. Copper deficiency can result in impaired iron metabolism.

Sodium and *potassium* interact with each other in controlling the amount of extracellular fluid in your body. When the sodium level is high and the potassium level low, the volume increases, leading to high blood pressure. Balancing these two minerals lowers your blood pressure. In addition, sufficient body magnesium is required for proper metabolism of potassium.

Zinc and *copper* compete with each other in various metabolic processes, and each one can block the toxic effects of too much of the other. A deficiency of each increases the toxic effects of other poisonous minerals, including cadmium, mercury, and silver (for copper).

Oxalic acid and *phytic acid* may bind various minerals, especially calcium, zinc, and iron, making them unavailable to us. We can secrete a digestive enzyme to break up phytic acid, rendering it harmless. The enzyme is also present in yeast and sprouting grains. Phytic acid is present in the seed coat of grains and legumes. Oxalic acid is found in tea, coffee, cocoa, spinach, rhubarb, dandelion, lambsquarters, chard, beet greens, sorrel, pigweed, and parsley, mainly in the form of calcium oxalate. This effectively binds the calcium in those vegetables, but little is left over to bind other dietary minerals, so the net effect is unclear. The concentration of oxalic acid in the leaves of rhubarb is so high that they are directly poisonous and should never be eaten. The stems are the only edible portion.

Of course, to a greater or lesser extent, all nutrients interact with one another in their effects on metabolism. These are the interactions that have been experimentally documented. Others remain to be discovered or verified.

Vitamin and Mineral Need

Vitamins	Role	RDA*		Sources/Comments
		Men	Women	
A (Retinol)	Vision, health of epithelial cells, cell membrane maintenance, glycogen synthesis, helps form infants' bones and teeth	1000 RE	800RE	Carotene in green and yellow vegetables is converted to retinol. Fat soluble, stored in liver. Other sources: butterfat, egg yolk. Toxic in doses far above RDA
D (Cholecalciferol)	Controls intestinal absorption and blood levels of calcium and phosphorus, mineralizing of bones	200 IU	200 IU	Best source is sunlight falling on skin. Other sources: dairy products. Fat soluble, stored, toxic in doses far above RDA
E (Tocopherol)	Protects many body chemicals from oxdizing (fatty acids, A, C)	15 IU	12 IU	Functions not fully understood. Accompanies poly-unsaturated fatty acids in foods. Lost in milling grain. Fat soluble, may be destroyed by freezing
K	Necessary for proper blood clotting			No RDA, abundant in foods, similar distribution to carotene. Also produced by intestinal bacteria
C (Ascorbic acid)	Affects virtually all metabolic processes, including protein formation, immune system, wound healing	60 mg	60 mg	Many claims being investigated. Fruits and vege-tables are main sources. Water soluble, heat- and oxygen-unstable
Riboflavin	Part of many enzyme systems, controlling protein, carbohydrate, and fat metabolism	1.6 mg	1.2 mg	Sources: Milk products, nutritional yeast, greens, grains, mushrooms, nuts, beans. Vegans take extra care. Water soluble, destroyed by light

Vitamin	Function	RDA*		Comments
Thiamin	Enzymes that metabolize amino acids and carbohydrates; nerve signal transmission	1.4 mg	1.0 mg	Pegged to calorie intake, 0.5 mg/1000 kcal. Sources: Yeast, beans, peas, nuts, grains, "enriched" white grain products. Water soluble, heat-unstable
Niacin	Energy-release enzymes, glucose metabolism	18 mg	13 mg	Pegged to calorie intake, 6.6 mg/1000 kcal. Body can synthesize from amino acid tryptophan. Sources: Dairy products, beans, peas, nuts, seeds, grains, yeast, avocado, mushrooms, greens. Lost in milling grain
Folic acid (folates)	DNA and RNA production, construction of amino acids	400 μg	400 μg	High consumption can mask B_{12} deficiency symptoms. Sources: Leafy greens, grains, yeast, legumes, avocados, oranges, bananas, cantaloupe
B_{12} (Cobalamin)	DNA and RNA production (with folic acid), maintains nerve fiber sheath	3.0 μg	3.0 μg	Synthesized by bacteria, fungi, molds. Sources: Milk, fermented soy and other vegetable products. Vegans should take care to get RDA. Stored in body
B_6 (Pyridoxine)	Many processes, including amino acid metabolism, energy release, hemoglobin synthesis	2.2 mg	2.0 mg	Sources: Greens, whole grains, legumes. Much lost in milling, and "enriched" white grains usually lack it. Water soluble, light- and heat-unstable
Pantothenic acid	Part of coenzyme A, used in metabolism of fatty acids, proteins, carbohydrates			No RDA, 5-10 mg should cover needs. Present in every living cell, deficiency unknown. Good sources: Grains, greens, seeds, legumes, egg yolk, milk, dates, sweet potato, cantaloupe, strawberries. Lost in milling
Biotin	Fatty acid synthesis, energy release, DNA synthesis, others			No RDA, deficiency unknown outside of lab. Synthesized by intestinal bacteria, also available in diet

*Applies to adults in good health.

Minerals	Role	RDA* Men	RDA* Women	Sources/Comments
Calcium	Mineralizes bone, blood clotting, muscle contraction, nerve signal transmission	800 mg	800 mg	World Health Organization sets need much lower, 400-500 mg. RDA probably reflects high protein and phosphorus intake, which promote calcium loss. Sources: Dairy products, molasses, sesame, greens, hard water
Phosphorus	Mineralizes bone, energy release, tissue construction	800 mg	800 mg	Intake shouldn't exceed calcium's, since too much phosphorus can cause calcium loss. Sources: Dairy products, grains, nuts, legumes
Magnesium	Mineralizes bone, energy release, fatty acid breakdown, amino acid activation, protein synthesis, DNA synthesis, neuromuscular message transmitter	350 mg	300 mg	Deficiency rare in healthy adults. Interacts with calcium and with sodium/potassium balance. Sources: Grains, greens, legumes, dairy, others
Sodium and Potassium	Interact to control extracellular fluid balance (and thus blood pressure)			No RDA, sodium intake far above need, potassium need linked to sodium intake. 400 mg is enough sodium to cover daily losses—we get 4000 mg or more daily. Sources: Sodium—practically everywhere; potassium—fruits, legumes, greens, molasses
Iron	Oxygen transmission and storage, enzymes	10 mg	18 mg	WHO estimates women who eat mainly plant diet need much more, up to 28 mg, because of lower absorbability. This amount is virtually impossible to get without supplements. Sources: Prune juice, legumes, millet.

Mineral	Function	RDA*		Sources
Zinc	DNA, RNA metabolism, connective tissue formation, immune system	15 mg	15 mg	some greens, raisins, dates, molasses, wheat, acorn squash, torula yeast, strawberries, potato, oatmeal, cooking in iron pots. May be more easily absorbed from animal source foods. Sources: Legumes, green peas, spinach, cocoa, bran, also grains, vegetables, dairy products
Trace Minerals				
Iodine	Thyroid hormone system	150 mg	150 mg	Iodized salt covers needs of all. Sea vegetables are another rich source. Overconsumption of salt and processed foods may give some of us too much iodine
Copper Selenium Cobalt Manganese Nickel Chromium	Varies	No RDA, but shown to be essential		Sources for most of these are soil, by way of crops. Concentrations vary in food according to where it's produced. May become depleted in intensively farmed areas
Flourine Silicon Molybdenum Vanadium Tin	Varies	No RDA, not yet proved essential, but may be		Sources: Soil and water. Vary locally, may become depleted in intensively farmed areas

*Applies to adults in good health.

RECOMMENDATIONS FOR SUPPLEMENTATION

First and foremost, we should all get most of our nutrients from a good diet. This is how our bodies have been designed, and this is how we should try to live.

On the other hand, there is no logical reason not to supplement the nutrients we may not get enough of. We should try to find an acceptable middle ground.

For vegans vitamin B_{12} need bears some examination, since there are few convenient sources of the vitamin in nonanimal foods. Bacterially fermented foods may contain abundant amounts of vitamin B_{12}—tempeh and kombu, for example—but these are not always easy to find. Soy milk and nutritional yeast such as brewer's yeast may be supplemented with added vitamin B_{12}, even though the yeast does not synthesize the vitamin on its own. A supplemental tablet may be a good idea if you have difficulty finding these sources of the vitamin. Riboflavin may be in short supply for vegans, so they should pay attention to their sources of this vitamin. Vegans should also take care that they get enough calcium, although their needs are probably not as high as the RDA of 800 milligrams.

Both lacto-ovos and vegans may be borderline in getting enough iron and zinc (so may nonvegetarians), especially if they have a greater need, as do children and women before menopause (for iron).

Based on all these considerations, you might consider supplementing your intake of zinc and iron to make sure you get the RDA. If you eat a poor diet, which we strongly suggest you try to change first, or if you have poor absorption of some nutrients, the ones that will run short in your diet first will probably be vitamin A and the water soluble vitamins, C and the B complex. If you use no dairy products and stay out of the sun, you may need vitamin D. Finally, if you don't use eggs or milk, you must make sure to include a source of vitamin B_{12} in your diet (or take a supplement) as well as riboflavin and calcium.

Supplementary vitamins can be protective, especially if you are under a lot of physiological or emotional stress. In addition, some drugs deplete your body's store of certain vitamins, particularly vitamin C. Of course, if you supplement your vitamins and minerals, do it within reason. More than double the RDA of most vitamins and minerals is probably excessive (see the listings for individual nutrients to see any special cautions). *Never* take more than the RDA of vitamins A and D, because they can be very toxic in the forms provided by vitamin pills.

Many people take vitamins because they don't want to go to the trouble of improving their diets, and they superstitiously believe the tablets will protect them from their own indiscretions. Others take them because they feel vitamins are good insurance against possible flaws in their individual metabolisms. You may want to take supplementary vitamins for these reasons. Don't supplement to ridiculous levels—it may do much more harm than good.

"Organic" or "Synthetic" Supplements?

Tough question. Your health foods stores owner will tell you that you must have bioflavonoids with your vitamin C, so you need an organic product (from a health foods store). What he may forget to tell you is that your bottle of "Vitamin C with Rose Hips and Acerola" is mostly synthetic vitamin C, flavored with rose hips and sour cherry extract. Vitamins are sometimes a gigantic scam, and their labeling often borders on fraud.

Truly organic vitamins are those surrounded by food. The nearest thing you can buy in tablet form are vitamins extracted from foods by a variety of processes not disclosed on the label. *This doesn't mean the product is inferior*—it simply means you don't know how that vitamin B6 or whatever got into that little tablet. The single advantage to using "organic" vitamins is that they are not as pure as the lab-synthesized versions—depending, of course, on how they were extracted. They may be "contaminated" with other nutrients that are certainly not present in the synthetic versions. Remember that we have no idea whether all the nutrients essential to human health have yet been discovered. The "impurities" present in foods and, to a lesser extent, organic vitamins may very well contribute to your health in a way not yet discovered. The best brands of organic supplements also avoid gelatin, saccharin, and artificial coloring and flavoring. Synthetics don't.

Supplements shouldn't be necessary except for a few vitamins and minerals, supplemented in limited amounts. Ideally, you should get your nutrition from your diet, not from a pill. If you take supplements, you must decide for yourself if the possible difference in nutritive value justifies the great difference in price between synthetic and organic versions of these very expensive products.

Even with vitamin supplements, read the label. Vegetarians should watch out for ingredients such as fish liver oil and bone meal, often used as sources of fat-soluble vitamins and calcium, respectively. Even though an item is found in a health foods store, it is not necessarily vegetarian.

GUIDELINES

Vitamins and minerals are essential nutrients that your body needs in relatively small amounts, ranging from a couple of micrograms up to a little over a gram a day.

Vitamins are complex organic chemicals that generally must be consumed in one particular form. Minerals are simple ions composed of a few atoms that can be taken in a variety of forms.

The best way to insure you get enough of almost all these essential nutrients is to eat a varied diet of fresh, whole foods.

Some minerals and the water-soluble vitamins can be lost by cooking foods in large amounts of water and then throwing the water away. A better way is to steam or quick sauté food, to preserve nutrients and flavor.

Other rules to preserve nutrient quality of food include:

Store fresh food in a cold, dark, comparatively moist place, and use within a few days.

Cook food in rather large pieces and cut up for serving, if possible.

Serve food unpeeled if possible (although peeling is a good way to remove most of a food's retained pesticides and other unwanted chemical pollutants).

Cut or bruised fresh fruits and vegetables lose nutrients rapidly—don't store them this way, but use them immediately.

Green leafy vegetables, fruits, grains, and legumes are rich sources of a variety of these essential nutrients.

PUTTING IT TOGETHER: FOUR EATING STYLES

6
Putting It Together: Four Eating Styles

So far, we've given you a great deal of information about how nutrition works. But how do you take all the numbers, percentages, and proportions and apply them to everyday life? What follows are four plans for those who want a convenient approach to help guide them through a busy day. It is not necessary with any of these plans to measure amounts of foods and calculate nutrients compulsively. It's just not that difficult to get good nutrition.

We have already discussed the components of a good diet and how these fit into a vegetarian diet. These components break down into two groups—those of which you should get enough and those of which you must not get too much. Vitamins, minerals, and complex carbohydrates form the first group. Fats and sugars are the major representatives of the second group. Protein straddles the dividing line—you should get enough, but not too much.

Once again, these plans are not compulsory. If you keep in mind the general nutritional principles outlined in earlier chapters, you should be able to live a healthy life as a vegetarian without giving it much thought at all. In fact, the first plan is to do just that.

THE LAISSEZ-FAIRE APPROACH

The term *laissez-faire* is a French phrase that means literally "Let . . . to do." More loosely constructed, it means, "Let them do as they please" or "Let them be." The "them" in this case is you. What we mean is that there are no binding rules, no timetables or schedules, no goals to meet. You only need two things: knowledge and good common sense.

125

The first rule for Laissez-faire eating is that you be nutritionally aware. You need a working knowledge of what your body requires and what different foods can offer. This kind of nutritional awareness is essential to any kind of healthy diet, vegetarian or not. You can't afford to go through life with the blind faith that if it's in the supermarket or on the menu, it's good for you. You should especially try to find out about the foods you like, that you eat often. If you often have an avocado in your salad at lunch, it would be a good idea to know what it gives you nutritionally. Remember the bottom-line reason we eat—to nourish our bodies.

The second rule is to remember these two concepts: variety and natural, whole foods.

Variety

Vary your diet. If you eat the same thing day in, day out, you're bound to be missing out on important nutrients. By eating a variety of foods, you will insure a sufficient cross-section of nutrients, including a full complement of essential amino acids. There is no perfect food that provides everything you could possibly need. Even within the major food categories like grains or vegetables there are many variations in the nutrients specific foods offer. Select different foods from each group over time for a good balance. If you find yourself concentrating on dairy products or pasta or just one or two vegetables, consciously try to bring other foods into your diet. Different grains (brown rice, millet, barley, wild rice, buckwheat) offer a wide range of flavors and textures, plus a variety of nutrients you may not be getting enough of by eating only whole wheat bread. When you eat beans, don't always have chickpeas. Try pintos or soybeans.

Varying your diet also helps you to moderate. As the Romans said, "Semper moderatus." This is the hardest rule of all to live by, because it touches on our emotional connection to food. Food can be a comfort, a psychological reward, a place to hide. Realizing that you've had enough when you want to keep eating requires a degree of restraint that few of us can muster. Our forefathers' instincts come through strongly when it comes to food. "When you can get food, eat as much as you can hold. After all, who knows when you'll eat again?" Most of us don't have the supply problems our forefathers had. Generally, the most severe problem we run across in the supermarket is that they're out of blue paper towels and we'll have to make do with yellow. Still, it is hard to fight instinct, especially when at one time it had a survival value. Now it just makes us fat.

Moderation also applies to the all-too-American philosophy of More Is Better. If a little bit is good for you, a lot should be great. For example, we overeat protein at a rate of double or triple our actual needs, theorizing that it will make us big and strong and able to fight off everything from the flu to the aging process. It just doesn't work that way, and it isn't healthy—the protein we waste has to go somewhere. It is excreted through our kidneys, putting a strain on them for which they were never designed. In addition, much of that protein comes hand-in-hand with an overload of saturated fat. And we know *that* isn't good.

Natural Foods

The further a food is from the way nature made it, the less good it does you. A corollary to this rule is the more Madison Avenue a food has in it, the less *food* it has in it. Packaging and ad campaigns seem to increase in direct proportion to the amount of processing to which a food has been subjected.

The perfect example is wheat flour. There was a time not too long ago when wheat flour was a nourishing, good-tasting staple. It was ground between stones from the whole grain of the wheat, and it provided good-quality protein, iron, calcium, zinc, some B vitamins, and vitamin E, not to mention plant fiber, complex carbohydrates, and excellent flavor.

Then the image-makers got hold of it. It wasn't fine enough or light enough, so they took out the bran and the germ (and most of the fiber, protein, minerals, and vitamins). It didn't keep long enough on store shelves or in bakery storage rooms, so they gassed it with bromine, heated it, and gave it various other "treatments." Stone milling took too long, so they developed the high-speed steel roller mill, whose high temperature all but eliminated the last vestiges of vitamins and other perishable nutrients. Then they baked it and called it bread.

Not long after all this commercial manipulation of a healthful food took place, people began to notice a change in their health. Bread just wasn't supplying the nutrition it used to. Finally, enough public outcry was raised to force the nation's big millers to do something. So they "enriched" the flour that they had just finished stripping of nutritional value. They replaced some of the vitamins and a small amount of iron. Only riboflavin is replaced in amounts equal to what was removed. The utter gall with which they use the word "enriched" is some indication of the cynical way food processors use the language to make us think we're getting something we're not. A similar logic would be to cut off both our legs, replace them with prosthetic limbs, and call us "enriched."

They now had the word at their disposal, and they could use it to dispel criticism of their product. After all, wasn't the bread "enriched"? How could it possibly be better?

By leaving it alone.

Eating whole foods may be the most complicated part of your adjustment to a healthier eating pattern. We grew up on advertisements for Cool-Whip and 7-Up, not to mention Wonder Bread. Our parents often made our lunches with Oscar Mayer bologna and Miracle Whip on white bread. Birdseye International Vegetables graced the dinner table, along with the Butterball pressure-basted turkey. We topped it off with Jello or Whip 'n' Chill.

Compared to these foods, whole foods such as fresh fruits and vegetables, brown rice, beans, whole-grain products, nuts, and seeds may pale at first. They don't have the flashy names, and they certainly aren't as brightly packaged. Sometimes they taste, well, *different*. Usually they taste better. But people have a natural resistance to the new (even if it's old, as in this case), especially when it comes to food. This probably has a survival purpose, like many other human tendencies. But will almost certainly get in your way in improving your diet, and that change has a survival value of its own.

Perhaps the secret is to adopt a certain spirit of adventure. This is something new, exciting, and nonthreatening, not to mention healthy. You can take it at your own pace. If you slip and eat (horrors!) a Twinkie, just start over the next day. Remember the poster with the idiotic smiling face grinning the New Age message down at you: "This is the first day of the rest of your life!" You have as many chances to succeed as you are willing to give yourself. There is no need for ultimatums. Just keep trying to choose your foods wisely.

If the millet casserole is just too awful to contemplate when it comes out of the oven, don't despair. Throw some spaghetti in the pot, cook up some tomatoes, garlic, herbs, and whatever else you have. It's easy, once you get the hang of it, and delicious.

In short, there is no such thing as "failure." We try again, not necessarily harder, but in a spirit of adventure. What, after all, is so exciting about Rice-a-Roni?

The rules of Laissez-faire vegetarianism are:

Be nutritionally aware.
Remember: variety and natural, whole foods.
Given the above, go with your instincts. Most important: Get enough calories, and don't eat too many empty calories (sugar and fat).

THE PERSONALIZED APPROACH

If Laissez-faire eating doesn't help you in deciding whether your lunch is nutritious enough, try the Personalized approach. In this plan, you structure your diet around the foods you already eat, consciously adding foods here and there to improve the nutritional value. This is really Laissez-faire with a bit of analysis thrown in.

It's a pretty good guess that you have certain eating habits, certain foods you prefer and eat often, preferences about what and where you eat. If you cook for yourself, there are probably a few dishes you cook often and a much wider repertoire that you prepare much more seldom.

The idea here is to go along with those preferences, habits, and constraints of lifestyle as much as possible and still be well nourished. The first step is to make a study of your eating habits.

Do you always eat at home? Do you eat out often? Do you have a weekly or monthly routine—Tuesday dinner at your in-laws, Saturday out with friends? Are any of your meals comparatively ritualized and set—"the usual" for breakfast or lunch? Do you cook or does someone else do the cooking?

Do you have strong likes and dislikes in food? How many of these stem from taste and how many from the unexamined habits of a lifetime?

Are you willing to experiment a little, or would you just as soon not be bothered?

Answering these questions will give you a certain awareness of your eating style—how, where, and what you eat.

Keep a record of what you eat for the next week, where, and who prepared it. There is a pattern of likes and dislikes, not to mention constraints, hidden in there somewhere.

Once you have made the list, analyze it. Use the Food Groups approach outlined later in the chapter or our general recommendations as a guide. Are you eating enough complex carbohydrates? Too much fat? Not enough vegetables? Pinpoint the weaknesses in your diet.

If you are eating too much of a particular food or nutrient, the solution is obvious: Cut down. What if you're not getting enough of something? If, for example, there aren't enough complex carbohydrates in your diet, make a list of foods you like that are good sources. Look at the Food Groups Guide in the appendix for ideas. A sample list might be: dried apricots, broccoli, bread, pasta, apples, pears, rice. Then make a point to eat more of those foods.

There are as many ways to modify a diet as there are people. Remember, they can be simple ways. You don't have to restructure your life. For example, if you want to increase the protein content of your meals, add nuts, seeds, chopped tofu, or grated cheese to just about anything. Eat some bread and cheese as a snack or yogurt as a side dish or dessert.

Go over the week's menu and annotate it, filling in the nutritional gaps with possibilities that could have improved your meals. Take into consideration where you were as well, so you can choose practical improvements. For example, at a restaurant you might not be able to ask for a handful of seeds; some grated Parmesan cheese probably would be available, though. Use your annotated list as a guide to how you can eat better in the future. In a few weeks, do a week's analysis again to see if you really have improved. If someone else cooks for you, a bit of psychology is in order. Don't go marching in and make a series of demands, as though you were holding hostages in a laundromat. Casually inquire what's for dinner, then ask if it might be possible to add some nuts to it or have a salad with it or whatever. Of course, this is an oversimplication for many people, but the essential point is to introduce the subject in a nonpressuring manner and offer to help out as much as you can. Be knowledgeable about simple alternatives, so you can offer ready suggestions.

Whatever you eat, and whoever cooks it, there are always simple ways to improve the quality of a meal. Tailor your modifications to your own nutritional needs. Some likely additions to casseroles, in salads, as snacks, on cereal, in sandwiches, ad infinitum are:

Fresh fruit slices	Seeds
Raisins	Cheese
Dried fruit	Cherry tomatoes
Nuts	Raw vegetables, pre-cut

Alfalfa sprouts

Sprouted wheat berries

Yogurt

Wheat germ

Unsweetened juices

Lettuce leaves

Pre-cooked beans and grains

When you're out:

Order juice or milk rather than soda.

Order baked potato (hold the sour cream) rather than french fries.

Order a salad.

Ask for oil and vinegar dressing rather than a creamy variety.

Order fruit, cheese, or yogurt instead of a sweet dessert.

Carry small packages of seeds or dried fruit to avoid buying empty calorie snacks.

Order new (to you) foods instead of "the usual."

Avoid rich sauces.

Ask for lettuce and tomato on sandwiches.

Order whole-grain breads.

For the Personalized approach, remember these points:

Be nutritionally aware.

Variety and natural foods.

Find the weaknesses in your diet.

List the foods you like that can round out your diet.

Make an effort to increase the nutritional value of your diet.

Structure it around the foods you already eat.

THE FOOD GROUPS APPROACH

Remember the Four Basic Food Groups from third-grade health class? For some strange reason, the health textbook included meat as one of them. It is time to correct the error. The *real* Food Groups are (for lacto-ovos) (1) Whole grains; (2) Nuts, seeds, and legumes; (3) Vegetables, especially dark green, leafy vegetables; (4) Fruit; and (5) Dairy products; *or* (for vegans) (1) Whole grains; (2) Nuts, seeds, and legumes; (3) Vegetables; and (4) Fruit.

These groups of foods combine to supply all the nutrition you could possibly need. They form the structure of the Food Groups approach to improving your diet. Once you know the groups and what is included in each, you shouldn't have too much trouble making sure you eat enough from each group in the course of a day.

Grains, legumes, nuts, and seeds are the staples of a vegetarian diet. This may be difficult for a person raised in our country to understand, because of the twofold dietary prejudice existing here—first that those foods are starchy, bland, and non-nutritious, and second, that the basis for a good diet is a high-protein food such as meat, or at least dairy products. Widely available representatives of the grain group *are* starchy and non-nutritious, but that is a result of the way they are processed, not a fault inherent in the food itself. Of course white rice is starchy. Starch is about all that's left once it has been hulled and polished and washed and parboiled. It has lost a quarter of its protein, two-thirds of its fiber, and significant amounts of other nutrients (although they may have been partly replaced with synthetic forms). And white flour—who would consider building a diet around that?

Grains and legumes in their whole forms provide excellent nutrition, high quality protein, minerals, vitamins, and complex carbohydrates. Remember that complex carbohydrates should make up at least 60 percent of your daily caloric intake. Lentils, for example, are composed by weight of 58 percent carbohydrates, 25 percent protein, and about 2 percent fat (the rest is mainly moisture, even in the dried beans). This translates to 68 percent, 29 percent, and 3 percent of the total calories. Lentils by themselves are excellent sources of carbohydrates and protein, and they are very low in fat. They also offer respectable amounts of iron, calcium, phosphorus, potassium, vitamin A, and niacin.

All the other members of these two groups provide similar nutritional value, although in somewhat different proportions. Whole wheat, for example, is somewhat higher in carbohydrate and much higher in fat.

Dairy products are good sources of protein, fat, and many minerals and vitamins, including vitamins D and B_{12}. They should be considered supplementary protein sources because of the high fat content that often accompanies their protein. (Of course, vegans eliminate this group entirely and depend on the other listed foods for their nutrition.)

We don't normally think of vegetables as a protein source, but they do produce good quality protein, even though in rather small amounts.

Perhaps more important, vegetables provide excellent complex carbohydrates and the entire spectrum of minerals and vitamins except B$_{12}$. This lack is made up through dairy products for lacto-ovos, while vegans should eat a fermented food such as tempeh, a food fortified with vitamin B$_{12}$, or take a vitamin supplement in order to meet the requirement.

Fruit's major contributions to your diet are vitamins (C and A), minerals, fiber, sugar, and pleasure. In fact, fruit can help you to avoid other sweets that you may have become accustomed to eating. Most of us have a highly developed sweet tooth, and a ripe piece of fruit can take the edge off of it, while providing nutritional benefits rare in other dessert foods.

The key, then, is to use grain- and legume-based foods at every meal. This does *not* mean a cinnamon bun and a cup of coffee for breakfast—that's the antithesis of a healthy vegetarian meal. Remember the rule listed in the Laissez-faire approach: ''Natural foods.'' This is essential. Try to remember that you are nourishing your body, for better or worse, with every food you put in your mouth.

If you get a quarter of your calories from non-nutritious highly refined foods, for example, you must depend on the other 75 percent of your food for 100 percent of your nutritional needs. That's taking quite a chance. You just can't meet those needs with a hamburger and a vitamin pill.

Surround those grain-based foods with plenty of fresh vegetables (especially leafy, dark greens), some dairy products, and some fruit. Unless you happen to love raw green pepper, the fruit may be your most important source of vitamin C. So don't pass it up.

These lists show our recommended distribution of the Food Groups in your daily eating.

For *Lacto-ovos*
- 4 servings of whole Grains (for example, a serving is 1 slice bread, ¾ cup cereal or cooked grain.)
- 2 servings of Legumes, Nuts, and Seeds (a serving is 15 grams protein: 4 tablespoons peanut butter, 1 cup cooked beans, ½ cup peanuts or sunflower seeds)
- 3 servings of Vegetables, including dark green, leafy ones (a serving is 1 cup raw, ¾ cup cooked)
- 2 servings of Dairy Products (a serving is, for example, 1 cup milk or yogurt, 1½ ounces hard cheese, ⅓ cup milk powder, 1⅓ cups cottage cheese)
- 1 or more pieces of Fruit, including a vitamin C–rich source

For *Vegans*
> Vegans can use the above guide, replacing dairy products with fortified soy milk, or:
>
> 5 servings of whole Grains
>
> 3 servings of Legumes, Nuts, and Seeds
>
> 4 servings of Vegetables, especially dark green, leafy vegetables
>
> 1 or more pieces of Fruit, including a C–rich source
>
> Be sure to eat a source of vitamin B_{12}, such as tempeh or kombu.

Remember these rules for following the Food Groups plan:
> Be nutritionally aware.
>
> Variety and natural foods.
>
> Learn the Food Groups for your particular diet and what's in each group.
>
> Remember how much of each group you should eat each day.

THE MENU APPROACH

The Menu plan is merely a variation on any of the other plans. The idea is to plan out a week's meals in advance, on paper. This method has several advantages, among them that you won't ever have to wonder what to make for dinner. Also, you can look at your plan for the week and decide if the meals you've planned are nutritious and balanced.

Once you know what foods you are going to prepare, you know exactly what you must buy on that week's shopping trip. For that reason, it's an economical way to decide what to buy, because you won't be tempted to buy things impulsively (at least, not quite as tempted). Marketing specialists will tell you that it's those impulse purchases that eat up your food budget fastest—that's what they're counting on when they try to influence your purchases through advertising and packaging. If you buy something you don't need, you're wasting twice—once for the cash you could spend on something you *do* need, and once for the product that may well be wasted. If you buy a food item that is heavily processed and equally heavily promoted, it's a third waste, whether you actually use it or not.

Planning your meals this way may also save time in the long run. You'll gain awareness of how much time you need on various days to spend preparing your food ("I have a class that night. It'll have to be something quick"), what you can or should prepare in advance, and what staples you should have on hand in case of emergencies. Although it won't prepare you to deal with any eventuality, it can help out a lot compared to the haphazard "system" many food shoppers use.

The following sample week's lacto-ovo menu shows you how it might work for you. Obviously, you won't choose to eat everything on the list—people's tastes vary. The list is included purely for purposes of illustration.

SUNDAY

Brunch	*Supper*
Pancakes with strawberries and yogurt, glass of fresh orange juice	Giant salad, including cheese, mushrooms, sprouts, tomatoes, scallions, nuts, raisins, leaf lettuce; bread

MONDAY

Breakfast	*Lunch*	*Dinner*
Cereal, toast with peanut butter, milk, fresh orange juice	Cornbread with spicy kidney beans, salad, pear	Mushroom-bulgur pilaf, broccoli with cheese sauce, salad

TUESDAY

Breakfast	*Lunch*	*Dinner*
Leftover pilaf scrambled with one egg, strawberries with milk	Grilled cheese on rye, side of sliced tomatoes, carrot and celery strips, a few roasted peanuts (who can eat only a few?)	Bean, rice, and cheese loaf, steamed stringbeans and slivered almonds, salad

WEDNESDAY

Breakfast	*Lunch*	*Dinner*
Bran muffins, cereal, milk, apple slices	Leftover bean loaf in sandwich with tomato and lettuce, milk	Spaghetti with sautéed zucchini and onions, salad of romaine and endive

THURSDAY

Breakfast	*Lunch*	*Dinner*
Cereal, milk, bran muffins, orange juice	Swiss on whole wheat with tomato and sprouts, chunk of fresh pineapple	Thick vegetable soup, pumpernickel bread, salad, a few nuts

FRIDAY

Breakfast	*Lunch*	*Dinner*
Yogurt shake with wheat germ and strawberries	Peanut butter and banana on whole wheat, glass of milk	Rice and vegetable casserole with sesame meal, panroasted Brussels sprouts with lime, coleslaw

SATURDAY

Breakfast	*Lunch*	*Dinner*
Fresh fruit salad with cottage cheese and whole wheat sesame crackers	Sliced avocado with chopped scallions, sprouts, and cheese on rye, side of sliced tomato	(out with friends) Indian food—samosa, papadum, vegetable curry, boiled rice, onion chutney

It may strike you from this menu that you'll be eating a lot of food. The grain- and legume-based diet has quite a bit of bulk, which is satisfying on its own. It does not have the concentrated calories of a high-fat diet, so you're not as likely to overeat. If you ate the foods listed until you were satisfied (not stuffed), you'd get all you need for good nutrition that week.

It may also seem that there is a lot of preparation involved, but all the dinners usually can be prepared in an hour, and most of the ingredients for the breakfasts and lunches either can be purchased already prepared or can be prepared in advance. For those without much time to spare for food preparation, there are, of course, quicker meals (see Chapter 13).

Remember these guidelines for the Menu approach:

Use any of the other three plans.

Plan menus a week at a time.

Analyze your list to make sure you're getting a balanced diet.

A FEW WORDS OF ADVICE

We have taken the rules of nutrition and structured them into our four plans. These are only vehicles for organizing nutritional information so it isn't overwhelming. You needn't go by any of our plans, except Laissez-faire eating. In fact, even nonvegetarians should adopt the rules of the Laissez-faire approach to make sure they get the best possible nutrition. It is so simple, it's not really a method or a plan.

Otherwise, you may mix different plans, take some things from one and add them to another, or build your own four plans, or twelve plans. Any aware vegetarian, from the most structured to the most laissez-faire, will get more than adequate nutrition. The most important thing is to choose your foods wisely within any plan. Here are some suggestions (for more about choosing foods, see Chapter 12). You'll notice that there are more items to avoid than to choose, but take heart. Those in the "choose" list are more general categories. The "avoid" list includes many refined foods (high fat, high sugar, low nourishment), and, as you know, they come packaged in every form imaginable.

Choose

Dark green, leafy vegetables

Raw or lightly cooked vegetables

Fresh or dried fruit

Skim milk

Low-fat cottage cheese

Low-fat yogurt

Skim milk powder

Seeds

Beans

Soybean products (like tofu)

Unbuttered popcorn

Whole grains (like bulgur, buckwheat, barley, rye)

Wheat germ

Whole grain bread, muffins, rolls, and crackers

Whole grain pasta

Hot or cold whole-grain cereals (granola, oatmeal, shredded wheat)

Unsweetened juices

Herbs and spices

Moderate

Cheese

Nuts

Natural nut butters

Creamed cottage cheese

Liquid vegetable oils

Eggs

Low-fat milk

Molasses

Avoid/Limit

Fried vegetables

Creamed vegetables and soups

Canned vegetables

Canned fruit in sugar syrup

Whole milk

Butter

Cream

Ice cream

Cream cheese

Evaporated milk

Whole milk yogurt

Milkshakes

White flour and white bread
Sugared cereals
Flavored crackers
Cakes and pastries, especially mixes
Breakfast cakes
Sweet rolls
Refined grains (like white rice)
Sodas
Alcoholic drinks
Sugared drink mixes
Instant breakfasts
Hydrogenated peanut butter
Salted nuts and other salty snacks
Mayonnaise
Hardened vegetable shortenings
Coconut, palm, and cotton-seed oils
Commercial vegetable oil blends
Margarine
Sweeteners (like sugar, honey)
Jams and jellies
Syrups
Commercial pies and puddings
Dessert toppings
Nondairy creamers
Cake frosting
Textured vegetable protein products
Instant anything

GUIDELINES

Be nutritionally aware.
Vary your foods.
Eat natural, whole foods.
Choose the best food that
     is available to you in a
     particular situation.

SPECIAL CASES

Pregnancy
Babies and Children
Athletes
A Weight-loss Diet

7
Pregnancy

Susan had always been careful to eat a balanced vegetarian diet. She knew she would have to be even more aware now that she was pregnant, but her doctor gave her a difficult time from the beginning, ridiculing vegetarianism and insinuating, as the months passed, that she probably had a B-complex deficiency due to a lack of red meat. As Susan put it, "It was a very emotional time, and I wanted to do everything just right for the baby. Looking back, I simply didn't ask enough questions." What she did end up doing was eating red meat occasionally to ease her conscience.

Any nagging little doubts people may have about vegetarianism become aggravated when it comes to pregnancy. The general concern is: Can a pregnant vegetarian eat a sufficiently well-balanced diet in the amounts needed? Susan, for example, was afraid she would have to eat too much to obtain all the extra protein and other nutrients required when eating for two. "How much milk can one person drink?" she asked plaintively.

Certainly it is understandable to be willing to sacrifice your principles a bit for the health of your baby, as Susan felt she was doing. The special needs of pregnancy do not, however, have to be met with a dose of meat or by drowning yourself in milk. Indeed, except for organ meats, meat is not one of the best sources of the B vitamins or any other nutrients except protein. It isn't a necessary source of anything, including protein.

The most important things to remember during pregnancy are to increase your calories and make every one count. That is the best advice for vegetarians and meateaters alike. And vegetarians don't have to consume any more calories (or milk) than do meateaters in order to meet every prenatal need.

The first thing you should do is find a doctor who is supportive of your needs and feelings. It is easy at this time to become intimidated by doctors, who supposedly know more than you. On the subject of nutrition, however, myths still abound in the medical profession, and many doctors still want to "play it safe." While we agree that caution is generally a virtue in doctors, "playing it safe" by eating meat is simply a case of not looking at the facts. Your doctor should be your ally. Make sure he or she is.

Pregnant vegans will get even more static than will lacto-ovos. They need even more gross protein since their sources are generally less digestible, and they have to take special care with several other nutrients as well. We will cover these needs point by point, later in the chapter. Just remember that every pregnant woman requires extra nourishment. You'll be fine as long as you are aware of your particular needs and eat accordingly.

The National Academy of Sciences recommends that you increase your calories by about 300 a day. At first this may seem like a great excuse for an extra piece of chocolate cake, but in truth, those surplus calories are not a carte blanche to do anything but eat a larger, more prudent diet. Even if we assume you ate a varied wholesome diet before, an extra 300 calories of similar caliber food will not simply take up the slack. The caloric increase is only about 15 percent, while certain of your other nutritional needs have gone up 50 and even 100 percent. Forget the cake and eat more leafy greens.

At no time is the effect of nutrition more important to the future health of your child than while you are pregnant. From the moment of conception, growth is taking place. For the first eight weeks it is rather slow, but critical, as the cells for the various organs, arms, legs, eyes, and ears are differentiating. Then, for the last seven months, growth is tremendous; the baby's weight will increase 500 times, its height about 16 times. Different organs will be developing at different rates. For example, the embryonic heart will function long before the lungs. Excellent nutrition is necessary at all times. If at any point you are malnourished, you could permanently affect the growth and potential of one or more of your baby's vital organs.

Meanwhile, the mother is growing a whole new organ—the placenta—where her own and her baby's blood vessels interweave so that nutrients can travel from mother to child. The amniotic sac fills with fluid to cushion the baby. The uterus and surrounding muscles get larger. The breasts prepare for lactation. The blood volume increases greatly.

During the first trimester, you will gain just a few (2 to 4) pounds, and calorie consumption will be somewhat lower than the pregnancy RDA. After that about a half-pound to a pound is usually gained every week, and the full 300 calories should be added. Try to spread it out over time as evenly as possible. A total gain of 24 to 28 pounds is ideal, no matter what your weight is to start out.

Never try to reduce or fast while you are pregnant. If you have gained more than you like, it is better to keep it on than to eat less than you should. Too little food will deprive you both of essential nutrients. Furthermore, the breakdown of fat results in ketosis, a slightly toxic condition that could damage the fetal nervous system.

On the other hand, too much extra weight will often cause high blood pressure and problems with delivery. All in all, it is best to start out as a healthy individual at a good weight. From there is is easier to be especially careful for the nine months of pregnancy, when you are directly responsible for the quality of your unborn baby's life.

To some extent, you would be the one to suffer first from any carelessness, since the fetus can draw what it needs from you, thus depleting your supply. It cannot, however, get everything it needs from a malnourished mother. Generally, whatever you're doing to your body, you're doing to the baby.

That is reason enough to abstain from smoking, caffeine, alcohol and other drugs, and food additives, not to mention the recent weighty evidence that such substances may cause birth defects. Caffeine, incidentally, is a major ingredient in tea, cola, and chocolate, as well as coffee. Avoiding drugs would certainly mean avoiding meat, with its concentrated residues of pesticides, hormones, and additives.

Diuretics are often prescribed by doctors to relieve swelling caused by fluid retention, or edema. They can have disastrous side effects, however, including dehydration, loss of appetite, and vomiting. It is generally unwise to take diuretics especially since edema is usually not serious—in fact, it is somewhat normal—unless it is a result of malnutrition.

Malnutrition seems to be the key to toxemia as well, a more critical condition characterized by swelling and high blood pressure. As long as you are getting an adequate diet, including sufficient protein, you needn't worry about this.

In Table 1 you can see the recommended increases for each nutrient while you are pregnant. Needs vary according to the individual, but these RDA figures are a good guide. We have also

Table 1 Pregnancy Needs Versus Normal Nutritional Needs

Nutrient	Normal[1]	Pregnant	Increase	%
Calories	2000	2300	300	15
Protein (gm)	44	74	30	68
Vitamin A (RE)	800	1000	200	25
Vitamin D (IU)	200	400	200	100
Vitamin E (IU)	12	15	3	25
Vitamin C (mg)	60	80	20	33⅓
Folic acid (μg)	400	800	400	100
Niacin (mg)	13	15	2	15
Riboflavin (mg)	1.2	1.5	.3	25
Thiamin (mg)	1	1.4	.4	40
Vitamin B$_6$ (mg)	2	2.6	.6	30
Vitamin B$_{12}$ (μg)	3	4	1	33⅓
Calcium (mg)	800	1200	400	50
Phosphorus (mg)	800	1200	400	50
Iodine (μg)	150	175	25	17
Iron (mg)	18	18+(supplement)[2]		
Magnesium (mg)	300	450	150	50
Zinc (mg)	15	20	5	33⅓

[1]Refers to 120-pound woman, aged 23–50.
[2]WHO recommends 28 mg iron for women getting 10% or fewer calories from animal sources. Supplementation required.

included the increases in terms of percentages to help you determine just how much you should alter your particular way of eating. What follows is a detailed guide to some of the more important of these nutrients during pregnancy. The others are really just as vital, of course, especially if you don't get them, so study the table and look at the previous chapters to give yourself a good grasp of basic needs and sources for nutrients we don't include here, such as magnesium and zinc.

CALORIES

As we said, pregnant women should eat about 300 extra calories each day in order to meet the higher demands for nutrients and energy. Supplying your body with extra calories to meet energy needs also spares the protein, which is now so vital in building tissue and supporting growth. Remember, eat more calories, not empty calories. The distinction is crucial.

PROTEIN

A significant increase in protein intake during pregnancy is needed to build all of the baby's body tissues plus the mother's uterine and breast tissues. It is also instrumental in the formation of the placenta. Protein is especially crucial in the production of brain cells, a factor likely to affect the mental development of the child. Because of the much greater volume of circulating blood now, protein also is needed for the increased synthesis of blood components like hemoglobin and plasma protein. It even helps regulate blood sugar, the body's source of energy.

The National Academy of Sciences RDA for pregnant women is 30 grams extra protein each day or about a 68 percent increase. Extremely young or active women, as well as high-risk pregnancy women, may need even more—up to 100 grams daily. With teenage women, this is extremely important because you are dealing, in effect, with the growth of two children.

Lacto-ovo vegetarians should have no problem meeting these requirements. The four cups of milk recommended for all pregnant women supply 40 percent of the RDA to start with; whole grains, nuts, legumes, seeds, and other dairy products can easily give the rest.

Vegans must be more careful. They need more gross protein because of the lower digestibility of plant proteins—probably about 90 to 100 grams. Consequently, their diet has to be very compact and well-planned—there won't be much room for anything but the necessities. Soy proteins are especially good at this time, for example, four cups of fortified soy milk. The addition of soy powder and soy flour to baked goods and casseroles is helpful. Tofu and tempeh are good, too. These plus a good varied diet should be fine. It would be wise to eat foods from several food groups, including grains, at the same meal (or at most within a few hours of each other) since you need a full complement of amino acids almost constantly at this time for new cell growth. Choose your soy products carefully, incidentally. Soy milk, for example, is sometimes a highly refined product with stabilizers and too much sugar. Look for a brand as natural as possible (Veg-E-Lac is one possibility), or make your own. Recipes are available in various cookbooks; several in the bibliography have recipes.

CALCIUM

We all know that calcium is a primary component of bones and teeth, and it is just as important in the formation of the bones and teeth of the fetus. If the mother doesn't take in enough calcium, the baby will take what it needs from her bones at her expense. Calcium is also important for the proper clotting of blood. It also apparently aids in vitamin B_{12} absorption and decreases the absorption of heavy metals, such as lead, across the placenta. Any surplus will be stored for milk production.

The RDA for calcium is 1200 mg during pregnancy, a 50 percent increase. Those four cups of milk will supply it, as will four of these calcium equivalents to one cup of milk: ⅓ cup nonfat instant dry milk powder, 1 cup yogurt, 1⅓ cups cottage cheese, 1½ cups ice cream, or 1½ ounces cheddar cheese.

If you have a milk intolerance, try yogurt, buttermilk, or hard cheeses like cheddar or Swiss for easier digestibility. Or try acidophilus milk, in which the lactose had been predigested by bacteria.

Remember, milk and milk powder can be added to baked goods, blender drinks, sauces, soups, and casseroles if you don't want to drink a quart a day.

Other sources of calcium include soybeans and other legumes, blackstrap molasses, figs, apricots, dates, ground sesame seeds, and dark leafy green vegetables such as broccoli and kale. Certain other greens contain oxalic acid, which binds calcium and inhibits its absorption. Try not to eat these foods (spinach, chard, beet greens, rhubarb) and your calcium sources at the same meal.

Vegans will be hard-pressed to find 1200 mg of calcium in their daily diets. Soy milk has but one fifth the calcium of cow's milk, and it would be extremely difficult to get it all from plant sources, even with careful planning. Look for calcium-fortified soy milk and consider taking a supplement.

Calcium supplements are more easily absorbed when taken on an empty stomach. Vitamin C helps, as does any acid medium such as fruit juice.

VITAMIN D

Vitamin D is important in helping your body to use calcium efficiently. Strangely, there are very few naturally occurring food sources for vitamin D; the best sources are the sun and fortified milk. The same four cups of milk that supply your calcium requirement contain the RDA for vitamin D, 400 IU. Vegans should check to see if their soy milk is similarly fortified. If not, or if you don't drink the milk, a supplement is recommended.

Be careful with a supplement, however. Too much can damage the major blood vessels in the fetus and be toxic to the mother as well. Only take the RDA, or spend some time in the sun each day.

IRON

During pregnancy your blood volume increases greatly in order to nourish the baby and support a higher metabolic work load. Iron is needed for this greater production of hemoglobin. Large amounts are also required for prenatal iron stores that the mother transfers to the baby for use during its first few months of life and uses to replenish her own red blood cells after the birth.

The RDA for iron is more than 18 mg, an amount that is very hard to get in any ordinary diet. Most doctors feel that all pregnant women should take a supplement of 30 to 60 mg elemental iron after the first trimester.

Even so, you should fill your diet with iron-rich foods: prune juice, dried fruits, yeast-raised breads, dried beans, wheat germ, and dark green vegetables. Oxalic acid binds iron as well as calcium, making foods such as spinach less valuable in this respect than Popeye fans have always believed.

Cooking in uncoated cast-iron pots increases iron content significantly, and vitamin C and acidic foods help absorption.

THE B VITAMINS

The B vitamins include thiamine, riboflavin, niacin, B_6 (pyridoxine), B_{12} (cobalamin), folic acid, and pantothenic acid. During pregnancy, they play a role in cell division and fetal growth, protein and carbohydrate production, and the prevention of anemia. They are generally found in whole grains, wheat germ, brewer's yeast, milk, nuts, and dark, leafy green vegetables. Don't count on enriched grains, breads, and cereals to take the place of the original whole grains, especially where B vitamins are concerned. Some have been put back in; others have not. Any way you look at it, you're being gypped by these foods.

A few of the B vitamins are especially important during pregnancy, particularly for vegetarians. A more detailed discussion of those nutrients is presented here. You will get enough of the others if you increase your calories and eat a healthy, compact diet that includes the foods noted earlier. A daily dose of brewer's yeast (if you can acquire a taste for it) wouldn't hurt, especially for vegans. It can easily be hidden in loaves, bread, and casseroles.

RIBOFLAVIN

Most Americans get their riboflavin from milk and other dairy products, so vegans should take special care to know where they are getting this vitamin. Good plant sources include dark or leafy green vegetables such as broccoli and asparagus, whole grains, mushrooms, nuts, and beans. Brewer's yeast is also an excellent source.

FOLIC ACID AND VITAMIN B_{12}

Folic acid is a special necessity during pregnancy. It is required every time a cell divides to make two other cells, and this process is going on rapidly in a developing fetus. For this reason your needs during pregnancy double from 400 to 800 mg. The result of a deficiency is anemia, which is especially troublesome during pregnancy, when your blood volume is increasing rapidly.

Luckily it is easy to avoid a deficiency and get all the folic acid you need. The best sources are dark green leaves such as spinach and leaf lettuce, followed by beans, green vegetables, oranges, and whole grains. Vegetarians should have an advantage over flesh-eaters in respect to folic acid, since it is present in foods that are more likely to show up in our diet. Many women take a folic acid supplement, and you may want to do so also if you feel your consumption of leafy greens isn't enough.

Vitamin B_{12} interacts with folic acid in controlling cell division and the copying of the genetic code in cell nuclei. Four cups of milk daily will supply the 4 mg of vitamin B_{12} in the RDAs; so will two cups of cottage cheese. Eggs and other dairy products are also good sources. A vitamin B_{12} deficiency can cause a similar anemia to that of folic acid, with equally severe consequences, apparently by impairing the function of folic acid. Because of this, B_{12} deficiency anemia may respond to a high dose of folic acid, but the original B_{12} deficiency may go undiscovered. That lack of vitamin B_{12} can continue to cause damage to the fetal nervous system as well as the mother's. For this reason, any diagnosis of pernicious anemia should be accompanied by a blood test to determine which vitamin is in short supply *before* starting a folic acid supplement to curb the anemia.

Vegan women should be especially careful about B_{12}, since nonanimal sources are hard to find and may be neglected in the diet even if available. Vegans should make absolutely certain they get the RDA for vitamin B_{12}, especially when pregnant. Unless you are eating large amounts of tempeh, kombu, and wakame—or have found a sufficiently fortified soy milk or brewer's yeast—take a supplement. Your higher intake of folic acid could mask the early symptoms of vitamin B_{12} deficiency, allowing nerve degeneration to proceed undiscovered.

So get enough vitamin B_{12} and eat your green vegetables.

VITAMIN A

Vitamin A is important to the development of all the cells that line the outer surfaces (skin, eyes) and inner cavities (mouth, digestive tract, vagina) of your body. It also regulates the stability of fat in all cell membranes. Your body requires vitamin A for its role in the formation of bones and tooth enamel.

The RDA for pregnant women is 1000 RE, a 25 percent increase from normal. Excellent sources are whole or fortified milk, dark, leafy green vegetables like spinach and broccoli, and deep orange fruits and vegetables such as apricots, carrots, and sweet potatoes. Keep in mind that vitamin A is sensitive to heat—up to 40 percent can be destroyed by high temperatures.

It is probably not necessary to take a vitamin A supplement. Be careful if you do, since vitamin A in concentrated pill form can be toxic. You needn't worry if you get it in abundance from your food.

VITAMIN C

How much vitamin C is truly beneficial is still being debated. The RDA for pregnant women is 80 mg, an amount that can be easily met by eating citrus fruits, cantaloupe, strawberries, sweet peppers, broccoli, and many other fruits and vegetables. Illness, stress, and smoking (which we pray you are not doing while you are pregnant, not to mention other times) all seem to increase the need.

Vitamin C is essential in the making of key hormones, the development of connective tissue, the formation of bones and teeth, the repair of wounds and fractures. It helps maintain sound cell and blood vessel walls, including that of the placenta. It also aids in the body's use of calcium, iron, folic acid, and vitamin A.

It is easy to see why people are tempted to take large amounts of vitamin C. Even if you usually take 1 gram doses, pregnancy may not be a good time to continue this practice. Overconsumption could cause the baby to require excessive amounts after birth. In that case, the child would become deficient eating normal amounts. On the other hand, you shouldn't abruptly cut your consumption, either before or during pregnancy. The best course is to cut back gradually to a lower level—the RDA is a decent guide—*before* you get pregnant. We realize this kind of planning isn't always possible, though.

SALT AND IODINE

Doctors used to recommend a low-sodium diet for pregnant women to prevent preeclampsia, an early stage to toxemia. More recent evidence suggests that such a diet may retard fetal growth. In fact, more sodium is needed when you are pregnant because it is diluted in the increased body fluids. Too much sodium is not the cause of toxemia; rather, a lack of protein is thought to be at its root.

Don't restrict your salt intake. On the other hand, don't start gobbling down potato chips. Maintain a happy medium and when you do use salt, use the iodized kind. Your need for iodine is higher, too, because of increased thyroid activity.

LIQUIDS

Drink plenty of liquids during pregnancy to maintain your natural increase of body fluids and help prevent constipation. Six to eight glasses besides the four cups of milk recommended would be ideal. Remember to stay away from coffee, tea, and soda; water and unsweetened vegetable and fruit juices are much better.

WHAT TO EAT

The Daily Food Guide will give you a good idea of the minimum you should be eating every day. Remember, individual needs differ. To insure that you are getting all the nutrients *you* require, vary the particular foods within each category from day to day. Even if you eat everything suggested in the guide, you may not be getting enough calories. If that is so, just eat more, plus a little butter and oil, if you wish.

SUPPLEMENTS

Whether you want to take supplements is a decision for you and your doctor. It seems to be good insurance if you don't overdo. Vegans, especially, may want to supplement their intake of calcium, riboflavin, and vitamins D and B_{12}, and every woman should take extra iron and probably folic acid. These may be included in a prenatal multivitamin, but don't assume that the manufacturers have taken care of your every need. Sometimes a manufacturer inexplicably leaves out some of the vitamins and minerals you require or the doses are inadequate or unnecessarily high. Check the label, and keep in mind that a vitamin pill will not take the place of a balanced, compact diet. Nourish your baby as carefully now as you plan to after he or she is born.

GUIDELINES

Increase your calories by 300 a day, and make them count toward the nutrients you need.

You should gain 24 to 28 pounds: 2 to 4 during the first trimester, half to one pound a week after that.

Don't reduce, take diuretics, or restrict your salt intake.

Avoid smoking, caffeine, alcohol and other drugs, and food additives.

Daily Food Guide for Pregnant Women

FOOD CATEGORY	Servings		EXAMPLES (PER SERVING)	Nutrients
	lacto-ovo	vegan		
Dairy	4	4 fortified soy milk*	1 cup whole or skim milk or yogurt 1/3 cup nonfat instant dry milk powder 1½ ounce cheddar cheese 1⅓ cups cottage cheese	100% calcium 40% or more protein riboflavin, vitamins A, B_{12}, D, phosphorus, magnesium, zinc,
Beans, nuts, seeds, eggs	2 or more	2 or more	15 protein-gram portions: 4 tablespoons peanut butter, ½ cup peanuts 1 cup cooked beans (¾ cup soybeans) 2 cakes tofu, ½ cup sunflower seeds 4 ounce tempeh, 2 eggs	protein, riboflavin, iron, magnesium, folic acid, vitamin E, thiamin, vitamin B_6, zinc (B_{12} from tempeh)
Whole grains	5	6	½ to ¾ cup cereal, slice bread, ¾ cup cooked pasta or grains like rice, bulgur, millet, wheat berries, 1 roll or muffin	protein, B vitamins, iron, vitamin E, magnesium, zinc, fiber, riboflavin, folic acid
Dark green or deep yellow or orange vegetables	2	3	1 cup raw, ¾ cup cooked portions: leaf lettuce, broccoli, spinach, cabbage, greens, asparagus, carrots, sweet potatoes, snap beans	vitamins A, C, E, B_6, folic acid, riboflavin, iron, zinc, calcium, protein, magnesium
Other vegetables	1	1	mushrooms, artichokes, beets, corn, etc.	magnesium, many others
Vitamin C-rich fruits and vegetables	1	1	1 stalk broccoli, 1 cup orange juice, 1 cup strawberries, ½ cantaloupe, 1 sweet pepper, ½ grapefruit, 1 orange, 1 mango, 8 Brussels sprouts, 1 cup kale	vitamin C, folic acid
Other fruits	1	1	dates, figs, apples, pears, pineapple, bananas, etc.	magnesium, many others

*If you prefer not to include the four cups fortified soy milk, you'll need 30 additional grams of protein. Be sure you know where your calcium, D, and B_{12} are coming from, too. Lots of dark green vegetables and tempeh are good choices to meet these needs, since they would supply calcium and B_{12}, respectively, as well as protein.

Getting enough protein is very important. Add at least 30 extra grams a day. Vegans need even more because of the lower digestibility of plant proteins.

All nutrient needs are higher. Especially important are calcium, iron, folic acid, and vitamins A, C, D, and B complex.

Everyone should supplement iron and possibly folic acid and zinc.

Vegans should consider supplementing calcium, vitamin D, riboflavin, and vitamin B_{12}.

Eat a balanced, compact diet that inclues whole grains, other good protein and calcium sources, and fresh fruits and vegetables.

8
Babies and Children

*A*s we have shown, the adult who takes no responsibility for his or her own nutrition will often pay the consequences in spades. Yet food has become such a complex issue in our world—emotional, economic, social, and political, as well as nutritional and medical—that getting down to the basics of nourishing ourselves simply and well is a tough proposition.

Sometimes it's hard for adults to believe that what they eat (and how much) affects how well their bodies cope. In certain ways this is similar to the smoker who can't make the connection between one more cigarette and cancer-ridden lungs. Obviously, there is much more involved for them than future health.

A great many of our feelings about food, nutrition, and health begin when we are young. A child's eating environment is probably just as important as the foods actually put on his plate. Essential connections are made now, and it is vital not to repeat the mistakes we battle from our own childhoods—that sweets are a reward, that vegetables are necessary evils that are "good for you" (so much for a favorable attitude toward nutrition), that cleaning your plate results in high praise.

Admittedly, some of our parents (and theirs) were misguided in their approaches, but even their mistakes were based on an instinctual and universal truth: Children need good food to grow well.

THE PROCESS OF GROWTH

Children must maintain their bodies the same way as adults and the same general rules of good nutrition apply to both. Beyond

154

that, everyone knows children have special needs regarding the growing process. "Drink your milk, you're a growing boy," is an old refrain.

The RDAs for various ages are listed in the appendices. Use the list as a general guide in determining your child's needs. The importance of meeting these needs is very apparent if you understand the actual process of growth, which involves an increase of cells in number and size. Basically, there are three stages. The first, *hyperplasia,* is a rapid increase in the number of cells through cell division. The new, smaller cells do not increase in size, however. In the second stage, *hypertrophy* begins, in which the cells get larger. They also continue to multiply, but at a slower rate. The third stage is marked solely by growth of the cells in size. By this time cell division has stopped, and the maximum number has been attained. The cells continue to grow from increased protein content (positive balance) until maturity. Growth then stops, and protein synthesis and breakdown come into equilibrium.

Almost every organ in the body follows this pattern of cell growth, from conception to adulthood, although each is on a different schedule. The first two stages are critical because these are the only times when cell division occurs. The number of brain cells, heart cells, and so on, is determined during these periods and is irreversible. Organs such as the heart, brain, kidneys, cartilage, and skeletal muscle can't regenerate later. (Of course others, such as skin cells, are continually lost and replaced throughout life.) If needed nutrients are not adequately supplied at these crucial times, the potential of these organs is limited. Because the timetables of the organs differ, a deficiency at one point may significantly affect the future functioning of the heart; at another time, the kidneys or other organs may be affected.

From the moment of conception through the first year virtually all the organs and tissues undergo intensive growth, including cell division. During these early stages the most elementary functions of each organ are determined. Malnutrition can have its most lasting effect on physical and mental development at this time. By the age of ten months, for example, the number of brain cells has been determined for life. There will not be another period of such rapid general growth until adolescence.

Overnutrition, incidentally, can have effects similar, though opposite, to undernutrition. A good example is the fat cells. Too many fat cells are thought to be a major problem in obesity control (or the lack of it). The two critical periods for fat cell growth are, predictably, early childhood and adolescence.

Once cell division has ceased (the third stage), the effects of deficiencies and overfeeding are usually more temporary. A particular organ may be smaller or larger for a time, but an appropriate adjustment in food intake will normalize things again.

Good nutrition is essential throughout the growing years. As we have described, growth is not uniform but rather comes in two growth spurts separated by a longer period of slower increases. Good external signs of these changes are the child's height and weight.

THE FIRST YEAR

Breast or Bottle?

Breast milk is obviously tailor-made for the human infant. Besides containing just about all the nutrients a baby needs, it has powerful antibodies programmed by the mother to fight infections and allergies in the child for months to come. The newborn baby, after nine months in a sterile sac, can certainly use the help until its defenses are better developed. One antibody, for example, immunizes the infant against intestinal disease, a major cause of infant illness and death. Breast milk also contains *bifidus factor*, a substance that favors the growth of friendly bacteria and crowds out more harmful organisms by providing an acid environment. Two proteins in breast milk inhibit certain bacteria by binding the iron they need to grow.

Mother's milk never causes milk allergy, as cow's milk sometimes does, and it may prevent or postpone other types of allergies for years. In fact, breast milk seems to have many beneficial functions. The fact that these are not completely documented is all the more reason to rely on breast milk: Until each factor is fully realized, it can't be duplicated in a formula. The immunological agents, for example, have not so far been reproduced chemically. Whatever the individual elements are, they seem to reduce the incidence of gas, diarrhea, eczema, and respiratory illness in babies. Certain natural chemicals are thought to stimulate organ development, while others aid greatly in the absorption of vital nutrients. Even the presence of cholesterol in breast milk seems to have a purpose by increasing the body's ability to handle it in the future.

On top of that, there is no preparation time needed. Breast milk comes out sterile and at just the right temperature. Most women experience breastfeeding as a pleasurable, close time between mother and child. It has physical benefits for the mother, too. Hormonal changes and infant sucking hasten the process of *uterine involution*, the return of the uterus to a nonpregnant condition. The production of milk may also use up much of the fat accumulated by the mother during pregnancy.

Unfortunately, toxic-waste chemicals such as PCBs can concentrate in fat tissue and breast milk. High concentrations can cause stunted growth and learning disabilities in children. Vegetarians need not be quite as concerned, since PCBs are found mainly in fish, poultry, and meat, although also in whole-fat dairy products. In a study by the Environmental Defense Fund, vegetarian women had approximately one half lower pesticide and PCB levels in their milk than did the average meat-eating woman. Probably long-time vegetarians would have less to worry about than would more recent converts, since chemical build-up in fat tissue takes quite a while to dissipate. Certainly women who are planning to become pregnant should lower their consumption of animal fats.

Industrial contaminants could concern anyone. If you live or work in a high-risk area (or are a relatively new vegetarian), consider having your fat tested about three weeks before the baby is due. If chemical pollutant levels in your milk are high, talk to your doctor. A good compromise might be to breastfeed for three months and then switch to formula or nurse once or twice a day with formula feedings the rest of the time. That way, your baby would get most of the benefits of breast milk while reducing any risks.

If a woman is very reluctant to breastfeed, for whatever reasons, the bottle is probably a better choice. A loving environment is the priority here, the benefits of breast milk notwithstanding. Certainly the freedom bottlefeeding offers the mother should not be underestimated. It also gives the father and others in the house more of a chance to interact with the baby. A child can grow healthy and happy drinking from a bottle. Commercial formula has been made nutritionally similar to breast milk, and that plus preventive medical care make it the best alternative.

If you are undecided, however, give breastfeeding a try. You can always switch to formula, whereas breast milk will dry up within days if you don't begin.

Nutrition for the Breastfeeding Mother

The mother is now supplying food for the infant through her milk rather than her blood. As in pregnancy, she is using her own stores as well as the nutrients from her diet. The production of milk, however, requires even more energy than does pregnancy—about 500 extra calories a day. Actually, it takes approximately 800 calories to produce the one quart of breast milk needed daily, but some energy is supplied from the fat stores of the mother. Of course, if weight gain was low during pregnancy or falls below normal during lactation, even more than 500 extra calories are necessary.

Given those extra calories, the same general rules of eating apply that applied during pregnancy. The food guide in the previous chapter is appropriate, as long as you remember to add 500 (rather than 300) calories in balanced, compact form. During lactation, the needs for zinc, iodine, vitamins A and C, niacin, and riboflavin have increased a little from pregnancy, while the requirements for protein and folic acid have dipped. You might want to take this into account if any of your sources were marginal. Also, drink eight to twelve cups of fluid each day, essential because of your own increased production of fluid. Milk, juices, water, and soup are good choices.

Finally, avoid all drugs unless specifically prescribed by your doctor at this time. Most, if not all, will appear in your milk.

How to Begin Breastfeeding

The first liquid to come out of the breasts is colostrum, a thick, yellowish premilk substance that is extremely rich in antibodies. Within three to six days, it will gradually resemble breast milk.

If possible, it is good to begin nursing your baby as soon as possible. The sucking reflex reaches a peak about one half hour after birth and does not peak again for a couple of days. The immediate establishment of mother-child contact is important as well.

The baby's sucking causes the release of hormones which

stimulate milk production and flow. In this handy little system, you can be sure that supply will equal demand. Be aware, though, that even minute changes in the hormone level can trigger the letdown reflex of milk flowing—a signal from the baby, a readiness on the mother's part is all it may take for milk to start dripping from the nipples. Likewise, stress can inhibit the flow. The mother will need a relaxed, supportive atmosphere.

Lactation should be fairly well established in a week's time, although first-time mothers may take a couple of weeks longer. Until that time, more frequent feedings may be necessary to stimulate full milk production. Remember that the infant's instinctual rooting reflex is to turn her face in the direction of stimulation, so don't put your hand on her cheek, pushing her toward the breast. She will naturally turn away toward your hand instead. Rather, let your breast touch her cheek, encouraging her toward it.

There are usually six to eight feedings a day about three to four hours apart. After two or three months, the proverbial 2 A.M. feeding can be stopped. A good general guide is to feed on demand within reason. It takes about ten minutes to empty a breast. Let your baby determine the length of time, however; everyone's needs are different. As long as he or she is gaining weight and seems satisfied, the odds are everything is just fine.

Bottlefeeding

If you have decided to bottle feed, it is best to use a commercial formula. Nutritionally, it is the most similar to breast milk.

Fresh cow's milk, as has been pointed out time and again, is more appropriate for the calf, with three and a half times the protein of human milk and a high concentration of butterfat. The protein is in a more complex, less easily digestible, form that stresses the kidneys, and the butterfat can't all be absorbed by the infant intestine, possibly resulting in a lack of adequate calories. Skim milk is no better a solution since it, too, would be deficient in calories and would lack the essential fatty acid, linoleic acid.

Homemade formula based on evaporated milk is somewhat more acceptable because the protein is more digestible than that in fresh milk. However, it is less nutritious and more time-consuming than commercially prepared varieties. Generally, homemade formula has stressful concentrations of protein and minerals and no vitamin C.

Commercial formula, on the other hand, has lower levels of modified protein and minerals and more carbohydrates, as in breast milk. The butterfat of cow's milk has usually been replaced with unsaturated vegetable oil. Look for brands high in the protein lactalbumin, the same protein in breast milk. If your baby shows a milk intolerence or you are bringing up your child as a vegan, soy formulas are equally good.

A major pitfall of bottlefeeding is overfeeding, which may lead to obesity. Unlike the nursing mother, the mother of a bottle-fed baby can see how much her child is drinking. This in turn may cause her to encourage him to finish the bottle, rather than trusting his judgment as the nursing mother must. The amount he should drink is based on his weight, activity, and growth rate. Typically, it is about two and a half ounces per pound of body weight. But use the baby's appetite as your gauge: If he drains his bottle and seems to want more, add an extra ounce the next day. Again, don't insist he finish it. As in breastfeeding, feed on demand within reason.

If you are diluting the formula at home, it is very important to use the amount of water specified. Too little water will produce a formula with higher concentrations of nutrients than the baby can handle; too thin a dilution will fill him up on liquid before his nutrient intake is adequate. Also, consider checking into the nitrate level of your water supply. In 5 percent of American communities, the levels are so high that the water shouldn't be used in formula preparations. If used, it could prevent sufficient circulation of oxygen in the baby's body.

Don't prop the bottle next to the baby to feed him. Hold your child close and feed him love as well as milk. It is worth the extra time for both of you.

Meeting the Infant's Nutritional Needs

For the first six months of life, all the nutrients a baby needs can be supplied by breast milk or commercial formula, with the possible exception of a few vitamins and minerals. This may be surprising when you consider that an infant more than doubles her weight during this time, and her need for calories, protein, and other essential nutrients is far greater than an adult's in proportion to body weight. Much of this goes toward the formation of new tissue, as well as the higher maintenance requirements of an infant. Everything takes more energy now. The heart rate, for example, is twice that of an adult.

The breast-fed baby may need supplements of vitamin D, fluoride, and iron. A stint in the sun could satisfy your baby's vitamin D requirement, but in many locales this is difficult and a supplement of 400 IU is usually prescribed. Her need for additional fluoride depends on whether your water supply has a sufficient amount—about 1 part per million. If not, supplementation may be recommended by your doctor to help your baby form cavity-resistant teeth. Don't play with the dosage, however; too much fluoride is poisonous. Finally, additional iron may be advised. Theoretically, a child is born with iron stores to last three to six months. This isn't always the case, though, and it is prudent to give your baby iron supplements or iron-rich foods after two months or so. This is in spite of the fact that the small amount of iron in breast milk is well utilized.

Commercial formulas are usually fortified with all the necessary nutrients, except perhaps iron. Be sure you use a well-known brand, preferably recommended by your doctor. Use iron-fortified brands if you prefer not to introduce solid (iron-rich) foods until later.

Weaning

Both breast- and bottle-fed babies should be given water between feedings. The need for more water could explain why your baby is crying, since infants are prone to dehydration. It is also a good way to introduce the bottle to breastfed babies—excellent preparation in case the mother is temporarily detained or must stop breastfeeding suddenly because of accident or illness. In fact, nursing mothers may want to use expressed breast milk or formula for one or two feedings a day. This has the advantages of freeing her, giving the father and others the opportunity to share in the feeding, and familiarizing the baby with getting nourishment from a bottle.

The details of when and how to wean your baby from breast milk or formula onto solid foods are largely an individual matter. Many mothers begin solids early on; others prefer to wait as long as possible. It is generally agreed that milk alone can no longer satisfy a baby's nutritional needs after six months. In large, fast-growing babies, it could be as soon as four months. There is no reason to start before the child obviously needs the extra nourishment. It seems foolish to try to improve upon natural provisions (or a facsimile). Early introduction of solid food may also predispose a child to allergies. A good rule of thumb is to provide additional food when the breast-fed baby is hungry more often than every two or three hours or the bottle baby wants more than a quart of formula a day. The baby will probably weigh about 12 pounds at that point and need the extra calories and nutrients. Keep a level head, though, and don't get confused between actual need and overeating. Obesity is a major problem in infants.

By the age of six months, solid foods should be introduced on a gradual basis. The usual order is iron-fortified cereal (rice or barley), fruits, bland vegetables, then other foods such as pudding, cottage cheese, and stronger-tasting vegetables such as cabbage and cauliflower. Wheat products are generally put off for a while, since wheat often causes allergy. Really, your baby's tastes will dictate what is eaten first. Start with a tiny amount, diluted to a thin, smooth consistency. A teaspoonful—or even half that—is enough. Introduce only one food at a time; if you notice diarrhea, a rash, or other symptoms, it will be that much easier to pinpoint the source. After about a week, you can try another food. Patience is the key. Just offer it again in a few weeks.

Slowly increase the amount your child is eating by teaspoonfuls. Eventually he will be eating several tablespoons a day along with breast milk or formula. Finally, at about a year (or later, depending), his diet will be mostly solid food.

During the period of weaning, no book can tell you exactly what to do when. You must trust your own and your baby's judgment. This is especially so when your child is breastfeeding and you can't measure how much is consumed. You'll know he isn't getting enough if he cries sooner than usual from hunger. For both breast- and bottle-fed babies, you can also use the RDA as a guide. From six to twelve months, calorie need is determined by multiplying your baby's weight in kilograms (2.2 pounds per kilogram) by 105. Assuming he drinks about a quart of milk a day (640 calories), any calorie need beyond that should be provided by additional food. As time goes by, the larger your baby becomes, the more food he will eat proportionately. But remember, don't force him to eat. These are only guidelines. Respect his individuality.

At about eight or nine months, you can gradually switch to foods with a coarser texture. Your baby may also enjoy something hard to teethe (or gum) on, such as a stick of celery or a stale crust of bread. Now is the time when children like to mess with their food, exploring textures and improving their manual dexterity. Patience.

When to stop breastfeeding is an individual decision, again based on you and your child. Your baby can probably tell you better than anyone. If fact, there seem to be certain periods when interest in the breast naturally lessens. These are ideal times to make the final break. Nine months is the average age when mothers stop, but there is nothing wrong with continuing for a year or two, even if it simply constitutes emotional support. Trust your child to tell you when he is ready to stop.

The same is true for bottle-fed babies. Although it is easier to make the transition from formula to cow's milk in a bottle, the desire for the bottle itself may persist. The sucking need is very strong and can continue into the second and third year. There is no reason to deny your child the secure feeling he derives from it. Breast-fed babies who are weaned early need a bottle, too. Let your child's need for sucking taper off at his own pace. Divide his liquids between bottle and cup for an easy transition.

You can introduce cow's milk and other dairy products after about eight months, when the baby can better handle its high level of protein. However, many infants display milk allergies which persist until the age of two or beyond. Never feed your baby more than a quart of milk a day, as it can crowd out other nutrients, especially iron. In fact, be sure your child has a good iron source, regardless. Vitamin C–rich foods should also be introduced early. By the age of one, children should be familiar with a wide variety of foods.

Vegans would be wise to breast- or bottle-feed for at least a year to insure a sound nutritional base. It is also important for vegan babies to get used to drinking fortified soy milk and eating dark green vegetables such as broccoli, lettuce, and kale, so that the change to solid foods will be smooth and healthy. Remember, children's needs are extremely high. The parents of vegan children must be very careful, and if they are, their children should be fine. Of course, vegan children can develop various deficiencies, as has been widely reported. The point is to avoid them by being aware of the pitfalls. We will point them out as we go along. Likewise, vegan children are reported to have a comparatively slower growth rate. However, there are indications that slower growth could mean longer life. Take your pick.

Commercial or Homemade Baby Food?

Commercial baby food is convenient, safe from bacterial contamination, and provides much variety for the consumer. Even the quality of these foods has improved recently, with no salt, chemical preservatives, or artificial flavors and colors. Many foods, however, still have added sugar and modified starch and, of course, none of the food is fresh. Commercial varieties also have less nutrient density—that is, they've been diluted with more water than homemade food usually has, then camouflaged with starch to improve the texture.

Fresh homemade food is quite easy to prepare with the aid of a blender, grinder, or food processor. It is just simple food puréed to an appropriate consistency. Don't add any salt, sugar, or strong spices to suit your palate; your baby enjoys bland food. As long as you cook and store it with care, it is a safe, nutritious, and economical way to feed your child.

Certain vegetables, especially spinach and beets, contain nitrates which sometimes are converted into nitrites during storage. Too high a level can be dangerous to an infant, because it interferes with hemoglobin production, so as a precaution, don't offer them (or carrot juice, another concentrated source) to your child before the age of eight months. You can limit nitrite production in these vegetables by keeping them refrigerated, and not storing them after they have been cooked, chopped, or shredded.

Another food to be wary of is honey. You probably wouldn't be feeding it to your child anyway since sugar, in whatever form, isn't a habit to encourage. Many babies have trouble digesting honey, and it has been shown to be a cause of botulism in infants. The Center for Disease Control in Atlanta recommends that honey not be given to infants one year old or younger.

Try preparing food at home for your baby whenever feasible. When it isn't possible, look for commercial varieties that don't sweeten with added sugar, thicken with modified starch, or attempt any other "improvements."

TODDLERS (AGES 1 TO 3)

By the time your child is one, she has tripled her birth weight and probably has about six teeth. Milk is still a primary source of nourishment, but solid foods have also come to the fore. It is at this point that growth slows somewhat; in fact, her growth rate is three times faster during the first year than the second. Even though it is slower and slightly more erratic, growth continues fairly steadily until adolescence. Within two years, by the age of three, your child will have grown about six inches, gained ten pounds, and will probably have all her baby teeth. She will grow from a rather dependent baby to a willful, independent, upright young child. In order to do that, she will be curious, assertive, and messy. Providing her with good nutrition will be, to put it mildly, challenging. Yet it is during these first few years that her ideas, feelings, and associations about food will be formed for a lifetime. It will be her emotional base.

Because she is now growing more slowly, you will see a definite decrease in appetite. Pound for pound, however, she still needs more nutrients than an adult. If you are careful, patient, and play it right, she will have no problem meeting nutritional requirements and growing at her own healthy rate.

Basically, the foods she eats should be chosen from the food groups mentioned in Chapter 6. In other words, children should follow your example in eating a varied, balanced selection of whole foods. These minimum guidelines are a good foundation for a lifetime of eating, and we will refer to them throughout this chapter. During childhood, it is only the amounts that will differ, increasing as one gets older. Certainly they will not always make up all the calories a child needs; size, activity level, and growth rate will determine that. Use the RDAs in the appendix as a guide, although your child's individual needs should be the final gauge.

Group	Serving
Milk and milk products (or fortified soy milk)	2-3 cups (3-4 school-age, 4 for adolescents.)
Whole grains	4
Vegetables, including 1 dark green	2-3
Fruit, including 1 C–rich	1 or more
Legumes, nuts, seeds	2

Young children, in general, are most likely to be deficient in vitamins A and C, calcium, and iron. A diet including the foods in this list should take care of the first three without any trouble. Iron, however, is a problem for people of all ages. Children are particularly susceptible if they drink more than a quart of milk a day, crowding out iron-rich foods. Be aware of your child's need for iron; make sure she has plentiful sources of it. Try sunflower or pumpkin seeds, raisins, dried apricots, roasted soybeans, and whole-grain baked goods. Consider supplementing. You may also want to supplement fluoride, if your water doesn't supply it, for decay-resistant teeth. Ask your doctor for guidance regarding the dosage, since even small doses of fluoride can be poisonous.

Vegans have to be particularly concerned about their children's sources of calcium, riboflavin, zinc, and vitamins D and B_{12}. Even vitamin A could be a problem during this finicky period, when children are often suspicious of vegetables. Fortified soy milk can provide the riboflavin and vitamins D and B_{12}, as well as some calcium. Experiment until you can find foods your child favors that are rich in each of these nutrients. You should also be careful to complement food groups in your child's diet, including grains with every meal. Growing children need a higher percentage (35 percent) of well-proportioned amino acids than do adults, and on a constant basis. Even a little soy milk with each meal could help satisfy this need.

Feed your child small amounts of simple food. If still hungry, she can always have more, whereas a large amount of food can be intimidating. You'll find that children at this age love finger foods, and this needn't be discouraged. In fact, you can use it to advantage by making available fruit slices, raw vegetable sticks, nuts, seeds, and dried fruit.

It is best to eat at regular intervals, so your child is neither too full to enjoy a meal nor so hungry as to be irritable. Mealtimes should be calm and happy and the food colorful and inviting. Remember that children, like all human beings, enjoy eating with others. Try to eat with your child, providing company and a role model.

This is the age when "no" becomes a favorite word. It is necessary for children to learn to assert themselves on the way to independence, and "no" is an excellent way for them to get attention. This will extend to likes and dislikes in food as well. Often a child will only eat one or two preferred foods for days at a time; sometimes she will refuse to eat at all. Remain calm and reasonable: This, too, shall pass. In the meantime, don't force food down your child's throat. One or two meals skipped will not damage a basically healthy child. Don't worry. When she is hungry, she will eat. Encourage variety by enjoying it yourself, serving new foods in small portions along with favorite foods, and avoiding confrontations that turn into power plays.

Vegetables may be particularly difficult to introduce. A few tips: Serve them raw or lightly cooked; use dips (like yogurt) for dunking raw "crunchies" into; encourage your child to help prepare them in the kitchen; don't introduce them when your child is in a foul mood; don't present them as if you expect her to dislike them; if she doesn't like them, remove them without a fuss and try again another time.

Snacking and desserts needn't be avoided if they are wholesome. For snacks, have on hand the finger foods we mentioned before, as well as unbuttered popcorn, peanut butter, cheese, and not overly sweet whole-grain baked goods. Likewise, desserts should be nutritiously made with whole grains, milk products, nuts, and fruit—and minimal sugar. Never use sweets as a reward.

If you offer a nice selection of whole foods to your child, you will all get through the first few years in good health—food jags, food hates, and erratic behavior notwithstanding.

PRESCHOOL CHILDREN (AGES 3 TO 6)

The preschooler continues in very much the same manner as the toddler, including fluctuations in appetite. This isn't a problem as long as he is getting a fairly balanced diet over a week or two. Generally, you can trust your child to respond to his own needs for growth and energy. Keep track of what is eaten, though. Bad habits can be as detrimental as unnecessary parental demands in the long run. No one ever said parenting was easy.

The preschool child is inquisitive and egocentric, like the toddler. Physically, he is less clumsy and socially, more verbal. He demands more freedom now but is still quite dependent on your approval.

His needs and preferences in food remain like those of the toddler, although the preschooler will eat larger quantities as his need for calories increases. Continue to offer small, appealing portions of simple foods. Keep in mind that simple doesn't have to mean dull. Rather, it means colorful, easily identified foods that your child can help prepare. Children can have fun and learn in the kitchen, as well as eat healthy food. Always be ready with seconds, but never insist he clean his plate. As surroundings become increasingly interesting to him, his desire for food may lessen. Don't be too demanding in terms of manners or behavior. A wiggly kid is a wiggly kid; it is best to accept that and let him leave the table when he is finished. Try to make mealtimes pleasant, and remember, your child is emulating you in ways that will affect him for a lifetime.

Even so, outsiders will have more and more influence—from well-meaning grandparents to television commercials. This is a good time to begin educating your child about nutrition—telling him about the connections between food and his body. It is not a good time to throw up your hands in despair and buy sugar-coated cereal. Don't allow yourself to be brow-beaten by your five-year-old. Let him select advertised foods that are nutritious, but if you give in and buy junk, you can't expect him to limit his consumption of it. It's a Pandora's Box.

Take him with you to the grocery store and introduce him to labels, ingredients, and the basics of nutrition. Let him help in the selection of nutritious foods that are good values. Emphasize the positive aspects of whole foods while not being deprecating or self-righteous about those you don't condone. Remember, his friends may be eating those foods. Try not to create conflicts that will limit him socially.

If someone—grandparent, friend, babysitter—gives him food you don't approve of, don't make a big deal out of it. Tell the person privately that you'd prefer your child not eat that food. Suggest an alternative for next time. In fact, always have wholesome food on hand so your child and his friends don't feel deprived (or hungry). Such foods include celery and carrot sticks, broccoli "trees," raisins, nuts, seeds, fruit, and small finger sandwiches. Involve your child in cooking simple snacks like unbuttered popcorn, pizza crackers, and whole-grain cookies (on occasion). Be firm about not having junk food in the house. If nutritious food is available and appealing, kids will eat it.

Add high-nutrient foods to soups, drinks, casseroles, bread, even cookies. Wheat germ, carrots, powdered milk, eggs, and oatmeal are just a few foods that can be added surreptitiously. Now is also the time to switch to low-fat milk. That way, your child still receives its benefits, while leaving more calories for foods rich in other vitamins and minerals, as well as fiber. Besides, why not set a pattern now that discourages the high-fat, high-sugar diet we adults are struggling against?

SCHOOL-AGE CHILDREN (AGES 7 TO 11)

The seven-year-old's natural preference for plain foods will gradually change over the next few years as she becomes interested in trying new things. Continue to use the food guide earlier in the chapter as the foundation for her diet. The milk serving should be three to four cups, and other serving sizes eventually match or surpass adult levels. Be sure she is eating sources of iron, calcium, and thiamin, as these are the nutrients most often missing from the diet at this age. The calcium is suspect only if the child won't drink enough milk. On the other hand, iron-deficiency anemia is commonly caused by too much milk taking the place of foods containing iron. So be careful that your child gets enough milk (don't forget yogurt, cheese, powdered milk, creamed soup, an occasional ice cream) but not too much (more than the equivalent of a quart). Vegans should be sure their children get the above as well as vitamins D and B_{12}, riboflavin, and zinc. Iron and fluoride are still the nutrients most likely to be needed in supplemental form.

Your child should be growing slowly and steadily during these years. Of course, each child has her own rate, and fluctuations in appetite continue. Generally, height increases 5 to 6 percent a year and weight 10 percent. The weight gain should come from nutritious foods and not the highly refined, sugary, fatty snacks displayed at a child's eye level in every supermarket. Healthy children are lean and strong, not flabby. In fact, sticky sweet snacks, including "natural" granola bars and flavored yogurt, contribute a great deal to two of childhood's major health problems: cavities and obesity. Children need those calories to build their bodies, not to start the process of decay.

It may be an uphill battle as your child spends more and more time out of the house. School, new friends, and all kinds of other activities become distracting and could affect when she is hungry and for what. It will be this way from now through adolescence, as your child takes much more of the responsibility for what she puts in her own mouth. At best, you can only maintain an excellent example at home, have nutritious, appealing food available at all times, continue your child's nutrition education in a calm, convincing fashion, and let her make her own decisions, without reprisals, when at school, friends', parties, the movies, wherever.

You could try to set certain rules and restrictions, but we all know about forbidden fruit.

Your child will probably have many questions if your eating style is significantly different from the others around her. Answer them, speak your mind, but don't get self-righteous or guilt-provoking. This is especially true of vegetarianism. If you push, your child will fight back all the harder, especially during this period. It is best to let a child make her own decisions, especially once she has left your watchful eye and is involved in the world on her own. She will let you know when you can no longer make all the rules. Eating a piece of meat, despite its hazards, is probably not as damaging to the soul as the conflict and guilt that come with disapproving parents. Certainly your child knows that you prefer she not eat meat, but if it's that important to her, so be it. It could be one-time curiosity or she may develop a taste for it. Discussions may be fruitful, but what seem like unreasonable demands by you will only be painful. You can only hope that your influence over the years has set a good foundation for future decisions, as is every parent's hope.

If your child does decide to become a meat-eater, you must resolve certain questions: Should you allow her to eat it in the house? Should you buy it for her and cook it for her? These are all individual decisions. They must be based on how far you are willing to go.

But let's assume she remains vegetarian. (That's more comforting.) Now you merely have to be concerned about refined, processed foods; candy; the bland, fiberless lunches in the school cafeteria; missed breakfasts; and vending machines offering an assortment of junk. As we said, it's an uphill battle.

If you have the time and patience, you might want to check out what sort of food is available at school. You might even try to improve the food system and nutrition education there. If you don't like what is being offered to your child, the least you can do is pack a good lunch from home. Be sure your child likes what you include or it will end up traded or in the garbage. If she tends to be late and skip breakfast, pack that, too, so she can eat it on the way, between classes, whenever. Despite her protestations, she will need the nourishment during the morning hours. Possibilities include: fruit, nuts, seeds, a peanut butter sandwich, whole grain muffins, a piece of cheese.

There is no denying that friends and television commercials can make Hostess Twinkies, Wonder Bread, and Kraft Macaroni and

Cheese seem very desirable, the ultimate children's food. Surely your child will taste them outside the house. You can only do your part. If your child associates whole foods with good feelings, she will return to them again and again.

ADOLESCENCE

The beginning of adolescence is marked by a second growth spurt—a tremendous increase in height and weight—as well as hormonal changes that affect every organ in the body. In girls it begins around age ten, in boys at twelve. Naturally there are variations. In each it will last for several years. The metabolic rate is greatly increased to accommodate such growth. Calorie needs soar, especially in active boys. Protein and especially calcium requirements are high also. Ironically, teenage diets are less well balanced than those of any other age group except, perhaps, older people.

The missing nutrients continue to be iron, calcium, and thiamin, with vitamins A and C, riboflavin, and folic acid not far behind. Of course, the more typically American your teenager's diet is, the more this is apt to be so. Soda, candy, and white bread do not a good diet make. Yet during these years when the need to conform to friends goes hand-in-hand with a need to rebel against adults, there is very little you can do but what you have been doing. Once again, set a good example. Have nutritious foods on hand. (Fortunately, most teens have huge appetites, if not regular eating habits.) Sneak in nutrient-dense foods when you are cooking. Platitudes, of course, will fall on deaf ears. You might, however, appeal to the natural obsessive vanity of your teenager. A balanced whole-foods diet is, after all, slimming and excellent for athletes.

Vegans can only hope that their teenagers have developed a liking for calcium-rich foods such as dark green leafy vegetables, fortified soy milk, and the others we have mentioned time and again. Also encourage your child to complement food groups—he or she needs a constant source of protein now for growth.

GUIDELINES

Childhood is marked by two growth spurts separated by a longer period of slower increases.

Pound for pound, children need more nutrients than do adults.

Breast milk is tailor-made for the human infant, containing essential nutrients plus powerful antibodies.

The lactating mother should follow the same eating guide as the pregnant woman, but she needs more calories and fluid.

Let the infant determine how much milk to drink.

During the first six months, the infant needs only breast milk or formula, plus, perhaps, supplements of vitamin D, fluoride, and iron.

Start feeding your baby solid foods when she needs more calories and nutrients than a quart of milk provides. However, milk remains the primary source of nourishment for another six months or so.

Introduce solid foods one at a time in small amounts.

Make baby food at home whenever feasible or choose commercial brands without added sugar or starch.

The growing years are characterized by fluctuations in appetite, food jags, and strong likes and dislikes.

Selections from the food groups guide can be the basis of a diet for a lifetime.

Set a good example and have nutritious, appealing foods on hand at all times. Be a positive influence.

Iron and fluoride may need to be supplemented throughout childhood.

Be sure your child gets enough calcium, iron, vitamins A and C, and thiamin.

Vegans should pay special attention to zinc, vitamins B_{12} and D, and riboflavin, as well. Vegan children should complement protein groups.

9
Athletes

To be stronger, faster, more graceful, more skilled than any-one has ever before been is a wish at least as old as the human race. The desire of the athlete is to transcend the limitations of the human body and thus become more than a mere mortal—to be a superman or—woman—or perhaps to redefine those limitations.

As a person trains and conditions his or her body, the gains are at first rapid and obvious: Things that were once difficult or impossi-ble now become easy, goals are quickly met and then surpassed, and the rush of excitement and exhilaration can carry over into all aspects of life and perspective.

As training and conditioning continue, however, they are met with diminishing returns as each person approaches his or her physical limitations. Smaller gains require greater effort. At this point real athletes are separated from individuals who simply want to be fit and healthy. Those whose goal is greatness in sports must be ready to work long and hard to condition their bodies for a particular competition.

The motivation is obviously strong to find the simplest and most efficient way of training to peak condition. Would-be runners attend seminars or seek out coaches whose methods promise that they will run more quickly and better than they could on their own. The search for the athletic Philosopher's Stone extends to drugs and diet as well. Athletes are especially vulnerable to the pitches of every drug and health-preparation huckster who ever cried the virtues of a favorite magical nostrum. There are more idiosyncratic eaters, dieters, pill-takers, and trainers among athletes than among any other group.

THE PHYSICAL NEEDS OF AN ATHLETIC BODY

The body's needs are generally straightforward:

Water to transport, lubricate, cool, and cushion
Energy to operate
Protein to grow, heal, and replace what is lost
Vitamins and minerals to replace what is lost
Rest and recuperation

All bodies differ in their needs for various nutrients, of course, but most of these differences stem from metabolic variations and not from life style or activity level.

Only water, energy, and rest needs are substantially different in athletes from the general population's needs. Yet athletes often insist on varying their intake of virtually everything they eat and drink, the way they sleep, and even the way their bodies use the nutrients supplied. Here we look at these needs, real and imagined.

Water

Without being too dramatic, we could say that water is the nectar of life. We tend to neglect its importance in our diet, but life could not go on for an instant without water. Every cell in our bodies is filled with water—in fact, water makes up 50 to 70 percent of our bodies by weight. Every single chemical reaction that takes place inside us is mediated by water.

We need to consume water constantly to replace what we lose through the four main paths of urination, elimination, respiration, and sweat and surface evaporation from our skin. The first two functions allow our bodies to get rid of poisonous waste products. The kidneys continuously sweep the bloodstream, concentrating all the toxins and excess blood chemicals in a smaller amount of fluid to be excreted as urine. They can't concentrate this solution beyond a certain limit, so urine necessarily has a comparatively large amount of water being discarded.

As food moves through our intestinal tract, water is removed from it along with protein, carbohydrate, fat, vitamins, and minerals. How much water remains after the waste is eliminated depends on how long it has traveled through the intestines and how much fiber and other water-holding materials it contains. The more nutritionally desirable, high-residue diet has a much shorter intestinal transit time and a much higher level of water-binding indigestible material, so more water is lost than with a less healthy low-residue diet.

Anyone who has been outside on a cold day is aware that we lose moisture through respiration. Those clouds of steam we exhale are almost 100 percent water vapor, and we lose a surprisingly large amount this way—as much as three fourths of a quart a day in men. These water losses are unavoidable because the moisture comes from evaporation from the huge surface area of the lungs, bronchial tubes, and pharynx. If you breathe faster or more deeply than normal, as during exercise, water losses will necessarily be higher through this route.

Finally, water is lost from the surface of the body constantly, and most of the time you're unaware of it. Skin is quite porous and permeable, especially for a molecule as small as water. Water continually migrates outward and leaves the body. Of course, sometimes glands in the skin release water in response to a high air temperature or a high body temperature. This response, which we know as sweating, tends to lower body temperature through the cooling effect of the evaporation of the surface moisture. When a liquid changes into a vapor, it takes with it a certain amount of heat energy, equal to the energy required for that change. Sweating is the very first example of climate control.

Athletes don't differ from the rest of us significantly in water loss through urination or elimination. Respiratory water loss, however, is related to the volume of air that circulates through our lungs, and body surface loss is related to body temperature, hence to the amount of effort we are expending. Both of these are much higher in someone who is exercising hard. Marathoners may lose more than a gallon of water during one race, even if the weather is not hot. Under hot, humid conditions the losses can be even greater. Runners have been known to lose 10 or 12 pounds in an afternoon, most of it as water.

It is difficult to keep up with that degree of water loss by drinking water casually. Thus, careful attention to water loss and replacement is crucial for athletes in training or in competition. If you become seriously dehydrated while exercising, a number of very dangerous changes take place in your body quite suddenly. Your muscles heat up so much that they can no longer contract, and you become paralyzed. Your body temperature shoots up, and can go above 110 degrees Fahrenheit. You become confused as your brain tissues literally start to cook in the overheated body fluids. Blood pressure drops dramatically, since there is no longer enough water to keep the blood volume up. Most body cells simply stop, because they are so dehydrated they can no longer carry out chemical reactions. These are the classic signs of heatstroke, and you can die without immediate medical attention.

The first requirement is to lower body temperature, quickly and decisively, by bathing the skin with ice, water, cold drinks—anything cold (and nontoxic). Since blood pressure is probably quite low, whoever is helping you should assure a continued supply of blood to the brain by elevating the feet and lowering the head in a prone position. If you are conscious enough to drink without choking, cold liquids should be drunk to replace body water loss. Try not to gulp quantities of water, but drink small amounts almost constantly. Hospitalization is almost always required after a heatstroke since other "aftershocks" can occur, including heart attack, stroke, and kidney failure, as well as heatstroke relapses.

Of course, this is the most severe consequence of water deprivation, since it can ultimately cause death. Other less severe consequences are also important to athletes. Dehydration can cause the body to tire more easily, cloud judgment, and destroy carefully trained muscles, among other things.

We obtain water from three sources: the liquids we consume directly, the liquid portion of our food, and the water released when we burn food for energy. When we exercise, we consume more energy, so it seems that we produce more water as a result of metabolic processes. This is indeed true, but the difference is insufficient to cover our increased needs. We must increase our consumption of fluids to cover the losses. The needs vary, based on activity level, temperature, and level of physical conditioning, but a good rule of thumb for moderately severe exercise (like running or playing handball) is a glass or two of water every 10 or 15 minutes.

Drinking water is not essential—it can be any liquid composed mainly of water. There are some strong reasons *not* to use any drinks that contain more than a small percentage of sugar or minerals, especially salt. Of course, you shouldn't use alcohol at all while exercising. Byproducts of alcohol metabolism tie up liver enzymes that are required to detoxify products of heavy exercise such as lactic acid. The liver and other organs work to capacity during hard exercise; there is no reason to monopolize their functioning with alcohol.

Fruit juice is an excellent supplier of water, because it is easy to drink and seems more thirst-quenching than plain water. It is a good idea to cut your fruit juice with water in about equal amounts, however, to cut the concentration of sugar. Fruit juice also provides some potassium, which may become depleted in muscles if they get very hot.

Energy

Athletes need food for energy. Any food provides energy from its carbohydrate, fat, and protein contents. Some of these food components are more appropriate as energy sources than are others.

Your body stores energy in two forms. Most of it is stored as fat, in deposits under the skin, around organs, and within muscles. Another smaller portion is stored as glycogen, a carbohydrate, in muscles and the liver.

Fat generally provides most of the energy for our ongoing physical processes—the energy demands of everyday life. To yield up its energy, fat is first broken down into glucose and fatty acids, which both go into solution in the bloodstream. Muscles can use both portions for fuel, while other organs must use glucose.

When your body is called upon to respond to some sort of emergency (like a 50-yard dash), this fat metabolism system is simply too slow to give the muscles the energy they require. For most of us, the energy source for this high-level activity is glycogen. Glycogen requires a minimum of steps in the body chemistry to be converted into usable form, and it is already distributed to the muscles before it is needed.

Extremely well-conditioned muscles seem to be able to make much more efficient use of the body's fat breakdown system, and they thus have a much greater reserve of energy. A significant improvement is out of the reach of most people, however, including many athletes.

Different diets vary in their effectiveness at helping muscles and the liver store glycogen. A high-fat diet is least efficient, a high-protein diet somewhat more efficient, and a high-carbohydrate diet most efficient. If the three different diets provided equal energy (calories), the high-carbohydrate diet would yield the highest levels of stored glycogen, and a small increase in stored glycogen can make a tremendous difference to an athlete in competition.

CARBOHYDRATE LOADING

In 1967, two Swedish researchers developed a special training diet for athletes who compete in sports that require tremendous endurance, such as long-distance running, rock climbing, cross-country skiing, or soccer. They found that if well-trained athletes radically depleted their body stores of glycogen through exhausting exercise and carbohydrate deprivation, their muscles would rebound when carbohydrates again became available and store as much as triple the glycogen they had before. This extra reservoir of glycogen could be decisive in competition. The system came to be known as *carbohydrate loading.*

As the researchers designed it, the program takes six days. On the sixth day before the particular competition, you train until you are exhausted. This depletes your muscle and liver glycogen stores. For the next three days you eliminate as much carbohydrate as possible from your diet, concentrating instead on protein and fat.

Three days before competition, you begin a high-carbohydrate, low-fat and low-protein diet, eaten in small meals throughout the day. Your muscles will immediately start storing this comparative overload of carbohydrate, in the form of glycogen. If all goes well, your endurance should be improved dramatically.

Carbohydrate loading is a one-shot method—you must plan carefully to prepare for a single competition. *It is not a good way to eat day in and day out;* in fact, it can be dangerous. We outlined in an earlier chapter why carbohydrate deprivation is dangerous—it results in a condition called *ketosis,* a high blood concentration of toxic ketones. Ketosis can cause dehydration and kidney damage, and is very dangerous for fetuses being carried by dieting mothers. The carbohydrate-overload portion of the regimen may be equally unhealthy, since blood triglycerides shoot up to very high levels when the dietary proportion changes suddenly upward. In addition, there is at least one recorded case of a forty-year-old runner who complained of chest pains during the loading phase of the regimen. He also showed an abnormal electrocardiogram, which might indicate some damage to his heart muscle or circulatory system.

Some muscle cells may break down during the deprivation and the loading phases, releasing large proteins into the bloodstream. These large proteins are hard on your kidneys, and they could exacerbate any kidney problems that may already be present. In addition, since the muscle cells actually swell with their extra load of glycogen, their volume becomes greater, requiring more potassium to keep the ion concentration up to normal levels. You can get this extra potassium from fresh fruits and vegetables.

This method of increasing endurance is new, so insufficient research has been done to prove its safety. Considering this, as well as the adverse effects described above, you should use this regimen *at most* two or three times a year to prepare for a specific event. These wide fluctuations in your food composition play fast and loose with your body chemistry, and they aren't in the best interests of your overall health.

TOTAL ENERGY NEED

A runner who trains by running 100 miles a week expends 9000 calories each week over those hundred miles, or nearly 1300 calories a day. This represents his or her extra caloric need, above and beyond the requirements for everyday living. All this energy must be supplied by food, unless the object is to lose weight. A person who could manage to run 100 miles a week probably doesn't need to lose weight, so we'll assume that the energy comes from food.

We have already stated that the ideal energy source is carbohydrate. Since carbohydrate gives 4 calories per gram, the 1300-calorie-per-day additional need works out to 325 grams of pure, digestible carbohydrate (about three quarters of a pound). If you got the extra calories needed in the form of protein, you would need 325 grams, since protein contributes exactly the same number of calories per gram as does carbohydrate.

Fat gives you 9 calories per gram, so if you wanted to get your extra energy need from this source, you would need only about 145 grams. We have already shown that protein and fat are inferior energy sources compared to carbohydrate, because of the extra requirements placed on your metabolism for their use. It actually makes sense to try to find these calories in the form of an energy source like carbohydrate, since the calories will serve no other purpose than energy.

Unfortunately, it is difficult to get pure carbohydrate in any but the most useless form—processed sugar or starch. A good compromise is to get your extra calories from natural foods composed mainly of carbohydrate. Examples include whole wheat bread, fruits and vegetables, pasta, rice and other grains, and legumes like chickpeas and lima beans. You could cover your extra caloric need by eating an extra loaf of bread a day or five and a half cups of cooked brown rice.

That is a lot of food. In fact, eating an unrefined, low-fat diet, you might have to spend a great deal of your time eating to maintain your caloric expenditure when running. You need a more concentrated calorie source, and the only one (besides alcohol) is fat. Although we hesitate to recommend that anyone increase his or her fat consumption, the fact remains that fat is the only food that concentrates a lot of calories in a form the body is able to metabolize efficiently for energy. Supplementing an unrefined low-fat diet with a small amount of fat can provide the extra calories your body needs to maintain your activity level. Good high-fat foods include nuts, avocados, olives, various seeds, soybeans, and chickpeas.

Keep these points in mind when you design your diet so you get the food energy you need:

Carbohydrate is the best energy source; however, it provides only 4 calories per gram.

Fat provides 9 calories per gram, but it is a less suitable energy source.

Try to get as much of your extra caloric need from carbohyrate, supplementing it as necessary with food fats.

Protein

"Muscle is meat—eat meat to build muscle." Even though this simplistic statement has been known to be false for nearly 100 years, many coaches and athletes—perhaps most—still act as though it were divine revelation. It simply isn't true. To build your muscles you must work your muscles. Extra protein can't accelerate the process; in fact, it's wasted. Still, training tables across the land are laden with steaks, cheese, and huge pitchers of milk, so football players and track team members can load up on "prime protein."

When an athlete starts a training period he or she must build extra muscle tissue. Although the muscle cells don't increase in number, their size and protein content do increase. Because the athlete's body is retaining protein, it is in positive nitrogen balance, and this increases his or her protein need somewhat. Since muscle tissue, even the leanest and toughest, is only about 20 percent protein, for every 5 pounds of lean muscle mass you gain, you increase your body's protein content about 1 pound. If, in your normal nontraining diet, you eat like most Americans (omnivore or lacto-ovo-vegetarian), you already get enough extra protein to build those 5 pounds of muscle in 10 or 11 days.

When you start to train, your caloric intake increases dramatically. Along with that caloric increase comes an increased intake of protein. You should get plenty of protein to cover almost any rapid weight gain from increased muscle mass, as long as you get a decent diet and enough calories.

Once you have built the necessary muscle mass, your body returns to nitrogen equilibrium, and your protein requirement returns to the normal level for your weight. Because of your increased caloric intake, you still get a relatively large amount of protein. Your body will burn this for energy, excreting the nitrogen portion in your urine. When your caloric intake is extremely high, you may get a protein overload even if you eat a diet proportionately lower in protein than before you started training.

This problem is multiplied by eating a high-protein diet. A training-table meal of steak, potatoes, green beans, bread, and milk can easily give over 100 grams of protein in a 1500-calorie sitting! If the other two (or three) meals give equivalent protein, an athlete requiring 4500 calories could conceivably get more than 300 grams of protein in a single day.

This protein overconsumption is more than wasteful—it's dangerous. We described in an earlier chapter the general dangers accompanying too much protein. Athletes are especially sensitive to the double load imposed by a low-carbohydrate, high-protein diet. A diet very low in carbohydrates can lead to muscle cell breakdown, which is bad for an athlete all by itself. Even worse, when muscle cells rupture, they release myoglobin into the bloodstream. This is the muscles' oxygen storage protein. Because it is a large molecule, the kidneys must strain to excrete it. Also, because iron is part of the myoglobin molecule, the body's loss of iron is increased.

The ketosis associated with a high-protein diet can also increase your chances of dehydration, since it increases urination. As mentioned earlier, dehydration is an athlete's worst enemy. In addition, the breakdown products of protein metabolism are similar to those of hard exercise. They can mimic the symptoms of fatigue and cause you to feel tired, even before your workout.

Obviously, protein is one of the last things an athlete need worry about, even as a vegetarian. Even so, if you eat a very idiosyncratic diet, particularly if it emphasizes either very low-calorie foods or very high-fat, high-sugar foods, you should analyze your diet to be sure you get enough calories and protein.

PROTEIN AS ENERGY FOOD

Of course, protein yields calories, just as carbohydrate and fat do. But many ads push it as somehow superior, giving more energy.

Several laboratory studies have demonstrated that protein is not used directly for energy, so high-protein foods *can't* give you quick energy. On the contrary, protein is digested more slowly than carbohydrate, and it must be deaminated and rebuilt into glucose before your muscles can use it at all. Those ads for protein supplements are misleading. In fact, they are expensive and worthless scams perpetrated on athletes to the tune of several million dollars a year. Protein supplements can't make you stronger, faster, or more muscular, or give you more energy or endurance, unless, of course, your diet is so poor that you are protein deficient. This is rare in the population in general, and unheard-of among athletes, whose primary concern is to care for their bodies. So save that ten bucks a can of Protein Booster will cost you, and spend it on 10 pounds of whole wheat spaghetti. It will take you a lot farther.

Vitamins and Minerals

At this point you may be starting to realize that athletes differ very little from the general population in the nutrient needs. Yet athletes are famous for swallowing dozens of pills a day, from kelp concentrate to 1200 IU of vitamin E. Most of these supplements are useless, at least physiologically. Their psychological effect is another matter entirely, though, because in a competition among well-trained, well-matched athletes, positive attitude can be the deciding factor. If you've loaded up on vitamins and you *think* they give you an advantage, your confidence will give you an edge over your competition.

Vitamins used this way are a psychological crutch. If you haven't started eating pills, don't. If you already down them by the fistful, try to cut back. They aren't doing you any good physically, and megadoses of some, especially the fat-soluble vitamins A and D, can be toxic.

That said, there are a couple of vitamins and some minerals athletes do need in slightly larger amounts. Thiamin and niacin are both required in proportion to caloric intake. Since athletes take in more calories than the rest of us, they need more of these two nutrients. However, both come in abundance along with the best sources of energy—complex carbohydrates. You need not place special emphasis on these if you eat a good diet with plenty of whole foods.

Because you sweat when you are training, you lose some minerals along with the moisture. In the past this was the justification for athletes to gobble salt pills, so they wouldn't become sodium deficient. However, sweat contains more water and less sodium proportionately than do body fluids, so when you perspire, you effectively *raise* your blood sodium level. Taking salt pills at this time is the last thing you need.

Of course, when you drink water to replace your losses, you then would need to replace the lost sodium as well, if the balance goes below the safe level. Since most of us get far more salt than we need in our diets, it is extremely unlikely that you would lose enough salt to throw off your body's ion balance. The next meal you eat will probably supply you with plenty of sodium, whether you salt your food or not. Medicating yourself with salt makes sense only when you will be losing and replacing more than a gallon of fluid (eight pounds) before your next meal.

In fact, there is some indication that the amount of salt excreted through perspiration is connected to the amount you take in. People with very low sodium intake simply have less salty sweat. This is the body's way of conserving its vital minerals. Conversely, very salty sweat may be your body's way of getting rid of excess sodium. If you get low on sodium, you'll develop a craving for salty food, whether you're accustomed to a low-sodium diet or not. This is another natural control on your mineral supply.

A much more important mineral is potassium. While sodium is found mainly in the fluids outside cells, potassium is found mainly inside cells, including muscle cells. When you exercise, your muscles heat up. Your body's adaptation to this excess heat is to try to carry it away in your bloodstream. When your muscles become overheated, they stimulate circulation in the nearby veins by releasing part of their potassium. The veins react by dilating to allow more blood to flow, thus drawing off the excess heat.

However, the blood also carries off the potassium the cells have released. Since potassium doesn't belong in your blood, your kidneys go to work cleaning the blood and depositing the potassium in your bladder. Once it is in your urine, you cannot reabsorb it. You may also lose some potassium through perspiration.

Since this system of "air conditioning" your muscles works on an emergency basis, it doesn't conserve potassium, and you lose quite a large amount. This can throw your mineral balance off unless the lost potassium is replaced. The best vegetarian sources of potassium are fruits, vegetables, and grains.

If, for some reason, you are not replacing the potassium you lose, you may suffer from a variety of physical and psychological maladies, including muscle cramps, depression, lack of energy, and (worst of all) poor training results. Your body has no automatic signal to tell you when it needs potassium as it does for sodium. You must supply your needs through a good diet, and you should remain aware of the physical results of workouts.

You also lose magnesium when you sweat, and the physical symptoms of too-low magnesium levels are similar to those of potassium deficiency—cramping and fatigue. The best sources of dietary magnesium are whole grains, nuts, and green leafies. Beer also supplies a small amount, so if you're in the habit of quaffing a few after a long run, beer is the best alcoholic beverage.

Rest and Recuperation

When you work your muscles, you hurt them. There is no way to avoid it. Your tissues are very happy to stay exactly as they are—if you want them to become larger or stronger, you have to stress them beyond their capacity so they will respond by enlarging.

For your body to do what you want—heal your slightly damaged muscles in such a way that they become stronger and more able to cope with stress—it must have time to heal. If you train hard day after day, your muscles won't have time to heal, and you won't get better. You may, in fact, get worse. If you continue to push your body without adequate rest, you can end up hospitalized, with a long road ahead just to return to square one.

The best way to avoid this is to insure adequate time to recuperate from unusual stresses before you repeat them. A day-on, day-off training schedule is probably best, especially if you are a beginner. This doesn't mean you work hard one day and loaf the next; if your body is well trained, it simply means you work hard one day and work less hard the next. The more conditioned your muscles become, the more constant exercise they require to stay in condition.

If you wake up still tired from the previous day's workout, today is a light day. Your body is telling you it hasn't had enough time to recuperate from the damage done yesterday. If you want to have a long competitive career, you must learn to listen to the signals from your body. Of course, if you wake up feeling great, today can be a heavy day.

PERFORMANCE VERSUS HEALTH

Athletes aren't necessarily healthy, especially professional athletes. In fact, far too many destroy their bodies in their search for performance. Too often, they must retire because their many injuries force them out, or because they have simply worn themselves out and become 35-year-olds trapped in 60-year-old bodies.

Among the many questionable health practices indulged in by athletes is a training method known as *peaking*. When you push your body to a high level of conditioning, you can't stay there forever. Your body has certain limits on what it is capable of doing. When you train, you must continue to push yourself further and further, or you will slip back. When you begin to reach your training limit, you simply can't push your body further. This is your competitive peak, and if you don't take advantage of it by timing it carefully to your competition schedule, you will lose it and drop back to a lower level of conditioning.

Skilled athletes are aware of their conditioning pace, and they know how to train for a specific event. If they have planned carefully, the peak of conditioning can be timed for their most important competitions.

This conditioning and deconditioning process does take its toll, unless you are very careful. After a peak, you need a rest period. Since your activity level has dropped precipitously, you must eat fewer calories to keep from gaining weight. You must keep your muscles toned with light exercise and plenty of stretching. A hard training period is often accompanied by an emotional high, and you may feel let down and depressed after your peak. Even your sleep may be disrupted.

You can offset many of these undesirable effects if you have a life outside of competition. When all your emotional energy is tied up in one part of your life, your psychological state is closely linked to the ups and downs of that one compartment of your being. If you have other outlets for leftover energy, your health will be better for it.

Drugs

Athletes take drugs. It is unfortunate but true that in the search for more power, shorter lap times, quicker reflexes, and greater endurance, many athletes dose themselves with chemicals. They may damage their health permanently in the process, and in many cases the effectiveness of these drugs is not at all clear.

The two types of drugs most commonly used by athletes are anabolic steroids and stimulants. Anabolic steroids are laboratory analogs of hormones produced in the bodies of adolescent males. These natural hormones have the effect of increasing muscle mass, and more than anything else, they contribute to the physical change from little boy to young man.

Athletes who take steroids believe the drugs will build their muscle mass and speed healing, thus accelerating the training process. No laboratory research has documented this effect, but athletes go on taking them because of the advantage they *might* confer.

Unfortunately, steroids have a potent effect on many parts of the body—not just the muscles—and these effects are often very damaging. Liver damage and perhaps cancer, sterility and testicular atrophy, growth interruption, elevated blood lipid levels, personality changes (aggression), undesirable hair growth in women, worsened acne, and increased blood pressure and blood sugar levels are some of the possible problems caused by steroids. The obvious conclusion is that they are not good for you. Whatever their positive effects on performance, there is no justification for their use because of the negative effects on overall health.

Stimulant drugs encompass everything from caffeine to cocaine and amphetamines. Caffeine, the stimulant in coffee, is closely related to theobromine, the stimulant in tea and chocolate. In 1976, Americans consumed 560 cups of coffee per person, on the average. Since many people don't touch the stuff, it is clear that the consumption is far higher for many others. Every cup of coffee has between 80 and 150 mg of caffeine, and one cup is sufficient to strongly stimulate the system of someone who isn't accustomed to the drug. With continued use, we become habituated to it, and many people become emotionally dependent on its stimulant effects.

Caffeine can also affect athletes, of course. Its effect is similar to that of the other central nervous system stimulants mentioned here—a sense of well being, increased heart rate, decreased sensitivity to pain. But caffeine is a lightweight compared to amphetamine—probably the most abused drug in athletic competition.

Oddly enough, it has been shown that amphetamine does not improve performance except in a simple, uncomplicated, repetitive task. It severely damages your judgment, however, and it can wreck your performance if you are called upon to make any kind of quick decision. Why, then, do athletes continue to take it? Because it makes them *feel* like champions.

Traded off against that feeling is the possibility of death from heatstroke or simple overdose, muscles damaged beyond repair through the drug's masking of pain, improper rest and consequent loss of conditioning, and simple fouling up when the chips are down. Amphetamine and other stimulants are no good, for your performance or for your health.

Don't take drugs.

GUIDELINES

Athletes must be careful of their water balance, total calories, and rest time.

Water is the most crucial nutrient for athletes, because they run a greater risk of dehydration than do the rest of us.

Athletes need sufficient extra calories to cover their higher activity level—carbohydrates are the best source.

Athletes don't need extra protein, beyond a very small increment for increased muscle mass, which is probably already in their diet from our national overconsumption of protein, even if they are vegetarian.

Thiamin and niacin are the only vitamins needed in increased amounts, and they increase automatically if calorie sources include grains, seeds, beans, and dairy products.

Don't take extra salt if you perspire heavily. You'll get

enough in your food unless your diet is extremely salt restricted.

Athletes should be sure to get enough potassium and magnesium—by eating fruits, vegetables, grains, and legumes.

If you must push your body hard, take care of it. Train properly, get enough rest, and channel excess energy while you recover from a peak performance.

Don't take drugs.

The best athlete's diet is simply *more* of a good whole-foods diet.

10
A Weight-loss Diet

*D*epending on their orientation, people invariably ask vegetarians one of two questions: "Don't you gain weight?" or "Have you lost much weight?" If they assume you've gained, it is usually based on the notion that carbohydrates are fattening and there's no way to eat beans and pasta and bread without getting fat. If they think you must be getting thin, they've probably associated thinness with being pale and weak, the supposedly inevitable consequences of what they suppose to be a low-protein diet.

In fact, of course, both assumptions are false, as we've shown in previous chapters. There are many myths surrounding weight control, usually about weight loss. They proliferate because we don't want to believe the facts. We'd prefer cutting out all carbohydrates or drinking lunch out of a can or eating a grapefruit with every meal. Anything but count calories. There must be an easier way.

There isn't. At least so far as we know, it's the same old rule: Reduce your calories, reduce your weight. More specifically, if you consume more calories than you expend, you will gradually gain weight. If you expend more than you consume, you'll gradually lose. It's that simple and, regrettably, that difficult.

Even so, there are no guarantees beyond that general rule. According to most sources, one pound of fat equals 3500 calories, so when you eat 3500 fewer calories than usual, you lose one pound. As we have said, however, nutrition is an individual science. You may gain or lose at a faster or slower rate than "normal," depending on your metabolism, how much you exercise, and the other variables of who you are.

189

DO YOU NEED TO LOSE WEIGHT?

Almost every diet book on the market includes the weight tables put out by insurance companies, which consider height, age, and bone structure before giving an "ideal" range of weights. Many people rely solely on these charts to decide what they should weigh. If they are above the ideal, they know they have to lose.

In fact, what we need to lose is fat, not pounds, even though they sometimes go hand-in-hand. To judge ourselves only by weight is deceptive, because it doesn't account for bone and muscle, which weigh more than fat but are much more desirable. (Face it, when we look at those insurance tables, we are *all* large-framed!) Many athletes, for example, would be considered overweight by the charts, yet they actually have a rather low percentage of fat on their bodies.

The question you should ask yourself is not "Am I overweight?" but "Am I overfat?" Percentage of body fat is the determining factor. Two people may weight the same amount, and one might be too fat while the other is fine.

The Pinch Test

One way to measure how "fat" you are is the pinch test. You can get a good idea of the total fat in your body by measuring the thickness of the fat under your skin in certain areas.

The easiest place is the back of the arm, halfway between the shoulder and the elbow. Find the spot while your elbow is bent. Then, using your thumb and forefinger, pull back the skin (or even easier, have someone else do it) while your arm is relaxed, hanging straight down. The fingers should have a light, steady hold while you measure the thickness of the "pinch." If it is an inch or more (a little less for men), you are probably too fat.

Of course, the very best guide is to stand naked in front of a mirror. Remembering that you are you—and not a fashion model—take a good look. It is more telling than a chart and more tailored to your needs than the most scientific pinch. The only trick to this method is objectivity. Give yourself a fair chance before asking for a refund on the mirror.

Once you've decided you have too much fat, the only way to get rid of it—short of increasing your activity immensely—is to lose weight. Thus, we have come full circle, back to the concept of weight.

Once you decide that you are too fat, you are also over the weight that is best for you. (We'll call it your "best" weight rather than the chart's "ideal.") Lose the weight, and you will lose the fat.

In effect, with no charts, you can only know how much to lose by losing it and seeing it is right for you. Before that, you can only estimate. Remember, if you increase your muscle mass but still keep down body fat, your best weight will be higher. Everything is relative.

WHEN IS IT A MEDICAL PROBLEM?

Unfortunately, most of the studies and statistics about weight are based on those generalized insurance tables. But based on the law of averages, they can still give us a good idea of our tendencies as a culture toward overweight and their medical implications.

Obesity has been associated with arthritis, gall bladder and liver disease, maturity-onset diabetes, cardiovascular disease, and cancer, among other ills. It complicates pregnancy and childbirth and is considered a surgical risk. It places an extra burden on the heart and circulatory systems. It decreases life expectancy.

The important question is when. When does overweight constitute a medical problem? Most of the answers, which seem to be educated guesses at this point, are in terms of those "ideal" weights. You use your own best weight as a guide (or estimate, if you haven't determined it yet) instead.

Most recent studies indicate that if you are mildly obese, about 10 to 15 percent above "ideal," that alone is not considered a health risk. One opinion even holds that it is healthiest to be 10 percent over ideal weight until the age of 30. The fatter you are, the riskier it is, however, until it does become a major factor in your health (or the lack of it). Even at the milder stages, it is uncomfortable, a psychological burden, and a social taboo. Although the evidence is not yet complete, a health risk probably exists if you are more than 15 percent overweight. At 25 percent above, it is a virtual certainty.

WHERE THE CALORIES GO

You lose weight by expending more calories than you consume. The kind of food you eat doesn't matter. When you eat it makes no difference. All that counts is the calories themselves. If you don't count them, they will add up all the same.

A calorie is a unit of energy. It was not devised to make people fat, but to measure the amount of fuel our bodies get from various foods. When we eat more food than our bodies require to keep going, the excess is stored as fat, whether from proteins, carbohydrates, or fats. If you have stored too much fat, you have eaten too much food—more than you need to fuel your body.

Like a car or other machine, our bodies need that fuel to work. We need it to jog, to lift a heavy object, to run up the stairs. But unlike other machines, our bodies do not turn off. Even when we are perfectly still, our hearts are pumping, our cells are working, our blood is circulating. We are always using some amount of energy. We need a constant supply in order to be alive.

This fundamental level of energy use is called our basal metabolism. We each have a different minimum energy demand, our own particular Basal Metabolic Rate (BMR) to maintain all of our involuntary body processes. Add to this our conscious work (activity level)—running up those stairs—and you can see where the calories go when they are needed.

HOW MANY CALORIES DO YOU NEED?

In order to figure out how many calories maintain your weight daily, you must determine your BMR and your activity level, and add the two. In both cases you can only estimate, of course. There are too many variables to arrive at a precise figure, unless you are tested in a laboratory.

Remember, a certain number of calories supports a certain weight. If you lose 10 pounds, you'll have to refigure (no pun intended) your caloric need in order to maintain your new lower weight.

Your BMR

Here's a general formula for BMR:

For women, multiply your weight in pounds by 11.
For men, multiply your weight in pounds by 12.

As an example, 24-year-old Lynn weighs 120 pounds. To figure her BMR, she multiples 120 by 11. The result, 1320, is the approximate number of calories demanded by her BMR just to keep her body running.

Individual variables can play an important role, however. Factors such as age and body type can make basal rates higher or lower than average.

BMR decreases with advancing age, for example. For every decade after age 20, you need at least 2 percent fewer calories to maintain the same weight as always. It doesn't seem like much, but it will add up if you don't cut those calories.

Thin or muscular people tend to have a higher metabolism. So do taller people, who have more body surface compared to body weight, resulting in more heat loss and consequently a higher BMR. On the other hand, fatter people are more insulated and tend not to lose as much heat.

What a cruel cycle it seems to be, when the fat get fatter while the thin stay thin. Taking this into consideration, add 5 percent to your BMR if you are thinner than average. Subtract 5 percent if you're fatter.

Your Activity Level

All people use a certain amount of energy simply going about their business during the day. They drive, they cook, they sit at desks, they work in factory lines. It is estimated that we use calories equal to 30 percent of our BMR for this basic daily activity level. Lynn would add 30 percent of her BMR of 1320 (396) to 1320 for a total of 1716 calories needed if she leads this fairly sedentary life. Many of us do, or close to it.

Others have opted for a more active life—running, playing tennis, taking a dance or exercise class. These people can afford even more calories per day, but it is difficult to determine just how many with any accuracy. There are charts, as you are probably aware, that tell how many calories you use in various activities. Still, people run at different speeds, are more or less aggressive in a game of tennis, may take a class in ballet or jazz dance. It is hard to estimate how much time you really spend in vigorous exercise. Rates vary from about 250 calories for a hour's brisk walk to 450 or more for an hour of moderate running. Again, these are averages that depend on your weight and how hard you actually work.

If this seems a bit ambiguous, it is. You can be sure that the longer and harder you exercise, the more calories you will burn. Just how many you burn can be estimated by charts but is basically guesswork.

If you count calories, you will discover soon enough whether your estimate for exercise is accurate. If your estimate is too high, for example, you won't be losing weight as fast as you thought you would. Indeed, you may not be losing at all.

In most cases, exercise can't take the place of diet if you need to lose weight. Most of us don't exercise that hard or long. Less exercise than usual, however, can be the subtle cause of slow gains, and exercise does give us a certain amount of leeway in terms of calories. It is important to our good health in other ways, too, keeping our bodies limber and strong and working efficiently.

Exercise is also perhaps the only answer for those who want to "spot reduce." It can't help you lose weight in a certain area, but it does firm up the muscles in that area. Spot reducing per se is a myth. Everyone loses weight from all of his or her body fat proportionately. One more plus: the benefits of a workout go beyond the activity itself, raising your BMR (thus the calories you burn) for up to 15 hours afterward. It can't hurt!

DECREASING YOUR CALORIES

If increasing your energy output is only a partial solution, the rest of the answer lies in cutting calories.

Theoretically, one pound of fat equals 3500 calories. In actuality, it varies from person to person for the same reasons BMR does. We have no way of knowing what a pound of fat equals for you, so we'll stick with 3500. In that case, if you eat 500 calories fewer a day, you'll lose a pound a week. If you cut your calories daily by 1000, you'll lose 2 pounds a week.

This works on a sliding scale. Since the number of calories your body uses is based more or less on your weight, the less you come to weigh, the fewer calories you'll need and the more slowly you'll lose, unless you cut more and more calories as you go along.

Say Lynn gains 30 pounds. At 150 pounds, she is eating 2145 calories a day to support her weight—a BMR of 1650 plus a basic activity level of 495. (Unfortunately, she is still leading a rather sedentary life.) She goes on a 1200-calorie-a-day diet—nearly 1000 calories fewer a day than the 2145 she was eating. At the beginning, she should lose almost 2 pounds a week. But as she approaches her goal of 120 pounds—maintenance level of 1716 calories rather than 2145—she's eating only 500 calories fewer than her maintenance level. Her weight loss slows to one pound a week.

If she changed her lifestyle to include an hour of brisk walking every day, she'd increase the rate of her loss quite a bit.

It would be unwise, however, for her to decrease her calories to fewer than 1200 a day. This is just about the minimum level at which she can get a balanced diet.

OUR DIET

We have devised a one- or two-week 1200-calorie-a-day diet with the intention that it be as satisfying as possible. No diet is truly satisfying, if only because you know you're on a diet. That aware-ness alone can make you want to eat more than usual.

Unfortunately, our bodies don't always tell us when to stop eating in time.

The part of the brain that controls appetite is called the *appestat*. One of its centers turns your appetite on, the other off. Both seem to react to the level of glucose in the blood to make decisions. When the level of glucose (the sugar product of digestion) signals that your body's needs have been met, you feel satisfied. This mental satisfaction may or may not work in conjunction with a feeling of fullness in your stomach. The point is that both proc-esses, satiety and fullness, take a certain length of time to occur. That's why dieters are advised to eat slowly. If they eat too fast, they get ahead of the signals and eat too much. (Obviously, this problem doesn't apply only to dieters.)

We have designed a diet that does the following:

Keeps calories to a safe minimum
Includes a variety of foods
Is easy to fit into your lifestyle
Tastes good
Has a good balance of nutrients
Is as filling as possible.

The nutrients are generally in the same proportions we recom-mend throughout this book. The only difference is that the amount of protein is higher proportionally because your protein need remains the same even when you decrease calories. (Remember, figure your protein need based on best weight.) The average breakdown for nutrients in this diet is: 19.9 percent protein; 62.6 percent carbohydrate; 17.5 percent fat. Although the diet should provide a nice balance of vitamins and minerals, take a daily multivitamin pill with iron to be sure.

The diet is designed for someone whose best weight is about 120 pounds. For those whose best weights are higher, add the foods in Number 9 of Rules on the days specified. This is necessary since protein needs are on a sliding scale according to weight. The additions will raise your protein intake sufficiently. On the remaining days, the protein is enough to suit just about anyone. Those with higher best weights may need to add a few hundred extra calories of complex carbohydrates for energy on those days. Fruit would be a good choice.

Stay on the diet for one or two weeks. Then stay off the diet for as long as you've been on it. During the interim, raise your caloric intake to that needed to maintain your best weight (BMR plus 30 percent). By doing this, you can stabilize at your new weight before going on to lose more, if you intend to.

The diet will be harder for people used to eating between meals, since it relies on three good meals with nothing in between. The fruit from breakfast can be eaten any time, if that helps. In fact, you can switch the meals as you wish. There are no tricks to this diet. It's simply 1200 calories a day and is balanced.

No diet is easy. You have to be somewhat hungry at least some of the time. These meals are fairly filling, and the diet is effective. Besides making you lose weight, it should help you improve your eating habits, including no between-meal snacks, since it is really a scaled-down version of a healthy style of eating.

RULES

1. Beverages: unlimited water, club soda, black coffee, tea.
2. Take a multivitamin with iron daily.
3. If you must eat between meals, munch on the old standbys: carrots and celery.
4. Substitutions: If you don't like one of the meals, feel lazy, or *must* eat at a restaurant, use another meal twice or, for any lunch, you can substitute ½ cup low-fat cottage cheese plus a reasonable amount (200 calories worth) of fresh fruit. For any dinner, you can

have 1 cup cottage cheese, fruit, and a small whole-grain roll or slice of bread *or* a medium-sized vegetable salad with 1 ounce cheese, 1 hard-boiled egg, and oil-and-vinegar dressing (not more than 1 tablespoon oil!).

5. Vegetables for sandwiches: tomato, mushrooms, sprouts, carrot, cucumber, scallions. Put these on your sandwich in moderation. They should equal only 40 to 50 calories total.

6. Interchangeable vegetables for dinner recipes (raw weight):

½   pound broccoli
½   pound cauliflower
6-7 artichoke hearts
¾   pound spinach
½   pound cabbage
½   pound mushrooms
¾   pound summer squash
¾   pound carrots
¾   pound tomatoes
½   pound green beans

When substituting, use your own taste and judgment regarding proportions.

7. Onions and garlic have been used liberally in the recipes because they are both flavorful and low-calorie. If you don't like or can't eat them, omit them and experiment with herbs.

8. Unless specified, milk means skim milk, mozzarella cheese should be part skim, cottage cheese uncreamed, and yogurt is low-fat.

9. This diet is designed for someone whose best weight is about 120 pounds. If your best weight is nearer to 150 pounds, add one of the following, separately or to any meal, on days when you eat meals 1, 2, 3, and 5. If your best weight is about 175 pounds, add two of the following on those days. The additions will provide the extra protein and calories needed for your size.

1½ ounces cheese (not cream
    cheese)
    or
1½ cups skim milk
    or
5   ounces fresh tofu

2½ cups cut broccoli
    or
½   cup creamed or dry cottage
    cheese
    or
1   cup lima beans

OR

1	egg		1 cup broccoli or cooked
	or		spinach
1	ounce cheese	PLUS	or
	or		½ cup lima beans
1	cup skim milk		or
			½ pound mushrooms

OR

Two from:

1 egg
1 ounce cheese
1 cup skim milk

THE DIET

BREAKFAST *(Every Day)*   **calories**

(a) 2 raisin-bran muffins*
       or
    2 slices whole grain bread or toast   175
(b) topped with up to ¼ cup unsweetened applesauce
    (plus cinnamon or nutmeg)   25
(c) ½ cantaloupe (or 1 cup whole strawberries,
    1 tangerine, 1 large peach, 3 apricots, ½ cup blue-
    berries, 1 small apple, ½ banana, 1 wedge honeydew,
    1 plum, or ½ cup raspberries)   50
(d) 6 ounces skim milk   60
                                                               310

LUNCH *(Every Day)*   **calories**

A melted cheese and vegetable sandwich*   309
    or
A vegetable cream cheese and tomato sandwich*   307
    or
A large salad* with 3 tablespoons avocado dressing*
    or 1½ tablespoons of vinaigrette*   305
                                                (average) 307

*Recipe follows.

DINNER (In Any Order)

1. Pasta with Broccoli Sauce*	526
2. Rice with Cheese Plus*	518
3. Potato-Mushroom Soup* and small dinner salad*	483
4. Vegetables with Cheese Sauce* and small dinner salad	502
5. Pasta with Tomato Sauce*	566
6. Mixed Vegetable Casserole* and small dinner salad	488
7. Eggplant Parmesan* and small dinner salad	511

RECIPES

(All recipes are for one serving, unless otherwise indicated.)

Raisin-Bran Muffins (30 Muffins)

2 tablespoons butter	½ teaspoon salt
2 tablespoons sugar	1 tablespoon vanilla
1 egg	2 cups whole wheat flour
½ cup honey	1¼ teaspoons baking soda
2 cups yogurt	1 cup raisins
1½ cups bran	

Cream butter and sugar; beat in egg. Stir in honey, then yogurt. Beat until uniform. Add bran, salt, and vanilla.

Preheat oven to 325°. Grease 30 muffin cups lightly with butter.

Stir flour and baking soda into batter with as few strokes as possible, making sure there are no dry lumps of flour.

Pour batter into cups and distribute raisins over the tops.

Bake 25–30 minutes, until lightly browned. Cool. Store tightly wrapped in refrigerator. Makes 15 two-muffin servings. These are best warmed in the oven first. The muffins will keep in the refrigerator for two weeks.

Melted Cheese and Vegetable Sandwich

Top-brown 1 ounce cheese on 1 slice whole grain bread. Add sliced tomato, sprouts, and/or any other raw vegetable (see Rules). Top with another slice of bread.

This should be easy to order in a restaurant, but remember, no mayonnaise or butter.

*Recipe follows.

Vegetable Cream Cheese and Tomato Sandwich
    2 slices whole grain bread
    ⅓ recipe cream cheese (below)
        sliced tomato or other raw vegetable (see Rules)

Vegetable Cream Cheese
    ½ cup uncreamed cottage cheese
    2 ounces cream cheese
    1 carrot, finely chopped
    2 scallions, minced
    4 radishes, finely chopped
Blend all ingredients until smooth and store covered in refrigerator. Makes enough for three Vegetable Cream Cheese and Tomato Sandwiches.

A Large Salad
A large salad can be bigger than you think. It's the dressing you have to watch: only 3 tablespoons Avocado Dressing or 1½ tablespoons Vinaigrette. Here's a sample salad. Substitute other vegetables for those you don't like, but don't use more raisins or nuts than are called for here. Keep in the lettuce and sprouts. Iceberg is excluded because it is less nutritious than darker, leafy varieties such as Boston, Bibb, or Romaine. Use substitute dressings (below) in a restaurant.

    1 to 2 small heads   1 small tomato
        lettuce (not iceberg)   1 tablespoon raisins
    2 scallions   6 walnut halves
    1 carrot   1 cup shredded cabbage
    1 cup alfalfa (or other)   10 radishes
        sprouts

Avocado Dressing
    1 large ripe avocado   ½ teaspoon salt
    1 sliver of garlic   dash of pepper
    ¼ cup yogurt   dash of chili powder
    3 tablespoons lemon
        juice
Purée all ingredients into a smooth dressing and store in refrigerator. Remember, 3 tablespoons is the serving size for a large salad; 1 tablespoon for a small salad.

Vinaigrette

½ cup olive oil	1 clove garlic
½ cup tarragon vinegar	2 tablespoons French mustard
	fresh pepper
	parsley

Blend all ingredients and store in refrigerator. Use 1½ table-spoons for a large salad; ½ tablespoon for a small salad.

Substitute dressings: vinegar, lemon juice, yogurt, herbs.

Pasta with Broccoli Sauce

1 cup steamed broccoli pieces	2 tablespoons Romano cheese, grated
2 tablespoons yogurt	¼ pound pasta
1 sliver of garlic	salt and pepper

Purée the broccoli (or save part and add later), yogurt, garlic, and cheese in a blender or food processor. Season with salt and pepper.

Boil the pasta. When done, drain it briefly and mix into the sauce. The hot pasta will heat the sauce.

Rice with Cheese Plus

1 cup cooked brown rice	1 tablespoon roasted sesame seeds
2 tablespoons grated Romano	2 teaspoons butter
2 tablespoons grated Italian Fontina	¼ cup hot skim milk
	½ pound broccoli, steamed
	2 tablespoons lemon juice

Stir together the hot rice, cheeses, sesame seeds, and butter. When blended, add the hot milk and stir again.

Serve with the broccoli, sprinkled with lemon juice and fresh pepper.

Potato-Mushroom Soup

1 tablespoon oil	1 pound potatoes, cubed
½ stalk celery, chopped	2 cups vegetable stock (except
2 onions, chopped	bean stock) or water
½ pound raw mushrooms	milk powder—enough to make
salt, pepper, parsley	1 quart reconstituted

In a medium-sized, heavy-bottomed pot, sauté the celery, onion, and mushrooms in the oil until the mushrooms release their moisture. Add the potatoes and stock, and bring the mixture to a boil. Add salt, pepper, parsley. Simmer about 15 minutes until the potatoes are tender.

Add the milk powder. If you use noninstant milk powder, first mix it into a paste with a small amount of the soup stock, then add it to the pot. Stir until well blended.

Purée all or part, if desired, and warm again. Or serve chilled.

Vegetables with Cheese Sauce

½ pound cauliflower
1 medium zucchini (6 oz.)
½ pound broccoli
1 medium tomato

1½ tablespoons whole wheat flour
1½ ounces Cheddar cheese, grated
½ cup milk (or a tablespoon more)
salt, paprika, cayenne

Cut the vegetables into bite-sized pieces. Steam the cauliflower, zucchini, and broccoli for a few minutes, then add the tomato. Steam until the vegetables are done to your liking.

Meanwhile, mix the flour and cheese. Heat the milk in a saucepan. When it's quite hot, add the cheese and flour mixture. Cook it *very carefully*, to guard against scorching, over low heat until it has thickened. Season with salt, paprika, a dash of cayenne.

Pour sauce over vegetables and serve.

Pasta with Tomato Sauce

2 medium onions, chopped
4 cloves garlic, minced
½ tablespoon olive oil
2 pounds tomatoes, chopped
¼ pound pasta

basil
parsley
oregano
2 tablespoons Romano cheese, grated
salt and pepper

Sauté the onion, garlic, and herbs in the olive oil until the onion is soft and the mixture is fragrant. Add the fresh or canned tomatoes, salt, and pepper. Simmer to desired thickness. Makes about 1 quart.

Meanwhile, for one serving, boil ¼ pound pasta. Mix it with 1 scant cup of sauce, and top with the grated Romano. You can store the remaining sauce for another day (for example, for the eggplant parmesan) covered in the refrigerator.

A quick alternative: Chop a ½-pound tomato. Add 1 teaspoon

oil, herbs, a pinch of salt, a touch of chopped garlic (use very little), 1 tablespoon lemon juice, fresh pepper. Pour over ¼ pound (dry weight) pasta, cooked. Top with 2 tablespoons cheese. This is especially refreshing in hot weather.

Mixed Vegetable Casserole

½ pound broccoli, chopped
1 zucchini, sliced
½ pound cabbage, shredded
1 onion, sliced
½ pound mushrooms, sliced
1½ cups fresh breadcrumbs
¼ cup raisins

½ pound mozzarella, shredded
1 egg
½ cup stock or water
½ teaspoon salt
¼ teaspoon marjoram
1 teaspoon oregano
fresh-ground pepper

Steam the broccoli, zucchini, and cabbage (about ¼ head) for about three minutes. Mix with the onion, the mushrooms, the breadcrumbs, raisins, and ¾ of the grated mozzarella. Press lightly into a 2-quart casserole. Mix together the egg, stock, salt, marjoram, oregano, and pepper and pour over the top. Cover with the remaining mozzarella.

Bake, covered, 30 minutes at 350°F.

Serves 3.

Eggplant Parmesan

4 ½-inch slices of a large eggplant
1½ cups tomato sauce (from the Pasta with Sauce recipe)
2½ ounces grated mozzarella
2 tablespoons grated Romano

Broil the eggplant on both sides until it's brown and hot. Place it in a shallow baking dish and top it with the hot tomato sauce. Cover the top with the mozzarella and Romano, mixed.

Bake at 375°F or broil until the cheese has melted and begun to brown.

Small Dinner Salad

1 small head lettuce (not iceberg) or less
1 scallion, chopped
1 tablespoon avocado dressing or ½ T Vinaigrette. (see Large Salad)

AFTER THE DIET—THE PSYCHOLOGY
OF GAINING AND LOSING

It is after the diet that the struggle really begins. Most dieters tend to gain back the weight they've lost because they haven't changed their eating habits to coincide with their new weights. Back they go to eating more than they need to maintain their thinner bodies.

One of the most important ways to get a handle on losing weight and keeping it off is to try to understand why you got too fat to start with. Even heredity seems to play a part. Statistics predict that if one of your parents is obese, you have a 40 percent chance of becoming so. If both parents have a weight problem, the risk doubles. Of course, this may be environmental rather than hereditary—your family might have had too much food around the house, snacked excessively, or just emphasized eating too much.

Your eating habits as a child also have an effect on your fat cells. Some studies have shown that at certain ages, fat cells multiply at a rapid rate. If you were overfed before you were two or ate too much at about the age of puberty, the number of fat cells in your body may have increased quickly, giving you a greater capacity than normal for fat storage. This would seem to handicap you for the rest of your life, since you would have that many more cells waiting to be enlarged.

But a large number of fat cells at most would make it *easier* for you to get fat. It wouldn't cause you to eat so much that they actually would enlarge. It seems more important to look at what might be creating your present situation: eating too much for your body.

In many cases, eating more than you need stems from a lack of perspective. Although food is basically the packaging for nutrition, there is no denying it is a source of emotional gratification as well. Our parents rewarded us with candy when we were good. We celebrate our holidays by feasting. We enjoy sharing our meals with others on any and all occasions.

People tend to eat when they're feeling happy and festive. Likewise, it seems to fill a need (by literally filling them up) when they're anxious, bored, or depressed.

Eating too much may be encouraged by a particular lifestyle. Often, married couples find themselves getting fatter as they settle down and stop worrying about attracting partners. Don't forget that as you get older you don't need as many calories, and most people tend to exercise less.

Social life often centers on restaurant-going, which means several courses and large servings. For some, including businesspeople and students, eating out is a way of life.

Besides, food tastes good. Cooking is an art in itself. We read cookbooks and take courses in order to better prepare tempting, delicious meals.

Food means comfort, sharing, sensual pleasure, even love. Is it any wonder we often overeat?

For those who do, it is hard to stop. A diet is a good first step, but it comes with its own built-in discipline in the form of rules and recipes. Learning to cut down after the diet takes another kind of awareness and self-discipline.

Reaching your best weight by dieting is definitely encouraging, however. After all, you don't have to lose anymore, and you can up your calories from diet level to support your new weight. Use the guidelines mentioned earlier in the chapter to figure it out. This is how you should eat from now on.

Get familiar with the calorie content of the foods you eat. If you like to eat 4 ounces of pasta for dinner, know that it has 420 calories. It may be inconvenient at first to look things up, but soon you'll know most of it by memory. If you feel you must weigh and measure portions, do so. Eventually, you'll have an eye for that, too.

Weigh yourself every day. If you gain a couple of pounds, cut down. If they don't come off easily, consider dieting for a few days. Don't let it get out of your control. It *is* in your control.

Learn to heed your body's signals. Eat slowly. Take a break between courses. Fill up on bulky, low-calorie foods like salad or celery sticks. Stop eating when you feel comfortable and satisfied, not stuffed. This is one of the most difficult things to do when you haven't for so long. Fight the desire to keep eating when you know you should stop. If you must, salt or pepper your food so you wouldn't dare eat another bite.

Avoid refined and fat-laden foods. The refined foods have too many calories and not enough nutrients. The fats in food have more than twice as many calories (9 as opposed to 4 per gram) as the proteins and carbohydrates.

If you are hooked on sweets or fried foods, it will be rough, but keep them to a minimum. If you just can't, consider giving them up altogether. Forever.

Exercise more. It can make a difference in keeping off weight, especially if you watch calories, too.

Don't be tempted to go on crash diets or use pills or machines. They are shortcuts that encourage quick loss and quick gain. Many don't work at all. When they seem to, it is often a temporary fluid loss. Don't be fooled, it's not worth it.

You are.

GUIDELINES

Determine whether you are too fat by how much body fat you have, not by how much you weigh.

You can only know *your* best weight by having reached it. If you don't know it yet, estimate based on your body fat.

If you are more than 15 percent overweight (overfat), it is likely a health risk.

Once you have decided you have too much fat, you need to lose weight.

If you expend more calories than you consume, you will gradually lose weight. A 1200-calorie a day diet is a safe minimum.

Once you have reached your best weight, determine how many calories you need to maintain it.

Determine how many calories you need by estimating your Basal Metabolic Rate (BMR) and activity level (at least 30 percent of BMR).

Understanding why you tend to overeat can be a big help in learning to stop.

IS VEGETARIANISM HEALTHIER?

11
Is Vegetarianism Healthier?

We have avoided dealing directly with this question so far, partially because we don't consider it germane to the main purpose of this book, but mainly because hard-and-fast answers are hard to come by. Of course, it is easy to make invidious comparisons with the normal American's diet—Americans overeat fat, protein, and sugar, not to mention all the synthetic nonfood garbage that has found its way into the nation's food supply. This must have an effect on health.

Since most of these factors have little to do with meat-eating per se, it hardly seems fair to compare a vegetarian diet to the standard American diet. That would be like an arm-wrestling competition between a linebacker and a five-year-old. Of course, vegetarians can eat a poor diet almost as easily as can meat-eaters. Every individual's diet is different, with different restricting factors.

Of course, it is also true that most vegetarians pay closer attention to the quality of their diet than do most meat-eaters. Many people have become vegetarian for the express purpose of improving the way they nourish their bodies, so the ranks of vegetarians are already swelled by a whole group of careful eaters. In addition, many of the junkiest foods are nonvegetarian—bacon, luncheon meat, Jello, chicken pot pie. There are some vegetarians who, admittedly, live on Sara Lee cake and Tab soda, but probably not as high a percentage as there are of meat-eaters. A vegetarian diet on its own is a statistical indicator that an individual is probably better nourished than the Average American.

The best comparison would be between a carefully planned omnivorous diet and a carefully planned vegetarian one.

In the discussion below, we will point up specific differences between vegetarian and omnivore diets and indicate differences between vegan and lacto-ovo diets as well.

DIETARY GOALS

In 1977 the Senate Select Committee on Nutrition and Human Needs published a set of Dietary Goals for the American people.* They were immediately attacked by various representatives of the food-producing industry as radical revisions of the way most Americans eat and "unadvisable" alterations to our diet of plenty. Even so, the changes the committee recommended were quite modest. They suggested a reduction in total fat from as much as 50 percent of total calories to 30 percent, divided equally among the three categories of saturated, monounsaturated, and polyunsaturated. Refined sugar should be limited to 10 percent of calories, and complex carbohydrate and natural sugars should make up 48 percent. The remaining 12 percent represented protein's contribution to this improved diet. The committee also recommended a decrease in cholesterol intake to no more than 300 milligrams a day and a sharp decrease in sodium intake—perhaps the two most radical departures from the standard American style of eating.

Note that the recommendations call for a protein intake far in excess of the already generous RDA. For a sedentary man—that is to say, a normal American male—the 12 percent of calories represents a protein intake 29 percent greater than the RDA. A sedentary woman would get 18.5 percent more than her RDA.

To achieve these goals, the committee recommended the following changes in the way Americans eat:

1. Eat more fresh fruits, vegetables, and whole grains.
2. Substitute skim or low-fat milk for full-fat milk (except for children).
3. Eat less animal fat.
4. Eat less refined sugar and foods high in refined sugar.
5. Eat less of the high-cholesterol foods (except perhaps eggs).
6. Eat less of high-fat foods and partially substitute polyunsaturated for saturated fats.
7. Eat less salt and salty foods.

*More recent dietary guidelines, such as *Dietary Guidelines for Americans* (U.S. Departments of Agriculture and Health and Human Services, February 1980), agree with the Select Committee's recommendations.

Other changes to achieve the goals included eating less red meat and full-fat cheese (whole milk cheese) and perhaps substituting low-fat variants of these.

We can use this as our ideal omnivorous diet. It restricts the least healthy ingredient of a carnivorous diet—animal fat. Its emphasis on fresh fruits and vegetables and fewer refined food products is heartening and excellent advice.

Oddly enough, we find that the diet begins to resemble a well-designed lacto-ovo-vegetarian diet, except for the relatively minor presence of meat. By deemphasizing meats and the general protein overconsumption characterized by meat-eating and by emphasizing fresh fruits and vegetables and whole grains, the entire complexion of the diet changes. Still, let's compare the two.

THE FACE-OFF

We must ask first: What are the inherent dietary advantages of each style of eating? Since the difference between the two diets is simply the presence or absence of meat in the diet, the question becomes What are the dietary advantages and disadvantages of meat?

For a diet that includes meat we turn to the National Live Stock and Meat Board, the industry group that acts as speaker for stockmen, slaughterhouse operators, and meat packers. The Meat Board is a very effective lobbying and public relations organization, and they have produced a series of pamphlets extolling the glories of meat consumption and implying that anyone who advocates eating less meat is either insane or plotting against the American Way of Life and the Health of the Nation. In their pamphlet titled "Meat and the Vegetarian Concept"—a collection of canards about vegetarians—we find these claims for meat as a nutrient source.

Meat is a primary source of "complete" protein.

Meat supplies substantial quantities of the RDAs for thiamin, riboflavin, niacin, vitamins B_6 and B_{12}, and zinc.

Meat is the best source of iron.

Meat supplies "vital phosphorus, potassium, and essential micronutrients, many of which cannot be duplicated in plant foods," such as vitamins A and B_{12}.

Let's look at these claims, one at a time.

Protein

Protein is the biggest red herring (so to speak) of the "eat meat" campaign. The Meat Board's pamphlet goes on to expand this notion. It first points out that Americans eat "only" 2.8 ounces of red meat a day per capita, but this is cooked meat, a reduction of more than 50 percent over purchase weight, and it includes every American, presumably including millions of vegetarians and infants and children, whose low or nonexistent consumption pushes the average even lower. In addition, the figures ignore consumption of other flesh, including 63 pounds a year per capita of fish and poultry, plus uncounted amounts of flesh from animals that have been hunted or caught by fishermen.

Having established this fake situation, the Meat Board then goes on to push the panic button. "Since some complete protein—including all of the essential amino acids—should be included in every meal, these figures indicate more meat, rather than less, is needed for protein in a readily available form." We will deal with the protein lie directly in a moment. First we'd like to point out that their impassioned plea for more meat so we can have more "complete" protein ignores the "complete" protein provided by dairy products. In fact, if one is comparing usable protein, dairy products provide protein of higher absorbability and biological value than does any kind of meat. Certainly, the Live Stock and Meat Board should advocate consumption of more dairy products rather than more meat if their main concern is that Americans get more "complete" protein.

As we've shown in the chapter on protein, however, the entire concept of "complete" versus "incomplete" protein is outmoded. Proteins are important as sources of amino acids. Different foods contribute different amounts of the essential amino acids to your body's amino acid turnover pool. As long as you get the necessary essential amino acids and your needed total amount of protein over a day or so, your body's protein needs are well taken care of. And an all-plant diet, as well as a diet including dairy products, is an excellent way to get the protein you need. You certainly don't need meat for that.

Various Vitamins and Zinc

Thiamin. Thiamin is one of the more difficult nutrients to find all in one place. We normally fulfill our needs from a variety of sources, and it is indeed found in many foods. Among meat products, the only standouts as thiamin sources are pork products, beef liver and kidney, and some shellfish. Other meats are somewhere around the middle of the continuum, better than some foods and worse than others as a source of the vitamin. To put it in perspective, one stalk of broccoli gives as much thiamin as does a three-ounce serving of beef (except the organ meats). Other superior vegetable sources include peas, beans, nuts, seeds, wild rice, and orange juice.

Riboflavin. Meat is indeed one of the best sources of this vitamin. Other rich sources include dairy products, especially fresh milk, and mushrooms. Dairy products give a lacto-ovo-vegetarian enough riboflavin, but other than the sources listed above, there are few excellent sources of the vitamin; rather it is found in small amounts in many foods. Vegans may have some difficulty getting enough riboflavin unless they pay attention to their sources. Deficiency is very rare, though, even among people eating a limited diet, and the symptoms are rather minor. This indicates that we may have an as yet undiscovered source that protects us from severe deficiency. No score for meat.

Niacin. Again, meat is one of the most concentrated sources. Since niacin is used for energy release, muscle cells must have especially rich stores. But the vitamin is found in so many foods that a concentrated dietary source hardly seems necessary except to account for other dietary insufficiencies. Pellagra, the disease of niacin deficiency, has virtually disappeared in this country because of a general improvement in nutrition and an increased breadth of choice for foods, coupled with fortification of many "white" grain products and cereals. Legumes, potatoes, fruits, seeds, and many grains are vegetable sources, and dairy products are also good sources.

Vitamin B$_6$. Meat is often cited as the primary source of this vitamin in nutrition textbooks and, indeed, in the standard American diet it does fulfill that role. When comparing calories per unit of the vitamin, a wide variety of vegetables, especially green vegetables and potatoes, rate as superior sources. The need for this vitamin increases with increased protein intake, so eating meat can actually increase your vitamin B$_6$ requirement if it boosts your protein intake significantly.

Vitamin B$_{12}$. Vitamin B$_{12}$ is required in truly infinitesimal amounts—a maximum of four micrograms (for pregnant or lactating women) according to the RDA. All animal protein foods provide the vitamin, and this is the most common source in the

American diet. However, vitamin B_{12} originally comes from non-animal organisms and is simply passed along in animal foods (meat and dairy products). Vegans have very rich sources in various fermented vegetable products (tempeh, kombu, etc.), but these are uncommon in the United States. The difference seems to be cultural: If a vegan were living in Japan, for example, the vitamin B_{12} question would never arise, since these vegetable sources are commonly eaten. People who don't eat sources of the vitamin obviously should take a supplement. There are relatively few vegan sources, but animal products don't represent some broad panoply of foods, either. In an ideal world where animal products were not consumed for food, people would very likely look askance at those who did not eat fermented vegetable products, citing the likelihood of a vitamin B_{12} deficiency to show that those foods must of necessity be included in the diet.

You need a source of vitamin B_{12}. Meat provides the vitamin; so do dairy products and several vegetable foods. Pick your source, it doesn't matter which you use in terms of your dietary need for vitamin B_{12}.

Zinc.   Meat is a good source of this nutrient, as are eggs, milk, and whole grains. Much has been made of the fact that whole grain contains phytic acid, which unites with various minerals, notably calcium and zinc, making compounds that may be indigestible for some people. The catch is that these *phytates* can be broken down by the enzyme *phytase,* present in the intestinal tract of people who are accustomed to a whole-grain-based diet. This makes the mineral available again. A generally adequate and varied vegetarian diet should have no lack of usable zinc, since most cases of zinc deficiency have appeared with other essential-nutrient deficiencies.

On the other hand, zinc is somewhat less absorbable from nonanimal sources, so vegans will have to take more care than lacto-ovos or omnivores that their diet provides adequate amounts. Since dairy products provide a suitable source for the many vegetarians who use them, meat can't legitimately get a score on zinc.

Iron

Iron plays a special role in the study of nutrition. It is the only nutrient often still deficient even when people get an otherwise adequate diet, whether omnivore or vegetarian. Women have a greater need than do men, and children's need is proportionately greater than adults'. In fact, adult men are the only group who nutritionists say consistently meet their iron requirements.

Meat is a primary source of iron in a highly absorbable form. Even so, only 10 percent of this iron makes it across your intestinal wall, because our absorption mechanism is apparently rather inefficient. Most of the iron in meat comes from the traces of blood left after the animal is slaughtered and butchered, although some of it is present in every muscle cell. The liver is the body's storage depot for iron, so it obviously provides the largest dose when eaten.

No plant sources approach meat as a rich source of iron, but beans, potatoes, green vegetables, dried fruit, molasses, winter squash, strawberries, tomato and prune juice, and some grains do supply large amounts of this mineral. Although spinach was once considered a good source of iron, it has been shown that spinach's iron is unabsorbable. Cooking food in iron pots can increase the iron content of the food significantly, especially acid foods.

A still unanswered question is why so many Americans don't get enough iron. A self-described "conservative" estimate claimed that two thirds of young American women are short of iron. The iron RDA for women in this age group is 18 milligrams, but even meat-eaters (the majority) don't get enough. Some nutrition writers say the reason is the lessened consumption of the many excellent vegetable sources listed above. Another reason may be the trend away from cast iron and steel as cooking media.

It is hard to determine how our prehistoric ancestors fulfilled their iron needs, since their primary foods were plants, and not much of them. Meat was a luxury, probably eaten seldom, so it couldn't have provided much of their requirement. Why did we humans evolve with a nutritional need that seems to be so hard to fulfill, whatever our diet? No one has a clear answer. While we fumble along, trying to understand, we must take care of our nutritional needs as best we can. In the case of iron, it seems that many of us, irrespective of our particular diet, need a supplemental source.

Phosphorus and Potassium

Meat provides both of these essential nutrients in abundance. However, the Meat Board's pamphlet implied, inadvertantly or not, that these minerals "cannot be duplicated in plant foods." Wrong. Primary sources of potassium are fruits and vegetables, equivalent to or surpassing meat. And every cell provides phosphorus, although in general muscle cells have more of it than do plant cells. Unfortunately for meat-eaters, meat provides miniscule amounts of calcium to go with its phosphorus. Calcium and phosphorous must be in rough balance in the diet to promote optimum bone mineralization. A disproportionately high phosphorus intake can cause bone calcium loss. Although some plant foods give lots of phosphorus with little calcium, this is not generally true of an all-plant diet, nor of one that includes dairy products. Meat represents a calcium drain in a diet because of its high phosphorus content.

Vitamins A and B12

The Meat Board says plant foods can't duplicate vitamins A and B12. We have already looked at the question in relation to vitamin B12. The claim is false on its face. But what about vitamin A?

What they say is literally true—you can't get vitamin A from plants. The chemical name for Vitamin A is *retinol,* and it is synthesized only by animals. The obvious conclusion, at least obvious from their dishonest presentation, is that you need animal products to get vitamin A. Nothing could be further from reality. Humans are animals, and they synthesize vitamin A from plant chemicals known as *provitamin A,* mainly the pigment carotene. Carotene is abundant in a wide variety of commonly available plant foods, such as carrots, spinach, and broccoli.

An added advantage of getting your vitamin A from plants is that you are less likely to get an overdose. Your body has certain physiological controls on how much carotene it converts to retinol, and thus on how much retinol is present in your body tissues. When you consume preformed retinol, your body has lost its control over its tissue retinol level, which can rise to toxic doses. Arctic explorers have become deathly ill from the retinol present in a single meal of polar-bear liver. While this delicacy is admittedly uncommon on most Americans' dinner tables, the example is still illustrative of the dangers of retinol overconsumption, even from natural sources.

ROUND TWO

The pro-meat forces have presumably taken their best shot, and have made a limited score on one count—iron. Now it's time to look at the picture from the other side. What's bad about meat (and good about a diet that avoids it)?

Meat is high in saturated fat.

Different meats provide moderate to high levels of cholesterol.

Meat is deficient in carbohydrates in general and fiber in particular.

Most commercially available meat is from animals raised with the use of antibiotics and growth-stimulating hormones.

Meat products as produced in this country may contain disease organisms such as salmonella and trichina. They must be handled and prepared carefully to avoid any risk of infection, and this careful handling seldom takes place.

Diseased and cancerous animals are butchered and sold as "wholesome."

A common curing agent called sodium nitrite found in many pork products and prepared meats unites with amines to make a powerful carcinogen.

Meats prepared according to standard cooking methods, including broiling, charcoal broiling, and even stewing, produce carcinogens and mutagens such as benzo(a)pyrene, malonaldehyde, and methylcholanthrene.

The minerals that accompany meat are generally acid in their effects on the blood, and this can lead to demineralization of the bones to return the blood to a normal acid-base balance.

Finally, several epidemiological studies have shown a statistical link between increased meat consumption and increased incidence of coronary heart disease and various cancers, particularly colon cancer.

Let's look at these issues in detail.

Saturated Fat

Meat and dairy products are the primary sources of saturated fat in Americans' diets. In fact, meat itself is composed totally of protein and fat, much of which is saturated fat. Fat accounts for 30 percent of the calories in very lean sirloin steak *after cooking,* and that is one of the leanest cuts of beef you can get. Of that 30 percent, nearly half is saturated, and only one fiftieth is polyunsaturated. The other common red meats are similar to beef in make-up, while fish and poultry are generally lower in total fat and give slightly more polyunsaturated fatty acids. However, no meats can approach an equal distribution of saturated, monounsaturated, and polyunsaturated fatty acids. The remainder of the diet must take up the slack for meat.

Beef is the meat of choice in this country, so we use it most often as an example in our illustrations. Of course, the other flesh foods eaten modify beef's impact on the diet. In terms of saturated fat and total fat, much depends on individual preferences—if you eat a lot of chicken or fish (assuming you eat flesh foods), your total and saturated fat will be much lower than if you eat various prepared meat products such as salami and sausage or the more fatty cuts of red meat, like prime rib. As we have shown above, one of the leanest cuts of red meat has precisely the maximum fat level recommended by the Dietary Goals. If that was the highest-fat meat you ate, you should have little trouble staying within the recommended maximum in the rest of your diet. Unfortunately, you must carefully balance off the other fat sources in your diet to make allowances for the heavy preponderance of saturated fatty acids in meat fat.

Of course, saturated fat is available from other places besides meat. Milk products have butterfat (full-fat milk and cheese, butter), whose distribution of fatty acids is as bad as that of meat. Egg fat found in egg yolk is about one third saturated, as the Goals recommend, but only one tenth polyunsaturated and the rest monounsaturated. A very few vegetable fats have tremendous amounts of saturated fat—coconut, palm, and cocoa. It is obviously possible to have a problem with saturated fat, even if you eat no meat. The only advantage for vegetarians is that saturated fat is easier to avoid—the saturated fat in meat is integral and can't be removed.

Since we're the home team and we're keeping the score, we'll give the meat people the benefit of the doubt on this issue. You *can* avoid most of the saturated fat in a meat-eating diet by carefully planning your diet and balancing your food sources. Careless vegetarians may have a problem equal to meat-eaters', so we won't chalk up a score for vegetarianism on this one.

Cholesterol

The Meat Board is cautious on this issue. They say that meat is not a primary source of cholesterol, although it does contain a certain limited amount. In comparison to eggs and butter on an equal weight basis, its content is relatively moderate. Of course, who eats three and a half ounces of butter as a serving? The fact is that any meat can be a major contributor to your day's cholesterol intake. Beef has 70 milligrams in every 100-gram serving. Meats like veal, which are lower in fat, are even higher in cholesterol. Organ meats are worst of all—liver, touted by the Meat Board as an excellent source of iron and vitamin B_{12} (which it is), has 300 milligrams in a single serving. If one of your two daily servings of meat happens to be liver, you are getting too much cholesterol. In fact, many organ meats have disproportionately high concentrations of cholesterol—brains, considered by some a delicacy, have incredible amounts, as much as 2000 milligrams in a three and a half ounce portion. Vegetable foods have none, and if a lacto-ovo-vegetarian switches to low-fat varieties of dairy products and doesn't eat too many eggs, it is easy to stay below 300 milligrams. Even so, since meat in general can't push you over the limit by itself, we won't claim a score.

Carbohydrate and Fiber

As we mentioned before, meat is all fat and protein. It has no carbohydrate at all, and certainly no fiber. Since the Dietary Goals call for 58 percent of calories from carbohydrate (48 percent from natural sugars and starches and 10 percent from added refined sugar), the rest of your diet must take up the slack for meat. Again, you must do a balancing act with the remainder of your diet to get the necessary carbohydrate. Vegetarians have no such problem, since even milk products contain some carbohydrate in the form of lactose. A vegetarian's diet gives protein, carbohydrate, and fat from the whole diet in almost every food eaten. Because a meat-eater gets his protein and fat in such a concentrated package, he must balance the rest of his diet with the meat to get his other necessary nutrients.

And meat is totally deficient in fiber. Fiber protects against colon cancer and high blood cholesterol, among other things, and this is especially important for someone who eats meat, as we show below in our description of meat's relation to cancer. How unfortunate it is, then, that the food that makes fiber so much more necessary should contain none of it.

Antibiotics and Hormones

Factory-farmed animals are fed antibiotics from the time they are weaned (or hatched) to the time they are slaughtered. The antibiotics, such as tetracycline and penicillin, are added directly to the animal feed, and fed to every animal in the feedlot, regardless of its health or sickness.

If you have ever received a prescription for tetracycline or penicillin, your doctor may well have told you to finish the prescription and take it exactly as directed, even if you feel better before the dosage period is over. The reason is that a certain blood level of the drug must be maintained for a certain period of time to be sure all the disease organisms have been killed. Otherwise, you may be killing the weak and susceptible ones, leaving the strong ones to return in a full-blown and much less treatable infection. Over repeated exposures, bacteria may begin to develop resistance to antibiotics if they aren't killed the first time around.

In addition, bacteria can transfer an acquired resistance from one to another, creating whole new strains of antibiotic-resistant infections. The effectiveness of any antibiotic depends on its being used forcefully and properly, and only when it is necessary, so bacteria will have as little chance as possible to develop a resistance.

No such care is taken with the drugs fed to meat animals. The doses are constant and relatively small, suitable only for the nuisance infections to which animals kept without fresh air and exercise are prone. Although required by law to make sure no antibiotics are in the flesh of their animals when they are slaughtered, many farmers sell meat with residues of powerful chemicals in it. These antibiotics enter your body and do exactly what they are supposed to do—kill bacteria. Because they are present in trace amounts, however, they simply further the evolution of tougher strains of bacteria through unnatural selection, weeding out the weak and especially vulnerable, as we described above.

Some people experience nausea or allergic reactions when they take certain antibiotics. If they suffer the same symptoms when they eat meat, they are unlikely to make the association with the antibiotics in it.

If this weren't bad enough, the animals themselves become individual factories on their own—factories for disease organisms resistant to treatment with the available and least physiologically stressful drugs. The situation became so alarming that the FDA proposed banning these two drugs (tetracycline and penicillin) as feed additives. Of course, the farmers and the pharmaceutical industry lobbied vigorously against the ban, and Congress blocked the action. You make your own decision. In two European countries where these drugs have been banned in animal feed, a 25 percent decrease in resistant bacteria infections has been reported.

Growth-inducing hormones represent another issue entirely. The most commonly used is called *diethylstilbestrol* (DES). This isn't really a hormone, but a synthetic analog that mimics the action of normally occurring hormones. It adds bulk and fat to the bodies of cattle and chickens, increasing the poundage and thus the price paid per animal. The use of DES is carefully regulated, because it is a powerful carcinogen whose effects last *even to the second generation* in humans. Animals must not be fed the drug fourteen days before slaughter, according to the Meat Board's pamphlet, so that any residues can be cleared out of the animal's system.

Slaughtered animals are not tested for DES, except for a few spot checks, so farmers have little inducement to switch their animals' feed two weeks before slaughter. In addition, no one can guarantee that the withdrawal period assures that not a single molecule of DES remains in an individual animal's carcass. Contrary to the Meat Board's view on carcinogens in general, there is no such thing as an infinitesimal amount of *any* carcinogen, particularly one as potent as DES. Carcinogens apparently do their dirty work by turning off a cell's growth control mechanism. The cell then grows out of control, forming a tumor. Only one cell need be affected, and only one molecule of a carcinogen is needed to do it. Of course, the statistical probability decreases as the concentration does, but it never reaches zero until the concentration reaches zero.

Finally, the chemical gives the meat-buying consumer no advantage. The hormone boosts weight, if it does so at all, by increasing fat, both around and in the flesh. Feedlot animals get very little exercise, so they are flabby anyway (read that "tender"). Their increased retention of calories simply means more fat on the body, not more muscle. DES is thus a high-tech meat extender, stretching the same amount of muscle tissue further by diluting it with flab.

So much for the benefit to the consumer.

Salmonella and Trichina

It is a standard rule that you have to cook pork thoroughly to kill the trichina organisms encysted in the animal's muscle. Far fewer people realize you can get trichinosis—complete with diarrhea, nausea, fever, stiffness and swelling of muscles, sweating, and insomnia—from ground beef as well. The disease organisms aren't picky about whose muscle they inhabit, and they are quite happy to go along for the ride when they are transferred from pork to beef through poor handling and sanitary conditions at local butchers. In the past few years more cases of trichinosis in the state of New Jersey have been traced to contaminated beef than to pork. The organisms can be transmitted on a knife, a countertop, hands, or in a meatgrinder (the most common).

Even when meat is contaminated with trichina, the organism can be killed by raising the temperature of the meat to 58°C (137°F). during cooking. Much evidence indicates this precaution is not always taken. Autopsies regularly report presence of trichina in from 1.5 to 4.5 percent of the population. Suits against restaurants alleging infections of trichina from poor food preparation are reported regularly. Recently, a group of famous and not-so-famous diners recovered damages from Trader Vic's Restaurant, in New York, claiming they got trichinosis from insufficiently cooked spare ribs.

Salmonella poisoning is not nearly as dangerous, although it appears to be much more common. The fever, cramps, nausea, and vomiting of the disease rarely cause any permanent harm to normal adults over the few days it takes to run its course, but infants, older people, and those who are already sick can die from the stress of dehydration and fever. The Center for Disease Control in Atlanta estimates that 2 million people get salmonellosis every year. Although salmonellosis can come from your water supply or even from improperly processed powdered milk, the most common source is poultry and meat. Meat is so often contaminated that public health services warn of handling it with bare hands and then touching your face before washing. Raw and cooked meat should never be prepared on the same surface, because the sterilized cooked meat could pick up the bacteria from the surface touched by the raw meat.

One other organism bears looking at: *Clostridium botulinum.* To destroy this dangerous bacterium in pork products, meat packers use sodium or potassium nitrite. We talk about this dangerous and potentially cancer-causing additive under "Nitrosamines."

Diseased Animals Butchered and Sold

The U. S. Department of Agriculture (USDA), the federal agency responsible for regulating the meat industry, reports that it is standard meat inspection practice to approve portions of animal carcasses for consumption *even when the rest of the carcass is condemned as unwholesome.* Meat inspectors routinely "retain" slaughtered carcasses when they show signs of disease. But when the "bad spots" are removed, like cutting a bruise out of an apple, the remainder is generally passed and given the USDA seal.

The diseases and disorders contracted by farm animals are many and varied, from tuberculosis to pesticide residues to cancer. Somehow the USDA's assurances of the safety of this method of cleaning up the product so it can be sold aren't completely convincing. Cancer victims know that simply removing a tumor doesn't mean the cancer is gone—they must submit to lengthy and debilitating treatment merely to increase life expectancy a couple of years, in some cases. In fact, surgical methods don't necessarily remove every single cancerous cell from a human or from any other animal.

Nitrosamines

You may have heard about the nitrite controversy. The meat industry claims that nitrites added to pork products and many prepared meat products such as bologna are necessary to prevent the growth of disease organisms in the meat and are harmless to humans. Critics claim that nitrites are there mainly for cosmetic purposes and that they can indirectly cause cancer.

Actually, nitrite is added to meat for both purposes—to make it look red and "fresh," and to block the growth of *C. botulinum,* the organism that causes the dread and often fatal botulism. *C. botulinum* seems to like living in dead meat (although it can also develop in improperly canned products), and as it grows it produces a potent nerve toxin, which accounts for the deadly effects of the disease—double vision, difficulty in breathing, muscle paralysis, and suffocation. The FDA approved nitrite as a meat additive because they felt the threat of botulism from meat products was so significant it overrode the dangers.

Recently, however, the FDA moved to have nitrite banned from meat products, claiming that other means were available to protect the public from botulism and that nitrites were implicated as a cancer risk. The ban was overturned in court.

The cancer risk factor in nitrites comes from the fact that nitrite combines with organic chemicals called *secondary* and *tertiary amines,* present in the intestine and in meat, to make *nitrosamines.* Although most responsible researchers agree that nitrosamines are dangerous, the Meat Board's pamphlet glosses over the risk: "never been shown to cause cancer in humans." They say this in spite of the fact that it has caused cancer in laboratory animals and even though potential carcinogens will *never* be tested on human beings. A chemical that causes cancer in one animal species usually, but not always, causes it in others.

We can't yet prove that specific chemicals cause cancer in humans. A conclusive research project on humans would be impossible, because it's unethical—in fact, it's abhorrent—to knowingly give another human being cancer. This certainly expresses rather succinctly the standards that should be applied to the meat producers' use of nitrite for curing.

The Agriculture Department noted recently that meat products now contain so little nitrite that the risk they pose is minimal. It is up to you to determine how minimal is minimal for yourself, but it is heartening to know that meatpackers have decreased their use of this dangerous additive.

Nitrite is also found in some vegetable products as well as in meats. Some vegetables, such as carrots and spinach, have a naturally high content of nitrate, a related compound. When these are stored unrefrigerated, particularly if they are chopped or ground and cooked, the nitrate is converted to nitrite. The concentration is so high that it can be directly poisonous, especially to infants, by interfering with hemoglobin production. Obviously, foods should not be stored this way for a variety of very good reasons.

If you eat vegetable foods that contain some nitrite, you don't face the same risk as from the nitrite in meats. Nitrosamines are formed when the nitrite combines with amines, available naturally in meat. Vegetables generally don't have these amines. Luckily, vitamin C can completely block the formation of nitrosamines, even when the necessary secondary and tertiary amines are abundant. Since vitamin C is common in many vegetables, it protects us from the nitrites they contain, even though our own intestinal contents can provide the amines to make the carcinogen.

The risk of cancer from nitrosamines is significant in meat treated with nitrite and nearly nonexistent in nonmeat foods. Since some strides have apparently been made in reducing the nitrite content of meats, and thus the danger, we'll be optimistic and not claim a score against meat on this issue.

Carcinogens from Cooking

You can avoid nitrite, you can avoid pesticide residues, and you can even avoid antibiotics and hormones by eating organically raised unpreserved meat, but how do you avoid the carcinogens you create when you cook meat?

Cooking meats at high temperature, for example, grilling or roasting, causes various amino acids and fat components to be converted into mutagens or carcinogens. Meat fat becomes *methylcholanthrene,* a potent carcinogen on its own and a cancer potentiator as well (helps other carcinogens do their nasty work more efficiently). One 3.5 ounce serving of charcoal broiled steak has as much *benzo(α)pyrene* as the smoke from *three packs* of cigarettes. Finally, during the digestion of meat, some of your bile salts form *malonaldehyde,* another mutagen and carcinogen.

Some would claim that these chemicals are safe until proven otherwise. After all, they have been shown to cause cancer in other species, not humans. The U. S. Congress, however, in the much-argued Delaney Amendment to the Food, Drug, and Cosmetics Act, stated that any chemical that causes cancer in any testing situation is unacceptable as a food additive. If food additives aren't safe under these conditions, are naturally occurring food components any more so?

You may think you can avoid these chemicals by not using high temperature, i.e., broiling or frying, to cook them. The alternative is stewing or slow-cooking. Even though this cooking method reduces the concentrations of carcinogens, you are still not safe. Recent research indicates that low temperature cooking produces another class of as-yet unidentified mutagens in meat. The longer a meat is cooked, even in water, the higher the concentrations become. The chemical or chemicals are powerful mutagens, according to the Ames bacterial mutagenicity test. A mutagen produces changes in a cell's genetic code. Although this is not proof positive of carcinogenicity, it is considered strong evidence.

Acid Ash

Meats, poultry, and eggs are classed as *acid ash* foods because their effect on the blood chemistry is to push it toward the acid end of the scale. When your body receives a load of acid ash, it must use its internal control system to keep the blood in a very narrow range on the acid-base scale. The most important part of the control system centers around calcium. Calcium tends to bond with acid ions (much of which are phosphate ions, mentioned earlier), neutralizing their acidity. In doing so, however, the calcium forms salts that are removed from the blood by the kidneys. This succeeds in removing the acid factors from your body, but it also succeeds in removing calcium.

It is crucial that your blood calcium level remain constant because calcium takes part in so many of the various metabolic systems in your body. When you lose calcium from your blood, it must be replaced from somewhere immediately. Luckily, your body has a huge reservoir of calcium in your bones, which it draws upon to balance your blood level.

The more acid ash you take in, the more calcium leaves. Meat, because it provides a particularly heavy acid load, drains more calcium from your body than do most other foods. Thus, you must consume much more calcium to replace your losses. If your losses are very heavy, your intestinal absorption can't keep pace with your replacement needs, and you have a calcium debt.

Meat-eaters apparently have a problem here. In a study that compared the relative bone density of matched omnivores and vegetarians, the vegetarians showed a very significant advantage. This apparently could be traced directly to the differences in diet, the absence of meat from their tables.

The implications of this problem are startling. Perhaps a lifetime of eating meat is the major cause of the brittle bones and slow-healing breaks of old age. Perhaps a vegetarian diet could reverse the process of chronic calcium loss, leading us toward a healthier old age.

Eggs also produce acid ash because of their high sulfur content. Since eggs are a part of a lacto-ovo diet, acid ash is not exclusively the province of omnivores. The study we cited above tends to indicate that calcium loss is more extreme in omnivores, but the dietary factor can't be ignored for vegetarians, so we'll refrain from claiming a point here. Keep in mind, though, that meat-eating is linked to lower bone calcium content.

Statistical Studies

A special branch of health statistics known as *epidemiology* compares the health records of entire populations and attempts to analyze the differences in their life styles that account for differences in their health. These studies generally can't prove links between habits and health, but they can make intriguing connections, which then bear further investigation.

Many studies comparing risk of heart disease and various types of cancer among different countries over and over found meat consumption as a significant factor.

Japanese people who immigrate to the United States begin to show an increase in the incidence of colon cancer over the course of a generation or two, as they slowly adopt the food habits of their new home. In Japan, where little meat is consumed, colon cancer is relatively rare. In the United States, colon cancer is the second worst cancer killer and meat is the "queen of the table." The researchers eliminated many variables, such as changes in pollution levels, and meat was one of the strongest indicators.

One study like this shows little beyond an interesting coincidence. The results have been duplicated, however, in comparisons among many countries. If countries are ranked on the basis of increasing per capita meat consumption, the incidence of colon cancer follows the same pattern. Meat consumption then becomes a very strong indicator of the incidence of colon cancer in a population.

The question arises whether this statistical linking of colon cancer to meat eating is more a factor of eating style (i.e., the high fat and sugar content of the diet and resulting obesity that are almost universally present with a high-meat diet, rather than simply the presence of meat. As it happens high fat consumption and obesity are both *independently* linked to increased colon cancer incidence. Still, meat-eating remains as a separate statistical risk in getting colon cancer.

Meat has similarly been linked to cancer of the breast and

prostate and to coronary heart disease. In one of the most striking studies, men from an American religious group (Seventh Day Adventists) that discourages smoking, consumption of alcohol, and consumption of meat showed a life expectancy more than six years greater than the general population's. Much of this increased life expectancy was due to their avoidance of smoking and drinking, but since not all Adventists are vegetarian, comparisons can be made between meat-eating and vegetarian Adventists, eliminating many of the other environmental factors that might affect the study outcome.

Lacto-ovo-vegetarian Adventist men have only two thirds the heart-disease mortality of their meat-eating coreligionists. Total-vegetarian Adventists showed only 36 percent of the heart disease mortality rate. These factors are in additons to the advantage all Adventists have in not smoking or drinking—meat-eaters still had only 64 percent of the mortality of the general population.

A similar trend can be shown for meat consumption and its relation to breast cancer. Adventist women who ate meat less than three times a week showed 85 percent of the incidence of breast cancer in the general population. Vegetarians had only 65 percent. Adventist women who ate meat more than five times a week, however, had a rate of breast cancer incidence well above that of the general population.* The main difference among the Adventist groups was obviously their intake of meat.

THE FINAL SCORE

You've seen the contest. Let's see how the sides fared.

Meat got a score on iron, although this point was modified somewhat (since most meat-eaters don't fill their need for iron any more than do vegetarians).

Meat got scored against heavily on these points: carbohydrate; fiber; antibiotics and hormones; trichinosis and salmonellosis; diseased animals; benzo(a)pyrene, malonaldehyde, methylcholanthrene, and other unknown mutagens; statistical links to colon cancer, breast cancer, and coronary heart disease. We gave away points on saturated fats, cholesterol, nitrosamines, and acid ash to be good sports, although the dangers are greater from these in an omnivore's diet.

*Reason unknown.

Home (vegetarians)	0	1	1	1	1	1	1	1	Total: 7
Visitors (meat-eaters)	1	0	0	0	0	0	0	0	Total: 1

HOW HARD IS IT?

Throughout this dietary comparison, we have assumed that a meat-eater's diet met the Dietary Goals set by the Senate Select Committee on Nutrition and Human Needs. Getting this good a diet is difficult for a meat-eater, however. It's not easy for a vegetarian, but we have certain innate dietary advantages.

We get our protein from our entire diet, not in a concentrated package that omits crucial carbohydrate. Remember, according to the Dietary Goals more than half our daily calories should come from carbohydrate. Since meat has none at all, the rest of the diet bears a heavier responsibility to provide it. Likewise, meat has no fiber. Although fiber is actually a carbohydrate, we can treat it as a separate nutrient because our bodies deal with it differently. Fiber is necessary for a variety of reasons, and again the rest of our day's calories must provide a disproportionately higher contribution of fiber to make up for meat's lack.

Meat has two main dietary components—protein and fat. About half that fat is saturated, and only a miniscule portion is polyunsaturated. Again, since the proportion is so far off the rest of the diet must balance it. Meats vary in their content of the different types of fatty acids, of course, as do all other foods. The general trend is toward a gross overrepresentation of saturated and monounsaturated fatty acids and a gross underrepresentation of polyunsaturated fatty acids.

In addition, many meat-eaters will find it difficult to lower their protein intake even to the excessively high levels proposed by the Dietary Goals. We have pointed out elsewhere the health disadvantages of a too-high protein intake. It is much easier to avoid on a vegetarian diet.

CONCLUSIONS

Meat is not a particularly useful part of a good diet. As a matter of fact, is has some powerful disadvantages, both from the point of view of its direct effect on health and from the point of view of trying to eat a well-balanced diet.

Whatever your reasons for becoming vegetarian, you can add health benefits to the list. Meat is simply not good for you.

GUIDELINES

We can't even compare the standard American diet to a vegetarian way of eating. Americans eat very poorly in spite of or because of their wealth and economic development. Thus we compare vegetarianism to an "idealized" meat-eating diet.

Meat is an excellent source of iron, which may otherwise be rather limited in the diet.

The other contributions of meat to your health include too much saturated fat and cholesterol, a carbohydrate and fiber gap, hormones and antibiotics, bacteria and parasites, various carcinogens and mutagens, a drain on your body's store of calcium, and an increase in your statistical risk of coronary heart disease and various cancers.

It is more difficult to eat a good diet when you include meat because it is more difficult to keep fat and protein to reasonable levels and increase carbohydrate and fiber consumption.

Wouldn't it be safer to supplement iron and skip the meat?

When you kill for food, your food will return the compliment.

DAILY LIFE

Shopping and Storing
Branching Out from Your Own Recipes
Eating Out—and Other Matters

12
Shopping and Storing

You can know an encyclopedia's worth about nutrition, but it is the boxes and bottles you finally buy that ultimately determine how well you are treating yourself. Put another way, once you know how to eat, it's important to know how to shop. They go hand-in-hand.

The first thing to realize is that you are up against a multibillion-dollar industry whose sole purpose is to convince you to "buy me." The advertising experts have tested what colors attract you, what size letters you like, what words you respond to. They have put together packages so they seem like just the things you need, whoever you are. Their foods are just like mother used to make, make your children happy, ease and enrich your life. Some of them appear on television or in magazines so often they seem like old friends, reliable and satisfying. These products mean to grab you at a level beyond nutritional sense and they often succeed. In fact, sometimes they make no nutritional sense at all.

It is up to you to sort through the words and decide what to buy—not an easy task when you are being emotionally manipulated. The best advice we can give you is to be informed and careful. That's not always easy, either. Sometimes foods seem to be what they are not. Ingredient labels are not always complete, and terms like "natural" are used indiscriminately. "Fresh" and "wholesome" are never literally true; indeed, Hostess Twinkies are advertised to be so. You can, however, buy the best that is offered. Usually, there is at least one fairly unprocessed choice. More than likely, you'll make compromises. It's almost impossible not to. But once you are informed, it is you who decide where to draw the lines.

READING LABELS

One important way to inform yourself is to read the labels of the products you buy. You might balk at first at the time and trouble involved, but once you make the initial effort, you know as a matter of course which brands or items are best. Just recheck periodically in case a change has been made.

Actually, if you eat most of your food in as whole and fresh a state as possible, reading labels isn't quite as necessary. It is the processed and ready-made foods that must be put in nutritional perspective. If you buy fresh string beans, for example, all you get is the vegetables themselves, their vitamins and minerals naturally intact. If you buy canned string beans, however, look for added salt, sugar, or citric acid, as well as the loss of some nutrients. Even seemingly whole, unprocessed foods like nuts and dried fruit sometimes have preservatives added.

Whether you want to eat foods containing additives is, of course, up to you and has little to do with vegetarian nutrition per se. Unfortunately, additives are often unnecessary replacements for things that have been removed or unhealthy additions that obviously weren't there to begin with. We recommend *Eater's Digest* by Michael F. Jacobson for an objective look at food additives. As we said, it is a matter of where you draw the lines. Certainly, additives don't contribute to your nutrition.

Labels provide a fairly good look at your options, although there is much room for improvement. The Food and Drug Administration's code of regulations sets the requirements that must be followed by food manufacturers. The rules are still rather incomplete, although they are changing for the better every year. Revisions have been suggested by the FDA, Department of Agriculture, and Federal Trade Commission, but some of these changes must be initiated and approved by Congress. With all the red tape and politicking involved, a major overhaul could take several years. The results would be worthwhile if all the ingredient and nutrient contents were required to be listed on the labels of all foods. Unfortunately, the food conglomerates would pass the extra costs along to shoppers rather than face a nip in profits, while smaller companies, among which are the most conscientious, might not be able to afford such changes at all. We hope any overhaul would address these problems fairly, keeping the consumer in mind.

As you can see below, the information on labels now is often incomplete or presented in a confusing format. With luck, it will change. Here's how it works as of this writing.

Ingredient Labels

Certain standardized foods, such as jam, mayonnaise, and ketchup, have actually been defined by the federal government. These "Standards of Identity" include the mandatory and optional ingredients a particular food may contain as well as the specified amounts or proportions necessary before the food name can be used. Because the mandatory ingredients must always be the same, they do not have to be listed on food labels. The optional ingredients, which include many additives, may or may not have to be listed. It all depends on the particular definition. The result is that you can never be sure exactly what you're eating, even if you have the federal code by your side.

That mayonnaise in your refrigerator, for example, *must* contain vegetable oil (not less than 65 percent by weight), vinegar or lemon or lime juice (not less than 2.5 percent), and egg or egg yolk. It *may* include salt, a sweetener, any spices or natural food flavorings that don't give a yellow, egglike color, monosodium glutamate, and calcium disodium EDTA or disodium EDTA (as a preservative). Of all the optional ingredients, only the EDTA must be on the label. Not much help for someone who is on a sodium- or sugar-restricted diet or is allergic to a particular spice.

Changes are being made all the time, however, and it is a good idea to keep up. According to R. E. Newberry, assistant to the director of the FDA's Division of Regulatory Guidance, the old standards are being revised to require declaration of all optional ingredients. Congress is also considering a bill that would call for listing of all ingredients in standardized foods. Some companies already do this voluntarily.

Standardized foods include margarine, milk chocolate and other cocoa products, flour, white and whole-wheat bread and rolls, milk and cream, natural and processed cheese, salad dressing, canned vegetables, canned fruit, and fruit juices, among others. If a food is labeled "imitation," as are some salad dressings and mayonnaise brands, it doesn't contain all the mandatory ingredients set by the federal government and is not, by definition, that food. "Imitation mayonnaise," for example, might not contain eggs. In this case, however, the "imitation" brand could well be healthier than its regular counterpart.

If a food does not have a standard of identity—a prepared cereal, for example, and most processed foods—all ingredients, including additives, must be listed on the label in descending order of predominance according to weight. Specific names must be used, except in the case of spices, natural and artificial flavorings, colorings, and chemical preservatives, which may be listed in those general terms. Even individual ingredients sometimes have definitions in the federal code. For example, the "eggs" in the mayonnaise ingredients can be dried, frozen, or liquid varieties.

Use of artificial flavors, colors, and preservatives, incidentally, must be stated on the labels of all, including standardized, foods. The only exceptions are butter, cheese, and ice cream, which for some reason don't have to list artificial colors.

Reading ingredient labels is especially important for vegetarians. Animal products pop up in the most unexpected places. Be on the lookout for gelatin, which is made from animal byproducts; animal shortening or just "shortening," which could be lard; mono- and diglycerides, which can come from either vegetable oil or animal fat; and beef and chicken stock, found in such innocent-seeming foods as vegetable soup.

Unfortunately, ingredient labels don't tell what percentage of a particular ingredient is present in a food. Furthermore, ingredients such as sugar are sometimes broken down into components like corn syrup, dextrose, and fructose and scattered throughout the listing, which can be very deceptive because there is no indication what portion of the food these sugars occupy. *Caveat emptor.*

Nutrition Labels

The FDA requires nutrition labeling for all foods that have been "enriched" with nutrients, such as many cereals, and all foods hawking nutritional claims or information, such as "twice as much protein." (The only exception is sodium content.) Included are foods made available for special diets, such as diabetic ice cream or infant formula.

All other nutrition labeling is voluntary, but if a food company does include it, labels must comply with the requirements set by the FDA.

The nutrition information label must include:
1. Serving size
2. Servings per container
3. Calorie content
4. Protein content
5. Carbohydrate content
6. Fat content
7. Percentage of U. S. RDA for protein, vitamins A and C, thiamine, riboflavin, niacin, calcium, and iron

The U. S. RDAs, formulated by the FDA, are based on the RDAs established by the Food and Nutrition Board. Needs were determined (and are periodically revised) for four groups: infants, children under four, children over four, and adults and pregnant or lactating women. For nutrition labeling, adults and children over four are usually considered, unless the product is aimed specifically at one of the other groups.

The fact that there are RDAs and U. S. RDAs can be confusing, but you'll probably come across U. S. RDAs only on nutrition labels. Just remember that the Food and Nutrition Board's RDAs are more current and are the basis for the U. S. RDAs. We use the FNB's RDAs in this book.

Nutrition labels may also include optional information about the amounts of saturated and polyunsaturated fatty acids, cholesterol, sodium, and other vitamins and minerals. It is obviously quite a help, although unusual, when the fat calculation, for example, is broken down this way. Unfortunately, it is not also done for carbohydrates. There is a substantial difference, after all, between 40 grams of complex carbohydrate and the same amount of simple sugar. So read labels and take advantage of the information you do find. If what you want or need to know isn't provided, here are several guidelines that might help:

1. Write to the manufacturer. Ask for the information you want and encourage a more complete labeling system.

2. Avoid foods that list sugar as the first or second ingredient.

3. If the ingredients sound like they come from a laboratory or the package brags about its vitamins and minerals, look twice. A reasonable amount of fortification, such as vitamin D in milk or iodine in salt, has undeniably been beneficial to those who weren't getting enough otherwise, but many food companies have gone too far, and vitamin-padded junk food is being peddled as "nutritious,"

a supposed alternative to real, whole food. You might as well take a vitamin pill and be done with it. Check the ingredients when possible to see how those nutrients are (or aren't) supplied.

4. To decide what percentage of calories in a food come from fat, multiply the grams of fat per serving by 9 (remember, 9 calories per gram of fat), divide that number by the number of calories per serving, then multiply by 100.

$$\frac{\text{grams of fat per serving} \times 9}{\text{calories per serving}} \times 100 = \begin{array}{l}\text{percentage of}\\ \text{calories from fat}\end{array}$$

If sugar is listed separately, as in many prepared cereals, you can do the same thing, only multiply the grams by 4.

$$\frac{\text{grams of sugar per serving} \times 4}{\text{calories per serving}} \times 100 = \begin{array}{l}\text{percentage of}\\ \text{calories from sugar}\end{array}$$

For example, 10 grams of sugar in a 110-calorie serving is 36 percent (10 grams × 4 calories per gram ÷ 110 calories per serving × 100 = 36 percent of calories as sugar).

5. If the nutrition label doesn't break down the fat content into saturated and polyunsaturated, look to the ingredients. Remember that coconut and palm oils, as well as animal fat, are highly saturated. Unspecified "vegetable oil" probably means coconut or palm as well, because they are cheap for the manufacturer.

6. If you avoid processed foods, you generally avoid the whole labeling problem. As a rule, the shorter the ingredient list, the more natural the product.

7. Remember that additional claims in big letters like "all natural" and "no preservatives" are usually advertising ploys and often deceiving. Take a closer look. "No preservatives" doesn't necessarily mean no additives, and "natural" can mean anything.

WHERE TO SHOP

Supermarkets

Many people think vegetarians do all their shopping in health food stores, and, indeed, some vegetarians wouldn't be caught dead in a supermarket. This may be a case of reverse bias, however. It is definitely possible to wade through all the processed foods bedecked in their brightly colored re-finery and find unadulterated food, including excellent brand-name products. Unless you insist on organic food, here are some of the foods you can find in supermarkets: dairy products, eggs, fresh fruit and vegetables, canned goods such as olives, cereals, grains, bread, molasses, raisins, dates, juices, ricotta, mozzarella, other natural cheeses, wheat germ, herbs, olive oil, cottage and farmer cheese. If your supermarket doesn't have a brand you want, ask for it and tell them why. If they don't respond, look into other supermarkets in the area. Some good qualities to look for in a supermarket: fruits and vegetables you can select individually, a cheese counter for a larger, fresher array of cheeses, a natural foods area, exemplary brands of many foods, prompt removal of damaged produce and expired products, a clean, well-organized store.

Produce Markets

Indoor and outdoor fruit-and-vegetable stands are popping up everywhere. They can be excellent sources of fresh produce, especially if they buy from local farmers and don't jack up the prices too much. They may even offer organic produce.

Talk to the owner about his or her sources. He or she may have contacts beyond the general wholesale markets, which can result in better quality food. If your market has farmland in back, this does not necessarily mean they grow their own. It could just be a part of their image, so check into it.

Prices may depend on where you live. They could reflect overhead rather than the availability of food. Compare prices around town.

Make friends with the owner. Get advice on what's in season, what's especially good today, which melon is perfectly ripe. A friendly owner may sell you items from the back room—fresher stock not yet for sale.

Produce markets often carry other types of food as well—gourmet products, nuts and seeds, dried fruit, and natural foods. You might find it one of the best places to shop year round.

Health and Natural Food Stores

The terms "health food" and "natural food" are frequently used interchangably. In fact, you probably don't know which term would be more appropriate for your local store. It could be—and likely is—a hybrid. Originally, however, there was a difference. Since the early 1900s, health food enthusiasts have relied heavily on protein, vitamin, and mineral supplements to try to improve their health. More recently, the natural foods movement came into being, espousing organic and naturally processed foods as the key. The result is that you can never be sure what you will find in your local health (natural) foods store. As in any other store, you should assume nothing, especially since neither movement is essentially vegetarian. In the freezer case, for example, you will find a wide selection of organic meats. Read your labels in this store, too.

The entire concept of organic food is controversial. Within the United States, there are at least 25 different standards for "organically grown" foods. Some health food stores even sell produce marked "organic" when it is not. Don't confuse "organic" with "natural." Organic refers to the growing conditions—no pesticides used, no chemical treatment. Natural refers to the processing of the food—no additives, no artificial color or flavor, no additional sugar. The apricots used in that "natural" juice were probably not organically grown unless the label says so. It gets confusing. Take raw milk, for example. Often the milk has been heat-treated—not pasteurized, but certainly not raw. The label doesn't tell you that, however.

Here, again, you must draw your own lines. Organically grown food is generally more expensive and not always available. It might not come in the forms you like and might not even by truly organic.

On the other hand, it has no synthetic chemical residues, with their inherent risks. There is certainly much to be said for food that is residue free. It takes a bit of extra effort to eat all organic food, depending to some extent on where you live. Get to know your retailer and his or her standards and sources of supply. If you are going to the extra trouble, at least make sure it's worth the effort.

Eating naturally processed (natural) whole food is easier, and we have recommended it throughout the book. Whereas organic food is not necessarily more nutritious (it is the pesticides that are being avoided here), natural food definitely is. As we said, many such foods can be found in your supermarket. Certain foods that can't are often found in natural or health food stores: dried fruit and seeds without preservatives, raw nuts, organic and vegetarian vitamin and mineral supplements, sea salt, raw honey, stone-ground whole grain flours, vegetarian soap and other cosmetics, jams made with honey, natural peanut butter, unrefined oils, bread, a wide selection of unsweetened juices, tamari, raw milk, rennet-less cheese, soy products, and organic food.

Sometimes the owner of the store will order in bulk for you with a discount of 5 to 10 percent. Look into it.

Mail Order

Mail order sources are a good, and often cheaper, way to buy natural and organic food, and you can send for just about everything you could find in a natural foods store. Deliveries are usually through United Parcel Service. Walnut Acres (see appendix) also has truck delivery in certain areas. Mail order is an excellent way to purchase: whole-grain cereals and bread, unsweetened juice, raw honey, bran, dried beans, whole wheat flour, raw nuts, dried fruit, salad dressing, soup, jam with honey, unrefined oils, seeds, ketchup, mayonnaise, and much else. Send for catalogues at the addresses listed in the appendix.

Co-ops

Joining a co-op is also a good way to buy wholesome food at low prices. Co-ops work in various ways, but the point is that a large group of people can order in bulk and pay wholesale prices by sidestepping the retailer. Try to find out about any such groups in your area. Word-of-mouth is probably the best way. Some co-ops even have established stores. If there is no co-op in your area, consider starting one. Your library probably has several books on the subject.

Specialty Shops

These shops include cheese, gourmet, and ethnic specialty stores that may carry items you can't find anywhere else, such as fresh pasta, chickpea flour, and chili peppers, as well as numerous spices. You will, however, pay extra because these foods are generally unavailable elsewhere. Even so, cheese shops offer a huge, international selection, and ethnic shops are very handy when you want delicacies from various cuisines. Italian and Mexican groceries are often good places to find canned beans without preservatives. You are more apt to find such shops in urban areas or where there is a large concentration of a particular ethnic group. Look in the yellow pages under "cheese," "gourmet," and "delicatessen" for possibilities.

SELECTING AND STORING FOOD

Generally, we suggest that you read labels carefully, and avoid refined and overprocessed foods, additives and preservatives of all kinds, including stabilizers, emulsifiers (except lecithin), bleaches, and dough conditioners, and foods with too much sugar and fat. Instead, look for whole, fresh foods—those closest to their natural state. As vegetarians, you must also look for animal products in the ingredients.

Air, light, heat, and moisture are the great destroyers of nutritional quality, so keep food well-wrapped in a cool, dark place or the refrigerator.

We don't have the space to advise you on the specifics of choosing and storing every kind of food. We have selected a few, however, to give you an idea of what to look for and what to look past. For a complete guide, we recommend *The Supermarket Handbook* by Nikki and David Goldbeck.

Flour

White flour is just whole wheat flour that has been stripped of the bran and germ and then chemically bleached and aged. The result is a product with much less protein and virtually none of the vitamins (B,E) and minerals (iron, phosphorus) of the original. White flour is then "enriched" in order to put back what was removed, albeit in lesser quantities. Sometimes, dough conditioners are added, too, so that the enriched white flour is "phosphated" or "bromated" as well. What is left is a battered and inferior wheat product that caters to the esthetic that white is pure and good. That always was a simple-minded theory.

Instead, buy whole wheat flour (preferably stone-ground, for the best preservation of nutrients) for making bread and such and whole wheat pastry flour for other baking needs. At the very least, use unbleached white flour, although there really is no reason to do so. Experiment, too, with other types of flours—rye, soy, buckwheat.

Store in a cool, dry place, well sealed, or, better yet, refrigerate to keep weevils out and flour fresh. Incidentally, one bay leaf stuck in the flour bag helps to keep bugs out.

Grains

Americans seem to have settled into a pattern of using only certain "starches"—rice and pasta, to be specific. There are whole new fields of grain to try, however, and they not only supply complex carbohydrates but protein and B vitamins, too. Stock your kitchen with millet, bulgur, rolled oats, and wheat berries, for starters. Buy them whole and unseasoned; there should be no ingredients listed on the package. Use them, basically, as you would rice.

As for rice, it has a story similar to that of wheat flour. White rice has been debranned and polished, then "enriched" to compensate for the substantial protein, vitamin, and mineral losses incurred in the process. In the fast-cooking varieties, the rice has also been chemically treated. Buy brown rice instead. It is available in most supermarkets, takes just a little longer to cook, and has more flavor and nutrients than its refined counterpart. "Converted" rice retains more nutrients than does plain white rice, but it is still not as good as brown.

Pasta is usually made with white flour, although a few brands include wheat germ and yeast in the ingredients. Choose those brands or imported Italian pasta like DeCecco brand, which is made with a high-gluten (higher in protein) flour. These high-protein pastas compensate somewhat in taste and nutrition for the fact that they are not whole-grain products. Better yet is whole wheat pasta, which is also available and is, of course, less refined and more nutritious. Pasta made from Jerusalem artichoke flour is another possibility—higher in protein and lower in starch, though. Both can be found in natural food stores, if nowhere else. Try them.

Store grains, tightly sealed, in a cool, dry place to avoid bugs.

Sweeteners

By now, almost everyone knows to avoid sugar. Refined white sugar is perhaps the worst culprit, since it has been stripped of all nutrients, with only sweetness and calories remaining. Vegetarians, especially, should avoid this product: Charred beef bones may have been used in the refining process.

Brown sugar, used in many "natural food" recipes, is merely refined white sugar with molasses added. Raw sugar also is not what it seems; only the final processing steps have been eliminated. Still, if sugar must be used, go with the raw (or turbinado) type. It has a tiny bit more to offer.

Honey is the traditional alternative to sugar. It is still mainly a source for sweetness, but was processed naturally by bees, which makes it more emotionally appealing, although morally questionable for some. Buy raw, unfiltered brands, which have not been heated and contain all the original traces of nutrients. Explore all the varieties—from clover to buckwheat. Still, use sparingly. It doesn't contribute to your health (and, as we mentioned earlier, has been shown to cause botulism in infants.)

Molasses, on the other hand, does contribute to health. Blackstrap molasses is the byproduct of sugar refining and contains all the iron, calcium, and B vitamins that white sugar doesn't. It has a very strong taste, however, and is usually used only as a partial replacement or flavoring. Try unsulfured molasses, too, for a milder treat with the same nutrients.

Another tasty sweetener is maple syrup. You can find a multitude of uses for it beyond pancakes if you think of it on a par with honey. Buy 100 percent pure, though—not the maple-flavored varieties. Just check the ingredients of the imitators to find out why. Canadian brands are preferable, because it is illegal there to treat the trees with formaldehyde to increase sap flow. Some New England maple processors say "no formaldehyde" on the label. Again, use sparingly.

We include jams and jellies in this section, too, since they usually contain more than half sugar. Jam is one of those foods with a standard of identity, and the federal code allows 45 percent fruit ingredients, 55 percent sweetener. Note the term "fruit ingredient" and don't assume that's fresh fruit unless they brag about it. The sweetener can be sugar, invert sugar, syrup, dextrose, corn syrup, or honey. Only the use of honey, strangely enough, must be stated on the label. Other "hidden" ingredients may be an acidifying agent (vinegar, lemon or lime juice, citric acid, fumaric acid), pectin (sometimes with preservatives of its own), sodium citrate, sodium potassium tartrate, and an antifoaming agent (butter, lard, margarine, cottonseed oil, mono- and diglycerides). The antifoaming agents alone should make vegetarians think twice. Your best bet is a natural foods brand made with honey and lemon juice. Read the label, though. Some say, in large letters, "made with honey," but a closer check of the ingredients list reveals the use of sugar and corn sweeteners as well.

Store molasses, maple syrup, and opened jams in the refrigerator. Keep honey and raw sugar in well-sealed containers at room temperature. And don't use any of them very often.

Nuts and Seeds

Nuts and seeds are best eaten right out of their natural packaging. Many people are unfamiliar with the raw product, however, having always eaten the "cocktail" varieties, which are roasted or fried in oil and highly salted. Even dry roasted brands add sugar, salt, and preservatives. No need. Nuts and seeds are perfect as they are.

Buy nuts in the shell, if possible. The shell is nature's way to individually wrap, keeping in freshness and nutrients. If you need large quantities and shelling would be inconvenient, vacuum-packed brands offer the best protection, despite the fact that you can't see what you're buying. Skip those brands with extra oil, salt, or preservatives. If you prefer your nuts roasted, try doing it at home instead. The heating process destroys the amino acid lysine, so set the temperature below 300°F and don't brown them much to minimize the effects.

Generally, follow the same rules for buying seeds: avoid the roasted, salted, preserved varieties. Seeds are usually hulled already. If you can't find them in your supermarket, try the natural foods store.

For nut butters, don't buy the commercial brands, which almost always contain a total of 10 percent salt, sugar, and hydrogenated vegetable oil. Instead, buy a natural foods brand or make it yourself by blending nuts with a touch of extra oil in a blender or processor. It tastes far better and is better for you. Don't limit yourself to peanut butter, either. Try walnuts, almonds, cashews, and pecans, too.

Store nuts and seeds, covered, in a cool, dark place. Opened vacuum-packed nuts and all nut butters should be refrigerated. After a few months, nuts may go stale or rancid. Check periodically.

Oils

Vegetable and nut oils are known for the delightful fragrance and flavor they add to cooked dishes and salads. Each one has unique qualities, from fruity, flavorful olive to mild, light sesame oil. Beyond their culinary virtues, most are low in saturated fats and high in polyunsaturates. The only ones to avoid are coconut and palm oil. They are high in saturated fat and cheap, so you will find them in many processed foods you should be avoiding. None contain cholesterol.

The commercial oils found in most supermarkets are usually extracted by chemical solvents such as hexane, a petroleum product. They are then often highly refined by chemical treatment, filtering, and bleaching to increase the oil's smoking temperature and add to shelf life. The processes destroy both flavor and nutrients.

The alternatives are cold-pressed and expeller-pressed oils. Cold-pressed oils use no heat and are basically limited to certain brands of olive oil. Expeller-pressed oils go through a screw-type press that does employ some heat. Unfortunately, many oils calling themselves cold-pressed are actually expeller-pressed. In any event, either type is preferable to chemical extraction.

Buy cold-pressed or expeller-pressed oils that are unrefined with no preservatives except, perhaps, vitamin E. Virgin oil is best. Avoid all-purpose blends with no particular flavor and cheap ingredients. Any preservatives will be listed on the label.

Store your oils in light-resistant glass jars in a cool place. It is best to refrigerate them once they've been opened. Always use pure vegetable, seed, and nut oils rather than hydrogenated or animal products.

Salt and Soy Sauce

Salt should be only sodium chloride, but most brands in the supermarket contain sugar, sodium bicarbonate, iodine, sodium silico aluminate, and preservatives. Pure sun-dried sea salt is often suggested as the alternative and is said to have greater amounts of trace minerals. The difference in nutrients is very minor, and we have heard that not all "sea salt" comes from the source it claims. On the other hand, sea salt doesn't have the additives listed here, either, except for magnesium carbonate to prevent caking. The best we can suggest: Whatever brand of salt you choose and whatever its source, make sure it is free of additives and sugar.

Soy sauce is a strongly flavored salty liquid seasoning that can often be used in place of plain table salt, especially in cooking. Check the ingredients, though. Real soy sauce, or tamari, is made from soybeans, water, salt, and wheat. Many imitations include caramel coloring, sugar, and preservatives.

Store salt in a tightly sealed container at room temperature. In humid climates, you can add raw rice to it to prevent clumping. Keep tamari in the refrigerator to avoid molding. Use salt and tamari very sparingly. If you are really hooked on salt, try low-sodium alternatives which combine sodium chloride with potassium chloride.

Milk

Almost all the milk available in supermarkets and elsewhere is pasteurized and homogenized. Pasteurization is a heat process that destroys harmful bacteria. Homogenization distributes the butter fat evenly throughout the milk. You don't need the fat—it's only there for taste.

Skim milk contains less than 1 percent fat. Low-fat milk has 1 to 3 percent fat. Whole milk has 3¼ percent or more. Protein, calcium, phosphorus, and B vitamins are present in all types. Unfortunately, the less fat there is, the fewer fat-soluble vitamins (A, D, and E) remain in milk. Skim milk is usually enriched with vitamins A and D, however, and we recommend it as a good way to cut down on animal fat. If you are drinking whole milk, switch to low-fat first for an easier transition.

Some people swear by certified raw milk, which has been government inspected to meet sanitary requirements but has not been pasteurized and thus retains the vitamin C, thiamine, and enzymes destroyed in the heating process. Some "raw milk" has been heat-treated, however, to a temperature just short of pasteurization. The nutritional difference would then seem to be minor.

Yogurt, a bacteria-cultured milk, is rich in all the same nutrients as milk. It's an extremely versatile food that is also kind to the digestive tract. (The bacteria cultures have broken down the lactose, or milk sugar, that many adults can't digest in regular milk.) Read labels, especially on the flavored yogurts, which sometimes contain artificial flavors, colors, and additives. Remember that even pure fruit preserves are more than 50 percent refined sugar.

Keep milk and yogurt in the refrigerator, preferably in tinted glass bottles to retain vitamins. If the bottle or carton is dated, buy and use accordingly. In any case, consume as soon after purchase as possible.

Butter and Margarine

Ideally you shouldn't use either butter or margarine. Separated fat, whether butter, oil, or margarine, is unhealthy because it is very calorically dense, it displaces important nutrients while providing little in the way of nutrition itself, and it may be dangerous to your health.

That said, we realize that most people do use one or the other and will continue to do so. You should choose the best, however, whatever you use. If you use very little, whether for spreading or cooking, use butter. Note that "very little" here means less than a pat a day (one pat of butter or margarine is half a tablespoon). Under these circumstances, the high saturated fat content of butter makes such a small contribution to your diet that it is offset by its lack of processing, preservatives, and other unnecessaries. Even so, substitute vegetable oil for butter whenever you can; for example, in cooking.

If your usual diet contains a large amount of fat, consider using margarine. This is difficult for us to recommend, because we are, if nothing else, philosophically opposed to the use of such a manipulated and altered foodstuff. But butter is just too high in saturated fat for you to entrust your arteries to it (or encrust your arteries with it, as the case may be). We can't state strongly enough that you should decrease the quantity of separated fat in your diet. You receive enough from whole foods to supply your needs without including any extra.

For butter users, the top quality is US Grade AA or US 93 Score sweet cream butter. There is no need to buy salted butter; the salt is there only to disguise off flavors. Did you ever notice that unsalted butter costs *more* than salted? That's because the unsalted has to be better quality—there is no salt to cover up poor taste.

In buying margarine, read the label carefully. Many packages list the grams of saturated and polyunsaturated fatty acids in a serving (usually a tablespoon, although that may be wishful thinking on the manufacturers' part). Almost all brands that supply such a list show 2 grams of saturated fat in a serving, which is equal to about 1 gram in a pat. The polyunsaturated fatty acid content ranges from about 3 to 5 grams per serving (1.5 to 2.5 grams per pat).

The ingredients are equally important. Many margarines use artificial flavor to try to imitate the taste of butter. They also commonly use preservatives and emulsifiers to maintain the product in salable condition as long as possible. Unfortunately, the more the oil is polyunsaturated, the more preservative is required to keep it from oxidizing and turning rancid.

If the label fails to tell how many grams of fat are polyunsaturated, you can still get an idea from the ingredients list. If the first entry is "liquid vegetable (or corn or some other specific name) oil," then the largest part of the oil in the margarine is polyunsaturated. If the first-listed ingredient says "hardened" or "hydrogenated," the margarine is much lower in polyunsaturated fatty acids. The presence of palm or coconut oil is a giveaway that the polyunsaturated content is low. Cottonseed oil is a common ingredient about which we have great reservations. Cottonseed oil is obviously a byproduct of the cotton industry. Since cotton is not grown primarily as a food crop, the same care is unlikely to be exercised in protecting consumers from pesticide residues. Since many pesticides are fat soluble, this question is even more worrisome.

A pat of butter provides a bit more than 3 grams of saturated fatty acids, and negligible polyunsaturated fatty acids. The very best margarines give only 1 gram of saturated fat and as much as 2.5 grams of polyunsaturated. Substituting margarine for butter in your diet can have a significant effect in changing your polyunsaturated/saturated ratio (P/S ratio) to the high side, especially if you now eat quite a bit of butter.

If you want to try for a middle ground while using the best ingredients possible, you can try blending butter and safflower oil, half and half. The saturated fat content will be decreased by more than one third, and the polyunsaturated content will almost equal the best margarine. The mixture will be nearly fluid at room temperature, so you'll have to keep it well chilled.

Cheese

The problem with using cheese for some lacto-ovo-vegetarians is that it is often made with an enzyme from the gastric secretions of calves and pigs. To further complicate matters, it is impossible to know for sure whether or not this enzyme, rennet, has been used in a particular cheese. Most natural food stores carry cheeses that specifically have no rennet, but unless the label of a cheese says so, the only way to find out is to write to the manufacturer and ask.

Always buy natural cheese rather than processed cheese, cheese food, or cheese spread, which are heated cheese blends laced with various additives. You will know a cheese is natural if the name is alone on the label or preceded by the word "natural." (American "cheese" is an exception.) Even natural cheese may have additives, however, as it has a standard of identity that includes these chemicals as optional ingredients. Some must be on the label; others may not. Here are a few guidelines:

Preservatives must be on the label.
The use of bleached milk will be on the label.
Imported cheeses are more apt to be free of additives.
Buy white Cheddar instead of orange, which may be artificially colored.
Buy soft cheeses, like cottage cheese and ricotta, that don't have added stabilizers listed on the label.
Be aware that most hard cheeses have a lot of salt. You can tell by the taste.
Store cheese, tightly wrapped in plastic wrap, in the refrigerator. Some, like Cheddar and cream cheese, may be frozen. Ask your retailer.

Bread

First and foremost, use whole-grain breads. If you have questions, anyway see our section on flour.

Whole-wheat bread, as well as white and raisin, has a government standard of identity. It can contain only whole wheat flour (for whole-wheat bread, that is); water; salt; shortening (including animal shortenings) with added emulsifiers such as mono- and diglycerides; milk or a milk product; egg; sweetener; dried yeast; and a host of other food and synthetic additives, most of which do not have to appear on the label.

Specialty breads, such as rye, pumpernickel, or sprouted grain, must list all ingredients. Many whole-wheat breads do so on a voluntary basis, as well.

We see no reason not to know what you're eating when you can. In other words, buy breads that have nothing to hide and tell you what is in them on the label. Don't be fooled by deceptive names with "old-fashioned" or "homemade" in prominent letters. Make sure the bread is free of dough conditioners like sodium stearoyl-2-lactylate, polysorbate 60, and others; mold inhibitors such as calcium or sodium propionate; emulsifiers such as mono-and di-glycerides (except lecithin); animal or hydrogenated shortening; and preservatives. Remember, a label may proclaim "no preservatives added" and add any of the things listed here that have other functions.

Instead, look for whole grains, honey and molasses (rather than sugar and corn syrup), and fresh dairy products on the label. Locally made French and Italian loaves are often made simply from flour, water, yeast, and salt. Your bakery could be a good source for all kinds of bread. Ask about their ingredients to be sure. Or bake your own.

Store bread in a plastic bag in the refrigerator. It should stay fresh a week or more. It can also be frozen for months with no ill effects.

Fruits and Vegetables

Try to use fresh produce whenever possible. The fact that it is seasonal seems to make each fruit and vegetable that much more delicious when it is available. Fruits and vegetables in season are at their peak quality and usually lowest price. In their freshest, raw state they are at their nutritional peak also.

Select your produce according to freshness, color, shape, and size. Pick those items that look in their prime—not wrinkled, wilted, or bruised. Try to find those of characteristic color and shape. A misshapen item is usually inferior in taste and texture as well. Medium sizes are generally favored. A too-large vegetable or fruit is often tough and not as tasty. Tiny ones may be immature.

The longer a fruit or vegetable sits, the more nutrients it loses. Chilling slows the process, but often you can't be sure how long your produce was out before or after refrigerated shipment. It is conceivable that frozen produce could be of higher nutritional quality. Here again, though, you don't know whether it was frozen at its peak or sat on a loading dock first.

Try to buy fresh produce according to the seasons and eat it as soon as possible. If what you want is not available, however, frozen is the next best thing. Here are some tips for buying frozen fruits and vegetables:

Don't choose packages that seem to have been even partially defrosted and then refrozen. Squeeze the package. If it squishes or is in one solid lump, chances are it was defrosted at one time. Stained packages are another tell-tale sign.

Buy plain fruits and vegetables, rather than those in a special sauce or seasoning.

Buy them in as whole a state as possible—preferably not peeled, diced, or julienned, which causes further nutritional loss.

Avoid the five-minute types of vegetables, which have been partially cooked, chemically treated, or both.

Avoid frozen potatoes, beets, and carrots, which most likely have been peeled with the help of a chemical treatment.

Look for frozen vegetables without added salt; fruit without added sugar.

Avoid additives. Check the label.

As for canned varieties, the fruits are better than the vegetables. Neither can begin to compare with fresh, however.

Buy canned fruit packed in its own unsweetened juice or water. Drink the liquid as well; it contains much of the nutrients. Avoid artificial colors, which will be listed on the label.

Avoid canned vegetables altogether, except for imported whole tomatoes, tomato puree and paste, artichokes, and olives, which often aren't available in any other form. Most other canned vegetables have been heated beyond recognition and usually contain additives as well. There are always better choices available in a fresh or frozen state.

Eating dried fruit is another good way to beat the season, if you're so inclined. Avoid brands bathed in sulfur dioxide to retain a bright, bleached color. Don't buy those with added sugar or preservatives, either. Both are completely unnecessary and will be on the label.

A shopping and storing chart for individual fresh fruits and vegetables follows. Remember to wash well or peel before eating, especially if you think something has been artificially colored or waxed on its surface.

FRUITS AND VEGETABLES CHART

For many fruits and vegetables, we suggest storage in the crisper of your refrigerator. However, if you notice that a food tends to wilt or dry out, keep in plastic wrap as well.

NAME	SEASON	CHOOSING	STORING
Apples	All year	Choose firm, unbruised fruit with intense color; avoid soft or punctured fruit, wax coating	Ripen a day or two at room temperature, then refrigerate in vegetable crisper
Apricots	June–July	Choose orange-yellow, plump fruit; avoid greenish, hard fruit	Ripen 2–3 days at room temperature, then refrigerate in crisper and use within a few days
Artichokes	all year; peak: March–May	Choose compact, plump, heavy globe with fleshy green leaves; avoid spreading leaves, leaves that are brownish or moldy	Refrigerate and use within a few days
Asparagus	March–June	Choose green, firm stalks with compact, closed tips; avoid angular or flat stalks, open tips	Refrigerate in crisper; Keeps up to 4 days
Avocados	All year	Choose bright, fresh-looking fruit, heavy for its size; avoid wilted or bruised fruit	Ripen at room temperature, then refrigerate. Sprinkle lemon juice on opened fruit to prevent discoloring and then cover
Bananas	All year	Choose plump yellow or green fruit; avoid bruises or splits	Ripen at room temperature, then refrigerate. Skin will turn brown, but fruit remains the same
Green beans	All year; peak: May–August	Choose fresh, green pods; avoid scars, discoloration	Refrigerate in crisper. Use as soon as possible
Lima beans	May–October	Choose fresh, well-filled dark green pods; shelled beans should be plump, tender, and green or greenish white	Refrigerate in crisper and use as soon as possible. Highly perishable

Item	Season; peak	How to select	How to store
Beets	All year; peak: June–October	Choose bunches with fresh tops; firm, well-colored roots small to medium-sized; avoid large, flabby, shriveled or rough beets	Remove tops and use as soon as possible or discard. Refrigerate beets in crisper
Blueberries	June–August	Choose plump, dry, bright blue berries; avoid shriveled berries, containers with stains	Refrigerate, covered, unwashed up to 3 days
Broccoli	All year; peak: October–May	Choose compact bud clusters, fresh green stalks and stems; avoid wilted, yellowed leaves, opened buds	Refrigerate in crisper and use as soon as possible.
Brussels sprouts	All year; peak: October–March	Choose firm, compact, bright green sprouts	Refrigerate in crisper and use as soon as possible
Cabbage	All year	Choose solid, heavy heads with few loose outer leaves; avoid yellow, wilted leaves with worm holes or blemishes	Refrigerate in crisper. Use within a week or 2
Cantaloupes (and persians)	May–September	Choose melons with a smooth, rounded, depressed scar at stem end; avoid rough stem end	Ripen 3–4 days at room temperature until fragrant and yellow, then refrigerate
Carrots	All year	Choose firm, smooth, well-shaped orange carrots; avoid soft, wilted, shriveled, cracked or rough carrots	Refrigerate in crisper
Casabas	July–November	Choose yellow fruit with slightly soft stem end; avoid dark water spots	Keep in a cool place

Item	Season	How to Select	How to Store
Cauliflower	All year	Choose clean, white, firm, compact head with fresh green leaves; avoid open flower clusters, spots, mold	Refrigerate in crisper. Use as soon as possible
Celery	All year	Choose crisp, thick, solid stalks with good heart formation; avoid very hard or soft stalks, seed-stems, discoloration	Refrigerate in crisper
Cherries	May–June	Choose firm, bright red to black fruit; avoid hard, light-colored, or soggy fruit	Refrigerate in crisper and use within 2 or 3 days
Chinese cabbage	All year	Choose crisp, compact heads; avoid wilted, yellowing leaves	Refrigerate in crisper. Use within a week
Coconuts	September–January	Choose heavy, full nuts that slosh when you shake them; avoid dry nuts, moldy or wet "eyes"	Refrigerate and use as soon as possible
Sweet corn	All year; peak: late spring, summer	Choose corn in fresh, green husks with thin-skinned, bright kernels, kept cool and out of the sun; avoid dry, strawlike husks, warm corn	Refrigerate and use as soon as possible
Cranberries	September–December	Choose plump, firm, highly colored berries; avoid shriveled, dull, soft or sticky berries	Refrigerate and use within a week or so. Can be frozen
Cranshaws	July–October; peak: August–September	Choose a golden yellow rind that is slightly soft and has a rich aroma; avoid watermarks	Ripen at room temperature, then keep cool and use soon

Item	Season	How to Select	Storage
Cucumbers	All year; peak: May–August	Choose unwaxed, well-shaped green cucumbers; avoid large, shriveled, yellow, dull cucumbers	Keep cool. Use within a few days
Dates	All year	Choose shiny brown, plump, soft fruits	Keep well wrapped. Refrigerate after opening package
Eggplant	All year; peak: August–September	Choose firm, heavy, lustrous eggplants; avoid wilted, shriveled, soft, flabby, scarred, or worm-injured fruit	Keep cool; Use as soon as possible
Endive (escarole, chicory)	All year	Choose fresh, crisp, cold greens, avoid dry, yellowing, wilted, or discolored leaves	Refrigerate in crisper. Use as soon as possible
Figs	August–October	Choose soft-ripe figs; avoid mushy figs with a sour odor	Refrigerate. Use immediately. Highly perishable
Grapefruit	Peak: September–April	Choose firm, springy, globular fruits; avoid soft, wilted, loose-skinned or pointed fruits	Keep at room temperature or refrigerate
Grapes	July–November	Choose smooth, plump, well-colored grapes firmly attached to stem; avoid sticky, soft, wrinkled grapes; dry, brittle stem	Refrigerate in crisper and eat within a week or so
Honeydews	All year; peak: June–October	Choose creamy yellow, velvety melons; avoid white or greenish rind, soft spots	Ripen 2–3 days at room temperature, then eat or keep in cool place
Kohlrabi	May–November; peak: June–July	Choose firm, crisp stem, green, fresh tops; avoid too-large stem	Refrigerate in crisper and use within a few days

Item	Season	Selection	Storage
Leeks	All year; peaks: September–November, spring	Choose fresh, green tops, medium-sized necks; avoid yellow, wilted, damaged tops	Refrigerate in crisper
Lemons	All year	Choose firm, heavy, rich yellow, fine-textured fruit; avoid off colors, shriveling, soft spots	Keep at room temperature or refrigerate
Lettuce	All year	Choose clean, crisp, tender heads, iceburg should be fairly firm; avoid seedstem, ragged brown leaves	Refrigerate in crisper and use soon
Limes	All year; peak: June–August	Choose bright colored, heavy fruit; avoid dull skin, brown spots	Keep at room temperature or refrigerate
Mushrooms	All year; peak: November–April	Choose firm, white mushrooms with slightly open caps revealing light-colored gills; avoid open caps, pitting, wilting, discoloration	Refrigerate in crisper. Use as soon as possible
Nectarines (peaches)	June–September	Choose smooth, plump, well-colored fruit; avoid hard, greenish, dull or shriveled fruit	Ripen at room temperature 2–3 days, then refrigerate and use as soon as possible
Okra	May–October	Choose young, tender, pods 2–4 inches long that snap easily; avoid dry, shriveled, discolored pods	Keep in a cool place and use soon
Onions	All year	Choose bright, hard, well-shaped onions; avoid seedstems, sprouts, moisture at the neck	Keep at room temperature or refrigerate

Item	Availability	Selection	Storage
Papayas	All year; peaks: May–June, fall	Choose well-colored (at least half yellow) smooth fruit; avoid shriveling, too much green, bruises	Ripen at room temperature, then refrigerate. Use soon
Parsnips	October–April	Choose smooth, firm, small to medium well-shaped parsnips; avoid soft, shriveled roots, discoloration, overlarge parsnips	Refrigerate in crisper
Pears	August–March	Choose firm, blemish-free fruit; avoid shriveled, misshapen, wilted fruit	Ripen at room temperature until slightly soft. Refrigerate when ripe, eat as soon as possible
Peas (green)	January–July	Choose well-filled evenly green pods kept cool; avoid off-colored, immature pods	Refrigerate in crisper and use as soon as possible
Peppers (sweet)	All year; peak: May–October	Choose fresh, firm, bright, thick-fleshed fruit; avoid soft or dull-colored fruit	Keep in a cool place
Pineapples	March–June	Choose large, heavy golden fruit with deep green, fresh crown leaves and rich fragrance; avoid brown leaves, discolored or soft spots	Refrigerate in crisper. Won't ripen. Use as soon as possible
Plums	June–September	Choose full-colored, plump, not hard fruit; avoid soft, discolored fruit	Ripen at room temperature 3–4 days, then refrigerate
Potatoes	All year	Choose fairly smooth, well-shaped firm potatoes; avoid sprouts, cuts, green color, wilting	Keep in a dark place away from extreme heat or cold

Item	Availability	Selection	Storage
Radishes	All year; peak: March–May	Choose fresh, green tops, smooth, well-shaped, crisp radishes; avoid pits, cuts, wilting	Remove tops and eat or discard. Refrigerate radishes in crisper
Raspberries	June–August	Choose plump, tender, intensely colored berries; avoid wet, moldy, mushy berries; stained container	Refrigerate, unwashed, in covered container. Use as soon as possible
Rhubarb	January–June	Choose crisp, firm, deep red stalks; avoid wilted, thin, flabby, or oversize stalks	Refrigerate in crisper. Don't eat the leaves; they are poisonous
Rutabagas	All year; peak: winter	Choose heavy, firm, smooth, rutabagas; avoid cuts or punctures	Refrigerate in crisper
Scallions (also shallots)	All year; peak: April–August	Choose fresh green tops, medium-size necks, young, crisp, tender; avoid wilted or discolored tops	Refrigerate in crisper and use as soon as possible
Spinach	All year; peak: January–May	Choose fresh, green leaves; avoid discolored, wilted, crushed leaves; seed stems	Refrigerate in crisper and use as soon as possible. Highly perishable
Squash, summer	All year	Choose tender, young, crisp, heavy squash; avoid soft spots, tough skin	Refrigerate in crisper. Use soon
Squash, winter	Fall, winter	Choose heavy squash with thick flesh, hard rind, avoid soft rind	Keep at room temperature

Item	Season	Selection	Storage
Strawberries	All year	Choose bright red, well-formed berries with stems still attached; avoid white or green areas, moisture, mold, misshapen too-large or too-small berries, stained container	Refrigerate, unwashed, in crisper. Use soon
Sweet potato	All year; peak: October–April	Choose firm, well-shaped, smooth potatoes with bright, evenly colored skin; avoid cuts, worm holes, shriveling, wet, soft spots	Keep in a cool, dry place
Tangelos	October–January	Choose heavy, firm, thin skinned fruit with light orange peel; avoid blemishes	Keep at room temperature or refrigerate
Tangerines	November–January	Choose heavy, deep orange fruit; avoid mold, soft or wet areas	Refrigerate in crisper. Highly perishable
Tomatoes	All year; peak: July–August	Choose smooth, plump reddish tomatoes; avoid bruises, soft spots	Ripen at room temperature in paper bag with banana or apple, then refrigerate
Turnips	October–March	Choose smooth, firm, small to medium-sized turnips; young, fresh green tops; avoid wilted, coarse, overlarge turnips; yellowed, wilted tops	Remove tops and use or discard. Refrigerate turnips in crisper
Watermelons	May–September	Choose firm, symmetrical fruit, deep reddish flesh, black seeds; avoid white or pale green underside	Keep at room temperature until cut or refrigerate

TIPS FOR SAVING TIME IN THE KITCHEN

Make a shopping list before going to the store, with separate sections for each store you plan to visit.

Shop once a week. If you store food properly, this should be no problem.

Have a garden. It is the ultimate in fresh, nutritious food and *the* alternative to shopping for and storing fruits and vegetables.

A windowsill herb garden is another fresh timesaver.

Whenever possible or practical, cook double or triple the amount of food you'll need for a meal. Refrigerate or freeze the rest and use for lunch, snacks, and quick meals. This is especially good for grains, beans, dressings, sauces, loaves, and soups. For sauces and soups, freeze in ice cube trays, then bag to control the amount you want to defrost.

A food processer is often well worth its price in time and effort saved.

Foods to have on hand for snacks and quick, nutritious additions to meals include:

Quick fruits: apples, bananas, seedless grapes, pears, raisins, dried fruits
Bean flakes
Wheat germ (for thickening, on casseroles or cereal)
Shelled nuts
Hulled seeds
Sprouts
Canned beans, tomatoes (whole, purée, and paste), olives, artichokes, chilis (check labels)
Unsweetened applesauce
Pasta
Cheese
Oatmeal (for thickening)
Bread
Popcorn (a quick snack)
Nut butters
Tamari
Whole wheat crackers
Fresh tomatoes, especially cherry tomatoes
Fresh snap beans
Dried herbs
Whole-grain bread, muffin, and pancake mixes (check label)

Prepared sauces (check label)
Frozen vegetables (check label)
Cottage cheese
Yogurt
Whole-grain cereals
Carrot sticks, other precut raw vegetables
Unsweetened fruit and vegetable juices

GUIDELINES

Be as informed as possible so you can make your own decisions and compromises.

Read ingredient and nutrition labels and compare them whenever possible to get an idea of where the nutrients are or aren't coming from.

Various types of stores can serve you in differing ways. Get to know the strengths and weaknesses of those in your area. Try mail order, too.

Avoid refined and overprocessed foods, additives and preservatives, foods with too much sugar, fat, or salt.

Buy fresh, whole foods—as close to their natural state as possible.

Air, light, heat, and moisture destroy many of the nutrients in food. Keep food well wrapped in a cool, dark place or in the refrigerator.

13
Branching Out From Your Own Recipes

*T*his is not a chapter full of unrelated recipes. There are cookbooks for that, good ones that cover everything from split pea
soup to fettucine Alfredo.* The only problem with those books is
that they leave little to the imagination: You choose a recipe, buy
the ingredients, try it. Eventually, you develop a repertoire of
dishes, but they are random selections, separate entities. They are
most suited to dinner parties and special occasions when you can
plan ahead. They usually don't tell you how to use the leftover
string beans in your refrigerator, nor do they often suggest possible
variations on a theme. They offer few guidelines on how to make
everyday meals quickly, inexpensively, and nutritiously.

This is an idea chapter. It is for those days (weeks, months) when
you don't want to fuss, when you want to use what's already in the
kitchen. It is for simple, everyday fare.

We've put together a series of guidelines for experimenting with
basic recipes. We've included traditional breakfast, lunch, and
seven types of dinners, one for every day of the week. These are
general types of meals that can form the foundation for a simple
vegetarian diet. Choose whichever ingredients you wish from the
lists of possibilities. You can use the guidelines again and again,
each time with a different result. Or you can do it the same way
everytime, if you prefer. And of course, if you have a gourmet
bent, you can dress them up to your heart's content. All can be
lacto-ovo or vegan.

Our guidelines are not the last word on cooking or planning
menus. Our main purpose is to show you that cookbooks needn't
be the last word, either. You can put together your own meals,

*See Suggested Reading in the Appendix.

using your own taste and judgment. It's all in the attitude: Nothing is sacred.

If nutrition is an individual science, cooking is a personal art. Everything depends on your style, your time, your particular taste buds. One of the most-asked questions of vegetarians is: Doesn't it take a long time to chop all those vegetables? The answer: Everyone makes his or her own compromises. If you have the time and inclination, chop them by hand. If you have the money and inclination, buy a food processor. If you have neither the time nor the money, buy chopped frozen vegetables, and so on. Our post-script: There is more to vegetarianism than chopped vegetables!

Measurements in the guidelines are purposely vague or nonexistent. Decide for yourself how much of something you want to put in. We're not promising foolproof results every time. By their very definition, these are not tried-and-true. Sometimes your judgment will be off. If you've used good ingredients, chances are it won't be too bad even if it isn't perfect.

This fearless cook method calls for you to cast aside your preconceived ideas about what goes with what. How about peanut butter salad dressing, for example? Or breakfast for dinner and dinner for lunch?

Of course, don't throw out the baby with the bathwater. Take your knowledge of technique or your favorite recipes for sauces—anything that will open doors. Leave behind the strictures and fashions—those pieces of advice that have become your golden rules. You might start simply by substituting one thing for another in a particular recipe.

If others are relying on you for meals and you are afraid to disappoint them, make a dish you know along with the one you don't. Then it won't be a total loss no matter what the outcome.

Because we've kept things open-ended, it would be best for you to have at least one basic cookbook handy, especially if you are a new cook. Our guidelines assume some knowledge of cooking. Remember, we have limited ourselves in this chapter to variations on a few traditional meals. These suggestions are just a smattering of the possibilities. They are ideas for you to fall back on or take off from. You can use a food in a way we've neglected to mention, or you can use our method to expand other basic recipes. Be as unconventional as you like.

Generally, keep in mind that there are three basic ways to invent great vegetarian meals:

1. *Vary traditional vegetarian dishes.* An example is to add chopped vegetables to macaroni and cheese. Or use Swiss cheese instead of Cheddar. Or both.

2. *Substitute or leave meat out in meat dishes.* Favorite replacements are cheese or beans, but anything goes. It is often the sauce that makes a meat dish special. Try bean Stroganoff or mushrooms paprika. Sometimes you can substitute so many things that all that is left is a basic concept—sauce over grain, for instance.

3. *Improvise.* Make things up. Eliminate all fear of comparison by being completely original.

Another good source for experimentation is ethnic food. Italian, Mexican, Indian, Kosher-diary, Middle-Eastern, and Chinese cuisines all include wonderful vegetarian dishes. These foods needn't be unfamiliar to you or reserved for special occasions just because you don't share a particular heritage. Try them in nearby restaurants or make them from cookbooks. You don't have to be limited by authenticity, either. Make up your own combinations and variations. As an example, try hummus, a pungent Middle-Eastern chickpea spread, rolled in a Mexican corn tortilla. Or mix Chinese stir-fried vegetables into a bowl of steaming hot Italian pasta. Why not?

BREAKFAST

Breakfast is usually a fairly routine meal because we don't have the time in the morning to be creative or complicated. The fancier traditional breakfasts, such as pancakes or eggs Sardou, are often reserved for weekend brunches. There is no reason we can't be creative on a simpler scale, if only by varying the topping on our cereal, or eating just the topping: fresh fruit, cheese, unsalted nuts, raisins and on and on ad infinitum.

Cooked or cold cereal: oatmeal, kasha, barley, bulgur, shredded wheat, granola, rice

Toppings: cinnamon, honey, butter, salt, pepper, milk, dried fruit, fresh fruit, seeds, nuts, wheat germ, juice, shredded coconut, maple syrup, applesauce, yogurt, jam, cottage or farmer cheese

Whole-grain bread, toast, muffins, pancakes

Toppings: fresh fruit, ricotta, jam, honey, cheese, maple

syrup, butter, nut butter, tahini, yogurt, applesauce, applebutter, cottage or farmer cheese
Sprinkles: nuts, seeds, wheat germ, raisins, dried fruit

LUNCH

Lunch can be a large midday meal or a fast snack. More often it means soup, salad, or a sandwich, usually on the run, in a lunch-pail, at a restaurant, or between errands at home. Ideas for soups and salads are presented in the dinner section. We've chosen the sandwich as the traditional lunch to vary as follows:

Sandwich on any whole grain bread, roll, croissant, bagel, crackers, pita

Mix and match hot or cold:

Cheese	Dressing
Carrots	Leftovers
Lettuce	Scallions
Olives	Pickles
Beans	Cream cheese
Chilis	Onion
Fruit	Sauces
Peppers	Honey
Coleslaw	Radish
Marinated vegetables	Nut butter
Other vegetables, raw or cooked	Cabbage
Hard-boiled egg	Banana
Chutney	Watercress
Cucumber	Egg salad
Cottage cheese	Seeds
Jam	Relish
Avocado	Nuts
Mushrooms	Herbs
Tomato	Sprouts

SANDWICH SPREAD

Start with: cooked beans, cream cheese, cottage or farmer cheese, semisoft cheese, nut butter, tofu, avocado

Add: chopped vegetables (radish, tomato, celery, carrots, scallions, etc.), ketchup, sauce, yogurt, ricotta, grated cheese, mayonnaise, cottage cheese, herbs, salt, garlic, onion, sprouts, tamari, dried fruit, honey, seeds, dried milk, mustard, lemon, chopped egg, tomato paste, butter, pepper, nuts, juice
Blend all or part.

SAMPLE RECIPE—BLACK BEAN SPREAD

2 cups cooked black beans
juice of ½ lemon
salt
½ clove garlic

3 scallions, chopped
pinch of dill
½ teaspoon basil

Blend all ingredients.

DINNERS

Dinner is usually considered the most relaxed meal of the day, a time set aside to enjoy food, family, friends, thoughts, conversation. For many of us, however, the days are so full that it is often difficult to find all the time and energy needed to plan, prepare, and enjoy a big meal. We turn to convenience foods in boxes and cans that promise us "enrichment" to ease our consciences. Many people wouldn't consider being vegetarian because "nothing is faster than throwing a steak under the broiler." For them, dinner is a matter of "What shall we defrost tonight?"

The following dinner suggestions will ease your way a bit as a vegetarian. They offer solid advice on what to have for dinner but with the latitude to use what is in your kitchen: leftovers, food from your garden or grocery store. Each can be a main or side dish, not to mention lunch, breakfast, or snack. We reiterate: These are a few ideas; there are hundreds.

Pasta

Pasta, despite its reputation, is a healthy, versatile food. Besides being delicious, whole grain pasta is high in complex carbohydrates, protein, and B vitamins. Try pasta with anything. Here are three versions.

PASTA WITH TOMATO SAUCE

Chop: onion, garlic, celery, carrot, nuts, olives, peppers, capers, parsley

Sauté: in olive or other oil

Add: mushrooms, broiled eggplant, zucchini, broccoli, any other vegetables, cooked beans, raisins, pignolias

Add: chopped fresh tomatoes or canned, puréed, or paste (or any combination)

Plus herbs: basil, oregano, salt, pepper, tarragon, nutmeg, bay leaf

Plus wine

Simmer: to desired thickness

Thicken or thin, if needed: cashew butter, tomato paste or purée, stock, water, wine

Stir in: Ricotta, cream, Parmesan, other cheese, pesto

Mix with cooked pasta.

Top with Parmesan.

Vegans: top with ground nuts, seeds

Minimum fat: simmer vegetables and herbs in the tomato, rather than in the oil. Leave out cheese.

SAMPLE RECIPE: PASTA WITH CLASSIC TOMATO SAUCE

1 large onion
2 cloves garlic
½ stalk celery
1 carrot
parsley
1 tablespoon olive oil
½ pound pasta

2 to 3 pounds fresh tomato, chopped
1 teaspoon oregano
½ teaspoon basil
6 tablespoons red wine
tomato purée

Chop onion, garlic, celery, carrot, parsley. Sauté in olive oil until wilted. Add tomato, oregano, basil, wine. Simmer 15 to 20 minutes. Thicken with tomato purée or paste, if needed. Toss with hot pasta. Top with Parmesan. Makes 3-4 servings sauce.

PASTA WITH VEGETABLES

Sauté or steam: zucchini, broccoli, asparagus, artichokes, mushrooms, string beans, onions, peas, carrots, spinach, peppers, celery, cauliflower, corn, eggplant, squash, tomato, beans, any other vegetables

Mix with (enough to coat pasta): raw egg, tomato sauce, oil, puréed

*Optional

ricotta or cottage cheese, yogurt, cheese sauce, pesto, tahini, lemon juice, butter, herbs, garlic, any sauce (if warming the sauce, don't overheat ricotta or yogurt or they will curdle)

Toss with hot pasta or layer with pasta and bake

Minimum fat: steam vegetables, mix with ricotta, yogurt, lowfat tomato sauce, or lemon juice and herbs

SAMPLE RECIPE: PASTA WITH BROCCOLI AND ZUCCHINI

1 bunch broccoli, cut up	1 tablespoon lemon juice
¾ pound zucchini, sliced	pepper
2 tablespoons olive oil	½ pound pasta
2 cloves garlic, sliced	

Partially steam broccoli and zucchini. Sauté vegetables and garlic in oil. Toss with hot pasta and lemon juice. Pepper to taste. Serves two.

PASTA WITH PURÉE

Purée: cooked vegetable(s) (broccoli, onion, artichoke hearts, asparagus, cauliflower, carrots, mushrooms, spinach, etc.); *herbs* (basil, parsley); *nuts; cooked beans* (chickpeas, cannelini, kidney, soy, black, pinto, lentil)

Add (to smooth): yogurt, ricotta, mozzarella, nut butter, wine, water, soup, milk, stock, oil, cream, butter, herbs, garlic, cheese, raw egg, tomato paste

Heat: if desired

Toss: with hot pasta

Vegans: use nut butter, oil, etc.

Minimum fat: don't sauté vegetables; use yogurt, Ricotta, wine, soup, stock

SAMPLE RECIPE: PASTA WITH CHICKPEA SAUCE

1 onion, chopped	6 tablespoons Romano cheese, grated
1 tablespoon olive oil	2 tablespoons tomato paste
2 cups cooked chickpeas	bean liquid or more yogurt
5 tablespoons yogurt	½ pound pasta
½ teaspoon oregano	
¼ teaspoon basil	

Sauté onion in oil. Purée onion and chickpeas. Add yogurt, herbs, Romano, tomato paste, Thin with bean liquid or yogurt, if necessary. Toss with hot pasta. (You may have more sauce than you need for the pasta.) Serves two.

Loaves

For a 9 × 5 × 3 loaf pan.

Loaves are a little tricky, but they are well worth the risk and usually salvagable, even if they don't work perfectly. Sometimes they turn out very soft. In that case, use as a spread or paté. Loaves are delicious in sandwiches, hot or cold. They are very easy to make, especially if you have a food processor.

Start with 3 to 5 cups: cooked, mashed *beans* (chickpeas, soy-beans, kidneys, limas, lentils, others); raw or cooked *vegetables* (broccoli, zucchini, mushrooms, carrots, potato, spinach, green beans, asparagus, cauliflower, sprouts, corn); cooked *grains* (brown rice, bulgur, oatmeal, whole rye, wheat, buckwheat, kasha, wheat germ); *nuts* (chopped or ground); *cheese* (grated)

Flavor with: up to 1½ cups chopped onion, celery, green pepper, cheese, tomatoes; up to 1 cup vegetable juice or other sauce; 1 to 2 tablespoons herbs, vinegar, lemon juice, tamari, garlic

Thicken, as needed, with: wheat germ, bread crumbs, flour, dry oatmeal, soy grits, rice, ground nuts. The more of these you use, the more noticeable they become. Don't end up with a "flour loaf," by thickening too enthusiastically.

Bind with: eggs (usually 2), beans

Pour into oiled loaf pan. *Bake* at about 350 to 375° for 45 minutes to 1 hour

Depending on the texture you want: purée any or all of it (beans and/or vegetables especially); sauté onions, herbs before-hand; the more eggs you use, the wetter your mixture can be (but not too wet!)

Vegans: Instead of eggs, beans are a good binder, as are mashed potatoes. Make a drier loaf.

Minimum fat: Avoid cheese and nuts. Don't sauté. Use 1 egg if possible.

SAMPLE RECIPE: SWISS LOAF

1 large onion	6 ounces V-8 juice
1 carrot	⅛ teaspoon nutmeg
1 cup nuts	1 teaspoon thyme
1 cup Swiss cheese (5 oz)	¼ teaspoon marjoram
1 cup wheat germ	¼ teaspoon tarragon
2 eggs	

In a food processor: Chop onion and carrot; add nuts and chop; add cheese and blend. Add rest of ingredients and blend thoroughly.

Without a processor: Mince onion and carrot; grind nuts; grate cheese. Blend all ingredients.

Bake uncovered at 375°F for 45 minutes. Let stand 10 minutes before serving. Delicious on sandwiches the next day.

Soup

Soup is simple to make and can be as plain or elegant as you choose. A chilled yogurt soup is wonderfully refreshing on a warm summer night; a hearty vegetable stew is equally comforting at the end of a cold winter's day. Make more than you need and have it for lunch, snack, or appetizer as well.

Sauté: chopped onion, garlic, peppers, carrots, celery, parsnips, celery root

Add: stock, water, wine, vegetable juice, yogurt

Add: chopped vegetables, raw or cooked beans, grains, pasta, herbs (add longer-cooking foods earlier)

Simmer (although yogurt will separate), don't boil, until done

For thick or cream soup: add or start with roux (a cooked mixture of fat and flour), cream sauce, cheese, cheese sauce, ground nuts or seeds, powdered milk

Purée: all or part of soup

Garnish with: croutons, raw vegetable slices, fresh herbs, cheese, sliced lemon, brandy

Minimum fat: Don't sauté. Use milk powder to thicken. Avoid cheese.

SAMPLE RECIPE: CHEDDAR-CAULIFLOWER SOUP

2 pounds cauliflower	1½ quarts milk
4 tablespoons butter	2 cups water
½ cup whole wheat flour	½ pound Cheddar cheese, grated
1 teaspoon salt	¼ teaspoon paprika
dash cayenne	

Cut cauliflower into buds; slice the stems. Heat milk and water in saucepan. Melt butter, add flour and salt to make a roux. Cook

*Optional

over very low heat. Add hot milk and water all at once. Blend. Bring to a boil. Cook, stirring, a couple of minutes. Add cauliflower. Simmer, covered, over very low heat until tender. Mix in cheese, paprika, and cayenne. Purée part if desired. Serves 5 to 6.

Casseroles

"Casserole" is a good catch-all word meaning "put it in a dish and bake it." Do just that.

Start with: cooked *beans* (pinto, kidney, chickpeas, soy, lentils, etc.); cooked *grains* (rice, bulgur, pasta, barley, millet, etc.); *raw or cooked vegetables* (cabbage, broccoli, tomato, potato, spinach, green beans, asparagus, corn, mushrooms, zucchini, squash)

Layer or mix in: hard cheese (cheddar, parmesan, jack, feta, swiss); *soft cheese* (cottage, ricotta, mozzarella, cream, farmer, brie); *nuts and seeds* (ground, chopped or whole); *fresh or dried fruit* (apple or pineapple slices, grapes, raisins); *wheat germ, bread crumbs*

Flavor with: raw or sautéed onion, green pepper, carrot, celery, garlic (or rub garlic on casserole dish), herbs

Moisten, if needed, with: milk, vegetable juice, stock, yogurt, wine, eggs, sauces, tomato (including purée or paste), soufflé batter

Top with: cheese, seeds, wheat germ, bread crumbs, mashed potato, pastry or bread dough, corn bread batter

Bake at 350°F ½ to 1 hour or longer, if necessary. *Uncover* last 5 minutes.

Vegan: Moisten with tomato juice or sauce, wine.

Minimum fat: Avoid cheese, nuts, eggs. Don't sauté.

Variation: Make the casserole a pie.

SAMPLE RECIPE: RICE PRIMAVERA

½ cup raw brown rice cooked with 1 bay leaf

1 8-ounce can water chestnuts (about 14 nuts), sliced

1 green pepper, chopped

1 onion, chopped

1 clove garlic, minced

1 tomato, chopped

¾ cup mozzarella cheese, grated

¼ cup Romano cheese, grated

1 tablespoon dried parsley

1 cup peas, fresh or frozen

2 medium carrots, grated

pepper

Mix all ingredients in 2-quart casserole. Bake uncovered at 350°
for 25 to 30 minutes. Serves 2 to 4.

Salad

Some people refer to salad as "rabbit food," but those people
haven't lived! Basically, a salad is a mixture of several foods
unified by a dressing. The ingredients may be raw, cooked, cooked
and chilled, marinated, or any combination of these. A salad doesn't
even have to include lettuce, that favorite food of our long-eared
friends.

Mix and match from these possibilities:

Lettuce
Green beans, cooked or fresh
Green or red pepper, cooked or
    fresh
Cauliflower, cooked or fresh
Tomatoes, big or little, sliced,
    whole, diced, peeled, etc.
Water chestnuts
Sprouts
Dried apricots, pineapple,
    raisins, currants, dates
Cheese
Citrus segments
Sliced oranges, lemons, limes
Cooked potato
Eggs—hard boiled
Raw turnip
Horseradish
Seeds
Rice, other grains
Spinach
Olives
Tofu
Capers
Endive
Pickles
Cucumber

Other greens — chard, beet
    greens, etc.
Mushrooms
Carrots, cooked or fresh
Broccoli, cooked or fresh
Cabbage, cooked or fresh
Beets, cooked, pickled, fresh
Onions, scallions, shallots
Hearts of palm
Bamboo shoots
Nuts
Fresh apples, pineapple,
    apricots, peaches, grapes,
    figs, melon
Cooked beans—kidneys, chick-
    peas, etc.
Peas
Herbs—fennel, parsley, basil,
    chives, garlic, oregano,
    curry, coriander, mint
Zucchini, squash
Berries
Corn
Watercress
Pasta
Radishes
Celery

Avocado
Asparagus
Croutons
Chinese cabbage

DRESSING

Start with: 1 to 4 times as much oil as vinegar (or lemon juice) totaling about a cup. Instead of oil, try nut butter or tahini plus an equal part water.

Add 1 to 2 tablespoons: prepared mustard; ketchup; chili sauce; chopped onion, scallion, chives, parsley; chutney; lemon juice; chopped egg; watercress; horseradish; tamari; vegetable or fruit juice

Season with: herbs, spices, garlic, capers, curry powder, sugar, honey, tabasco (add fresh herbs shortly before using)

For a different flavor, add in larger amounts: puréed vegetables, juice, tofu

For a creamier dressing, add: tomato paste, cream cheese, cream, sour cream, grated cheese, avocado, yogurt, nut butter, egg or yolk, mayonnaise, tofu, ricotta, tahini

SAMPLE RECIPE: CREAMY VINAIGRETTE DRESSING

½ cup olive oil	pepper
¼ cup white wine vinegar	2 cloves garlic, minced
2 tablespoons prepared mustard	1 tablespoon parsley, chopped
salt	3 ounces cream cheese

Blend all ingredients. Makes about 1¼ cups.

Stuffed Vegetables or Pastry

Vegetables good for stuffing include green peppers, eggplant, onions, cabbage, squash, tomatoes, and mushrooms. You can also fill crêpes, turnovers, biscuits, or other pastry.

STUFFING

Start with: vegetable pulp, other vegetables, nuts, cheese, beans, hard-boiled egg, seeds, raisins, other dried fruit

Flavor with: onions, garlic, green pepper, herbs

Thicken with: bread crumbs, bread cubes, pasta, grains, nuts, nut butter, cheese

Moisten with: sauce, stock, wine, lemon juice, vinegar, ricotta,
    yogurt, egg
Heat, if desired.

SAMPLE RECIPE: STUFFED ZUCCHINI

4 zucchini, split and partially steamed	curry powder to taste
3 scallions, chopped	⅓ cup raisins
½ tablespoon olive oil	¼ cup pine nuts, chopped
	½ to 1 cup fresh bread crumbs

Scoop out and chop zucchini pulp. Sauté scallions and curry
powder in oil. Add raisins, nuts, zucchini pulp. Simmer covered,
on low heat. Add bread crumbs. Stuff zucchini shells with mixture.
Bake at 350°F for ½ hour. Serves 2.

Flavored Grains

An herb here, a vegetable there can change the whole feeling of a
grain dish.

Start with: rice, whole or cracked wheat, buckwheat, kasha, corn,
    wild rice, millet, barley
Sauté, alone or with: curry, cumin, pinch of saffron, dried mush-
    rooms, onions, scallions, green pepper, salt, pepper, herbs,
    garlic, molasses, vinegar, lemon juice, soy sauce, fruit juice
Add (at least twice as much): stock, water, wine, tomato or other
    vegetable juice, milk, rosewater, herb tea
Add: peanuts, cooked beans, scallion tops, nuts, raisins, dried
    fruit, cheese
Bring to a boil
Simmer until liquid is absorbed
Toppings or mixers: cooked vegetables, yogurt, grated cheese,
    whole or ground seeds

SAMPLE RECIPE: RISOTTO MILANESE

2 onions, sliced	5 cups stock
2 cloves garlic, chopped	½ teaspoon saffron
1 tablespoon butter	½ teaspoon salt
1 tablespoon oil	pepper
2 cups brown rice	Romano cheese, grated
½ cup marsala	mushrooms, sautéed

Sauté onions and garlic in oil and butter. Stir in rice. Sauté until golden. Add stock, wine, herbs. Bring to a boil. Reduce heat. Cook until liquid is absorbed. Top with cheese and mushrooms. Serves 4.

TRYING NEW FOODS

Certain foods are out of the mainstream in the United States, although many of them are used widely in other parts of the world. They are tasty and versatile, once you get to know them. Hence, a brief introduction, for those of you who have skipped over them in recipes because they were unfamiliar. Try them and see what you think.

Bean flakes.   These are partially cooked and rolled beans, processed in this way to shorten cooking time. Use anywhere you would use regular beans. They provide a unique texture to casseroles and soups. They are found in health food stores.

Bulgur.   Whole wheat that has been parboiled, dried, and cracked, this is a staple in the Middle East. Use interchangeably with cracked wheat or any time you need a grain. It is a good source of B vitamins and iron and can be found in supermarkets and health food stores in several grain sizes.

Kasha.   This is cracked buckwheat, barley, or millet. Use in grain recipes.

Millet.   This small, light-colored grain, used heavily in Africa, Japan, and China, provides low-gluten protein, iron, lecithin. Try it in soups or grain recipes, as hot cereal, in place of rice.

Miso.   A creamy black paste made from soybeans, barley, water, salt, and koji rice (a fermented rice), this salty seasoning is used often in soups and sauces. A good source of B_{12}, it is found in health food stores, oriental groceries.

Soy milk.   A white liquid extracted from soaked soybeans ground with water and strained through cheesecloth, this can also be made from soy flour. It is available in powder form. Use instead of milk. It can be found in health food stores. The kind sold in drugstores is often heavily sugared and stabilized with chemical emulsifiers.

Sprouts.   Seeds, beans, and whole grains can be sprouted by a soaking-and-draining process that takes several days. Sprouting increases the nutrient content of the food. Add to sandwiches, salads, casseroles or stir-fry with other vegetables. Sprouts are easy to make at home and are also found in health food stores, some supermarkets, and produce stands.

Tahini. This is made from hulled sesame seeds ground to a paste. Use it in sauces, dressings. Tahini is found in health food stores and Middle Eastern groceries. This is the best way to get the nutrients in sesame seeds, since we can't easily digest them unless they are physically broken down beforehand.

Tamari. This soy sauce made from soybeans, grain, salt, and water by a natural fermentation process is the excess liquid drained off miso. It is very salty, so use sparingly on grains, in soups, casseroles, even on popcorn.

Tempeh. These white cakes or patties made from cooked soybeans (sometimes with additional legumes, seeds, grains) are bound together by *Rhisopus* mold. It can also be made from peanuts, wheat and soy, okra, others. Tempeh is usually sliced and fried. It is good in sandwiches, casseroles, sauces and is a good source of vitamin B_{12}. You can find it fresh, refrigerated, or frozen in health food stores.

Tofu (bean curd). This soybean cheese made from soy milk is high in protein, low in fat and calories and has a bland taste. It picks up other flavors easily. Use tofu in soups, dips, dressings, or fried or broiled. It is sold fresh or vacuum-packed at health-food stores, produce stands, oriental groceries, some supermarkets. If fresh, store in water, covered, in refrigerator.

GUIDELINES

Vary traditional vegetarian and meat dishes with substitutions and additions to suit your taste and imagination.

Don't hesitate to invent meals from scratch.

Rules were made to be broken in the kitchen; don't be limited by preconceived ideas about food.

14

Eating Out—
and Other Matters

1. *I travel a lot and eat many of my meals in restaurants. Can you give me any advice that will save me time and trouble?*

There are certain kinds of restaurants that invariably have meatless dishes: Italian (eggplant parmesan, manicotti, cheese ravioli, fettucine Alfredo), Mexican (cheese enchiladas, rice and beans, guacamole, bean burritos), Middle Eastern (hummus, stuffed meatless grapeleaves, falafel, salad with feta cheese), Kosher-dairy (blintzes, potato pancakes, vegetarian "chopped liver," borscht), Indian (assorted vegetable curries), and natural food restaurants are a few. If you are given the choice, these are the types of places you'll want to frequent. Even at restaurants where a meatless entrée isn't offered, however, there are usually plenty of salads and side dishes to choose from.

It is important to remember to ask specific questions. Always call a new restaurant first or ask to see a menu before you are seated. If you call, be specific about what you do and don't eat. People are not always sure what a vegetarian can eat, and understandably so, since vegetarians themselves define the word in various ways. Often, the maître d' will immediately suggest a vegetable plate. It may not occur to him or her that manicotti is vegetarian (at least for lacto-ovo vegetarians). Don't be afraid to make your own suggestions, or, by all means, have the vegetable plate if you prefer.

Get used to the idea that menus are shorter than they look. Rarely will there be more than two or three entrées for you. And if you can find only one choice, *make sure* they are serving it that day.

When you are ordering, always double-check to be certain the dish you want is meatless. Even at the kinds of restaurants mentioned here, the tomato sauce could have a beef base or the beans could be cooked with pork. Be specific, right down to whether a chicken stock was used in the vichyssoise. Do this even if you have had the dish somewhere else. Remember, chefs may have varying interpretations of even the most classic dishes. By making it clear that you can't eat meat, you are also reserving the right to send back any "mistakes." Don't be shy when that happens. Inevitably, every so often it will.

Generally, you will find that waiters and waitresses are very interested in vegetarianism and are careful to bring you the right thing. They will usually check with the chef about ingredients and substitutions. They won't mind answering your questions; in fact you may find yourself answering a couple as well.

If you come across an obnoxious waiter, do your best to ignore it and find out what you need to know. If the person is completely uncooperative, ask to see the manager and/or leave.

Above all, don't avoid eating out because you are vegetarian. At the very least, you are increasing the awareness of restaurant owners and employees. At best, you are enjoying a delicious vegetarian meal.

2. *What is the best way to make the change to vegetarianism?*

We suggest easing into it for a while, unless you are an all-or-nothing person who would lose momentum by changing slowly. In either case, don't give yourself ultimatums that may be self-defeating. We all do that—the old New Year's resolution routine—ten promises to yourself never kept in which you set yourself up for failure. So go easy.

For those who favor a gradual change, give yourself several weeks (or more, if you need them) to adjust to a new way of thinking and eating. And don't start during a holiday that is symbolized by feasting with loved ones. Here are some ways you might start:

Read enough so you have a good foundation in nutrition.

List the meatless meals you already cook.

Read cookbooks and select recipes you are eager to try.

Cut out all red meat first.

Eat two or three meatless meals a week, gradually adding more.

Take inventory of your refrigerator, freezer, and cabinets.

Separate meat and vegetarian food. As you eat up your meat supply, don't buy more.

Start reading labels carefully, and don't buy food that contains any meat or meat products.

Order meatless meals at restaurants, choosing the restaurants with that in mind.

If you have vegetarian friends, don't be shy about asking questions. On the other hand, don't be unduly influenced by someone else's lifestyle. There are all sorts of vegetarians.

Be clear about why you are doing this, especially if you are afraid you'll be tempted by meat.

At first, tell people you're cutting down on meat. When you're sure, say you're a vegetarian. That way you won't lose face if you decide not to do it, nor do you further its unfortunate image as a fad.

3. *I'm a vegetarian, but my wife isn't. How can we best arrange our meals?*

Eat as many meatless meals as your wife will agree to. When she does want meat, however, plan your meals so there will be as little extra cooking to do as possible. This usually means she will have one extra meat dish and eat smaller portions of the salad and casserole that may comprise your dinner. If she prefers a more integrated dish like beef stroganoff (rather than the typically compartmentalized meat, potatoes, and vegetable approach), choose a vegetarian entrée that can also make use of the noodles she is cooking for hers. Or make a dish in which you can add the meat last (to her portion only, of course), such as spaghetti sauce or a Chinese stir-fry mix.

This should work out well if you both cook. It merely requires a bit of advance thought. If only one of you cooks, however, there could be problems.

If it is your wife, don't expect her to know how to feed you right off the bat. Do your own research and be ready with suggestions and a helping hand.

If you do the cooking, the vegetarian part is easy. The matter then becomes: Can you handle cooking meat for your wife? If you can't, and that is understandable, some renegotiation with your wife is in order. After all, it is not particularly fair to suddenly insist she find her meat elsewhere. That's what it will boil down to, though, if she doesn't start cooking it herself. It's a touchy situation that requires all the compromising to be done by her. Be aware of that as you discuss the possibilities with her; these could include tradeoffs in other areas.

Above all, don't put her down for not changing along with you. Your different eating habits could easily become a point of contention between you. Don't let that happen if there is any way to avoid it.

4. *Can I feed my dog a meatless diet?*

Yes, you can, but remember that a dog's needs are different from a human being's. For example, dogs need at least 1.25 grams of protein per kilogram of body weight (and as much as ten times more for pregnant, lactating or growing dogs). With this higher protein need, your dog will not do well on your table scraps and leftovers. It will take more effort and planning than that. A typical vegetarian mixture might include eggs or cheese, a tablespoon of oil, nutritional yeast, cooked vegetables, grains, and milk. You'll have to experiment, though, to see what he or she likes. For specific nutritional requirements, consult your veterinarian or a complete book on the subject.

Cats, incidentally, are somewhat more difficult to feed. They need even more protein than dogs, preformed sources of vitamin A, niacin, and the amino acid taurine. Cats also seem to require a weekly dose of fish oil, although the evidence on feline nutrition is not all in, and research is still being done in many areas.

5. *My parents are always put out with me on holidays because I don't "share in the traditions." What can I say or do so they will accept my decision?*

The important word here is *share*. Your parents may feel hurt or even rejected if you don't eat what they consider symbolic of celebration such as turkey at Thanksgiving. Try to fill the gap by emphasizing those rituals in which you do participate. For example, don't insist on an entirely different kind of meal. Instead, eat what you can from your family's traditional spread—sweet potato pie, peas, turnips, rolls, cranberry sauce. There will probably be plenty, but if you don't feel that the side dishes will be enough or you'd like to share a new tradition with them, make an additional casserole yourself—something that can serve as your entrée and another side dish for them.

Whatever you do, don't deride their traditions by becoming indignant or self-righteous about the fact that they are eating meat. Participate just as you always have and don't draw attention to what needn't be more than slight changes if the attitude is right.

If they still can't accept it, it's probably a more basic problem, rather than one that just crops up on holidays. All you can do is try to make things as convenient and comfortable for them as possible, and stick calmly to your decision.

6. *Can vegetarians eat fish?*

This subject comes up again and again. It is a strange issue of semantics, because it really centers on what a "real" vegetarian is.

The "official" definitions of various vegetarian societies describe three types of vegetarian:

Lacto-ovo-vegetarians eat no fish, fowl, or red meat.

Lacto-vegetarians eat no fish, fowl, red meat, or eggs.

Strict vegetarians, or vegans, eat no fish, fowl, red meat, eggs, or dairy products.

A person who eats fish but no fowl or red meat is simply that—a person who eats fish but no fowl or red meat. "Semi-vegetarian" will do also.

7. *I sympathize with the reasons people become vegetarians, but I don't like most vegetables. Any hope for me?*

The first thing you should realize is that everyone, meat-eater and vegetarian alike, has a similar need for vegetables. They are a vital source of vitamins, minerals, fiber, and other carbohydrates. Certainly, it is possible to be either a vegetarian or a meat-eater and not eat vegetables. The point is it's unhealthy in both cases. If you really can't stand any vegetables, make sure you eat a varied diet in other respects, including lots of fruit, and take a vitamin/mineral supplement daily.

Try first, though, to open your mind and taste buds a bit. There are so many different kinds of vegetables, you probably haven't even heard of them all! Experiment. You may be pleasantly surprised, especially if your dislike of vegetables started with mushy string beans in the school cafeteria. Fortunately, the cooking of vegetables has generally taken a turn for the better as people have become more aware that vegetables are a delicious part of a meal and not just an unappetizing lump that is "good for you." You don't necessarily have to eat them steamed and unadorned. Try them simmered in sauce, baked in a casserole, ground in a loaf, stir-fried in a wok. Vegetables are wonderfully versatile.

In any event, a dislike of vegetables needn't stop you from being a vegetarian unless *all* you like is meat. Eat grains, nuts, seeds, beans, pasta, bread, fruit, dairy products, eggs, and generous servings of any vegetables you do like.

8. *How should I handle dinner invitations?*

Recently, we saw this Ann Landers column in our local paper:

Dear Ann Landers:
During the last year, for health and philosophical reasons, I have gone on a vegetarian diet. Most of my friends and relatives are aware of my new eating preferences, but some are not.

How do I respond to a dinner invitation from people who may not know? Should I say, "I am a vegetarian," when I accept the invitation—thus obligating the hostess to provide me with an alternative if she plans a meat dinner? Or should I say nothing, and try to bluff my way through the meal?

—*Grains and Greens*

Dear G and G:
If the hostess doesn't know you well enough to prepare a vegetable plate, you don't know her well enough to impose the inconvenience. So, fake it, friend.

We have several things we'd like to say to Ann.

Certainly, at a large dinner party, a vegetarian should simply eat whatever meatless dishes are offered. A light meal before the party would also be a good idea.

When invited to a more intimate dinner, a vegetarian should definitely inform the hostess beforehand that he or she doesn't eat meat. We find it much more of an imposition to let the hostess cook an elaborate meat dinner for you that you can't eat.

If the hostess asks for suggestions, be ready to name several simple, familiar dishes—quiche, pasta, a vegetable casserole—or offer to bring one of the dishes, if you are so inclined.

Telling your hostess beforehand saves you from feeling you must eat some of the meat or push it around your plate "to be polite." "Faking it" at a small gathering is uncomfortable, eating it is unnecessary.

If your hostess "forgets," don't feel you must eat the meal. Explain that you can't, but that the mistake is perfectly understandable. You'll have a double serving of salad, rice, and vegetables instead. We think this is the best policy. We have a friend whose mother continually "forgets" she is trying to be a vegetarian. Our friend eats her mother's meals anyway. We think her mother would stop "forgetting" if our friend refused to eat the meat.

Finally, Ann, wise up. Vegetarians aren't limited to vegetable plates!

9. *Do all vegetarians eat natural foods?*

The only thing vegetarians have in common is they don't eat fish, fowl, or red meat. Other than that, a vegetarian can be a junk food junkie, a health food nut, a pizza freak, or a fruitarian.

A natural foods vegetarian, however, is the popular stereotype. It evolved because those who are vegetarians for health reasons tend to buy the most nutritious food they can find—natural food. Likewise, people who eat natural food are very health oriented, and that often leads them to a meatless diet. As a result, much of the literature and many of the food products overlap, and certain stores cater to both groups.

Nevertheless, you will find plenty of vegetarians buying TV dinners and cake. And you will see stacks of organic meat in many a natural foods freezer. The two concepts do not necessarily go together.

10. *Is the macrobiotic diet healthy?*

It depends on what version of the diet you are talking about. Certainly at its highest, supposedly ideal level, +7, it is a nutritional disaster and extremely dangerous. At some of the lower levels, it can be as adequate as any diet if you get enough calories and follow the principles of a balanced diet. This means combining your philosophical beliefs with a more common-sense approach than that encouraged by macrobiotics founder George Ohsawa, who at that time advocated a brown rice regimen and little consumption of liquids. At its worst, macrobiotics can result in dehydration, malnutrition, emaciation, and possibly death. But most knowledgeable practitioners of macrobiotics now ignore the more extreme of Ohsawa's recommendations, and the diet they practice combines the philosophic teaching with nutritional realities. On the plus side are low serum cholesterol, low blood pressure, and no weight problems. Of course, you can get those advantages on a regular vegan or lacto-ovo diet.

11. *I'm going abroad for several weeks. Should I make any preparations now?*

Most airlines offer vegetarian meals upon request, so don't forget to put in your order when you make your reservations. If you are going by boat, call or write to see if any special arrangements will be necessary.

For each country you are visiting, learn all you can about the cuisine. There are probably certain dishes you can be fairly sure about ordering. Learn how to order them in the language. In each language, if nothing else, learn to say: "I am a vegetarian. Do you have something I can eat? I can eat absolutely no fish, fowl, or beef, but I can eat all vegetables, nuts, fruit, cheese, milk, eggs, pasta, rice, and bread." It might also be helpful to know how to say: "Does it have any meat in it?" and "Is it fried in lard?"

If you have time, write to a vegetarian society in each area and ask for any information they can give you. You may be able to contact them through your local society. Order the *International Vegetarian Health Food Handbook* from the Vegetarian Society of the United Kingdom Ltd., Parkdale, Dunham Road, Altrincham, Cheshire, WA14 4QG, Great Britain. It lists vegetarian societies, restaurants, and hotels worldwide.

12. *I became a lacto-ovo-vegetarian for ethical as well as health reasons. Is it hypocritical for me to wear leather?*

A hypocrite, according to Webster's Dictionary, is one who affects virtues or qualities he does not have. A lacto-ovo-vegetarian, according to official definition, is one who eats no fish, fowl, or red meat. You can be, therefore, a lacto-ovo-vegetarian who wears leather but is not a hypocrite. Ethically, however, it is undeniably inconsistent. Unfortunately, in a world as complex as ours, it is virtually impossible not to be.

By becoming a vegetarian, you have taken a big step in avoiding unnecessary slaughter. It is logical to assume you will do whatever you feel you can toward this end. Will it be to eschew flesh foods only? To eat milk but not eggs? To not wear leather but set roach motels under the sink? To not use the roach motels but light candles made with pork fat? There may be animal products in glue, medicine, book bindings, toys, soap, rugs, tires, and photographic film, to name a few.

You can only make whatever decision seems possible, feasible, or even necessary for your life. You must draw your own lines.

APPENDICES

Food and Nutrition Board, National Academy of Sciences—National Research Council

Recommended Daily Dietary Allowance, [a] *Revised 1980*

	Age (years)	Weight (kg)	Weight (lb)	Height (cm)	Height (in)	Protein (g)	FAT-SOLUBLE VITAMINS Vitamin A (μg RE)[b]	Vitamin D (μg)[c]	Vitamin E (mg α-TE)[d]
Infants	0.0–0.5	6	13	60	24	kg × 2.2	420	10	3
	0.5–1.0	9	20	71	28	kg × 2.0	400	10	4
Children	1–3	13	29	90	35	23	400	10	5
	4–6	20	44	112	44	30	500	10	6
	7–10	28	62	132	52	34	700	10	7
Males	11–14	45	99	157	62	45	1000	10	8
	15–18	66	145	176	69	56	1000	10	10
	19–22	70	154	177	70	56	1000	7.5	10
	23–50	70	154	178	70	56	1000	5	10
	51+	70	154	178	70	56	1000	5	10
Females	11–14	46	101	157	62	46	800	10	8
	15–18	55	120	163	64	46	800	10	8
	19–22	55	120	163	64	44	800	7.5	8
	23–50	55	120	163	64	44	800	5	8
	51+	55	120	163	64	44	800	5	8
Pregnant						+30	+200	+5	+2
Lactating						+20	+400	+5	+3

[a] The allowances are intended to provide for individual variations among most normal persons as they live in the United States under usual environmental stresses. Diets should be based on a variety of common foods in order to provide other nutrients for which human requirements have been less well defined. See text for detailed discussion of allowances and of nutrients not tabulated. See below for weights and heights by individual year of age.

[b] Retinol equivalents. 1 retinol equivalent = 1 μg retinol or 6 μg β carotene.

[c] As cholecalciferol. 10 μg cholecalciferol = 400 IU of vitamin D.

[d] α-tocopherol equivalents. 1 mg d-α tocopherol = 1 α-TE = 1.49 1 IU

[e] 1 NE (niacin equivalent) is equal to 1 mg of niacin or 60 mg of dietary tryptophan.

[f] The folacin allowances refer to dietary sources as determined by *Lactobacillus casei* assay after treatment with enzymes (conjugases) to make polyglutamyl forms of the vitamin available to the test organism.

Designed for the maintenance of good nutrition of
practically all healthy people in the U.S.A.

WATER-SOLUBLE VITAMINS							MINERALS					
Vitamin C (mg)	Thiamin (mg)	Riboflavin (mg)	Niacin (mg NE)^e	Vitamin B-6 (mg)	Folacin (µg)	Vitamin B-12 (µg)	Calcium (mg)	Phosphorus (mg)	Magnesium (mg)	Iron (mg)	Zinc (mg)	Iodine (µg)
35	0.3	0.4	6	0.3	30	0.5[g]	360	240	50	10	3	40
35	0.5	0.6	8	0.6	45	1.5	540	360	70	15	5	50
45	0.7	0.8	9	0.9	100	2.0	800	800	150	15	10	70
45	0.9	1.0	11	1.3	200	2.5	800	800	200	10	10	90
45	1.2	1.4	16	1.6	300	3.0	800	800	250	10	10	120
50	1.4	1.6	18	1.8	400	3.0	1200	1200	350	18	15	150
60	1.4	1.7	18	2.0	400	3.0	1200	1200	400	18	15	150
60	1.5	1.7	19	2.2	400	3.0	800	800	350	10	15	150
60	1.4	1.6	18	2.2	400	3.0	800	800	350	10	15	150
60	1.2	1.4	16	2.2	400	3.0	800	800	350	10	15	150
50	1.1	1.3	15	1.8	400	3.0	1200	1200	300	18	15	150
60	1.1	1.3	14	2.0	400	3.0	1200	1200	300	18	15	150
60	1.1	1.3	14	2.0	400	3.0	800	800	300	18	15	150
60	1.0	1.2	13	2.0	400	3.0	800	800	300	18	15	150
60	1.0	1.2	13	2.0	400	3.0	800	800	300	10	15	150
+20	+0.4	+0.3	+2	+0.6	+400	+1.0	+400	+400	+150	h	+5	+25
+40	+0.5	+0.5	+5	+0.5	+100	+1.0	+400	+400	+150	h	+10	+50

[g] The recommended dietary allowance for vitamin B-12 in infants is based on average concentration of the vitamin in human milk. The allowances after weaning are based on energy intake (as recommended by the American Academy of Pediatrics) and consideration of other factors, such as intestinal absorption.

[h] The increased requirement during pregnancy cannot be met by the iron content of habitual American diets nor by the existing iron stores of many women; therefore the use of 30–60 mg of supplemental iron is recommended. Iron needs during lactation are not substantially different from those of nonpregnant women, but continued supplementation of the mother for 2–3 months after parturition is advisable in order to replenish stores depleted by pregnancy.

Dietary Standard for Canada
Recommended Daily Nutrient Intake—Revised 1975*

Age	Sex	Weight (kg)	Height (cm)	Energy[a] (kcal)	(MJ)[b]	Protein (g)	Thiamin (mg)	Niacin (NE)[f]	Riboflavin (mg)	Vitamin B₆[g] (mg)	Folate[h] (µg)
									WATER-SOLUBLE VITAMINS		
0-6 mo	Both	6	—	kg x 117	kg x 0.49	kg x 2.2(2.0)[e]	0.3	5	0.4	0.3	40
7-11 mo	Both	9	—	kg x 108	kg x 0.45	kg x 1.4	0.5	6	0.6	0.4	60
1-3 yrs	Both	13	90	1400	5.9	22	0.7	9	0.8	0.8	100
4-6 yrs	Both	19	110	1800	7.5	27	0.9	12	1.1	1.3	100
7-9 yrs	M	27	129	2200	9.2	33	1.1	14	1.3	1.6	100
	F	27	128	2000	8.4	33	1.0	13	1.2	1.4	100
10-12 yrs	M	36	144	2500	10.5	41	1.2	17	1.5	1.8	100
	F	38	145	2300	9.6	40	1.1	15	1.4	1.5	100
13-15 yrs	M	51	162	2800	11.7	52	1.4	19	1.7	2.0	200
	F	49	159	2200	9.2	43	1.1	15	1.4	1.5	200
16-18 yrs	M	64	172	3200	13.4	54	1.6	21	2.0	2.0	200
	F	54	161	2100	8.8	43	1.1	14	1.3	1.5	200
19-35 yrs	M	70	176	3000	12.6	56	1.5	20	1.8	2.0	200
	F	56	161	2100	8.8	41	1.1	14	1.3	1.5	200
36-50 yrs	M	70	176	2700	11.3	56	1.4	18	1.7	2.0	200
	F	56	161	1900	7.9	41	1.0	13	1.2	1.5	200
51 + yrs	M	70	176	2300[c]	9.6[c]	56	1.4	18	1.7	2.0	200
	F	56	161	1800[c]	7.5[c]	41	1.0	13	1.2	1.5	200
Pregnancy				+300[d]	1.3[d]	+20	+0.2	+2	+0.3	+0.5	+50
Lactation				+500	2.1	+24	+0.4	+7	+0.6	+0.6	+50

*Dietary Standard for Canada, Bureau of Nutritional Sciences, Food Directorate, Health Protection Branch, Department of National Health and Welfare, Ottawa, 1975.

[a]Recommendations assume characteristic activity pattern for each age group.

[b]Megajoules (10⁶ joules). Calculated from the relation 1 kilocalorie = 4.184 kilojoules and rounded to 1 decimal place.

[c]Recommended energy intake for age 66+ years reduced to 2000 kcal (8.4 MJ) for men and 1500 kcal (6.3 MJ) for women.

[d]Increased energy intake recommended during 2nd and 3rd trimesters. An increase of 100 kcal (418.4 kJ) per day is recommended during the 1st trimester.

[e]Recommended protein intake of 2.2 g/kg body wt. for infants age 0-2 mo and 2.0 g/kg body wt. for those age 3-5 mo. Protein recommendation for infants 0-11 mo assumes consumption of breast milk or protein of equivalent quality.

[f]NE (niacin equivalent) is equal to 1 mg of niacin or 60 mg of tryptophan.

		FAT-SOLUBLE VITAMINS					MINERALS			
Vitamin B$_{12}$ (µg)	Vitamin C (mg)	Vitamin A (RE)[i]	Vitamin D (µg cholecalciferol)[k]	Vitamin E (mg-d-α-tocopherol)	Calcium (mg)	Phosphorus (mg)	Magnesium (mg)	Iodine (µg)	Iron (mg)	Zinc (mg)
0.3	20[i]	400	10	3	500[m]	250[m]	50[m]	35[m]	7[m]	4[m]
0.3	20	400	10	3	500	400	50	50	7	5
0.9	20	400	10	4	500	500	75	70	8	5
1.5	20	500	5	5	500	500	100	90	9	6
1.5	30	700	2.5[l]	6	700	700	150	110	10	7
1.5	30	700	2.5[l]	6	700	700	150	100	10	7
3.0	30	800	2.5[l]	7	900	900	175	130	11	8
3.0	30	800	2.5[l]	7	1000	1000	200	120	11	9
3.0	30	1000	2.5[l]	9	1200	1200	250	140	13	10
3.0	30	800	2.5[l]	7	800	800	250	110	14	10
3.0	30	1000	2.5[l]	10	1000	1000	300	160	14	12
3.0	30	800	2.5[l]	6	700	700	250	110	14	11
3.0	30	1000	2.5[l]	9	800	800	300	150	10	10
3.0	30	800	2.5[l]	6	700	700	250	110	14	9
3.0	30	1000	2.5[l]	8	800	800	300	140	10	10
3.0	30	800	2.5[l]	6	700	700	250	100	14	9
3.0	30	1000	2.5[l]	8	800	800	300	140	10	10
3.0	30	800	2.5[l]	6	700	700	250	100	9	9
+1.0	+20	+100	+2.5[l]	+1	+500	+500	+25	+15	+1[n]	+3
+0.5	+30	+400	+2.5[l]	+2	+500	+500	+75	+25	+1[n]	+7

[g]Recommendations are based on estimated average daily protein intake of Canadians.

[h]Recommendation given in terms of free folate.

[i]Considerably higher levels may be prudent for infants during the first week of life to guard against neonatal tyrosinemia.

[j]1RE (retinol equivalent) corresponds to a biological activity in humans equal to 1 µg retinol (3.33 IU) or 6 µg β-carotene (10 IU).

[k]One µg cholecalciferol is equivalent to 1 µg ergocalciferol (40 IU vitamin D activity).

[l]Most older children and adults receive vitamin D from irradiation but 2.5 µg daily is recommended. This intake should be increased to 5.0 µg daily during pregnancy and lactation and for those confined indoors or otherwise deprived of sunlight for extended periods.

[m]The intake of breast-fed infants may be less than the recommendation but is considered to be adequate.

[n]A recommended total intake of 15 mg daily during pregnancy and lactation assumes the presence of adequate stores of iron. If stores are suspected of being inadequate, additional iron as a supplement is recommended.

Mean Heights and Weights and Recommended Energy Intake[a]

Category	Age (years)	Weight (kg)	Weight (lb)	Height (cm)	Height (in)	Energy Needs (with range) (kcal)		(MJ)[b]
Infants	0.0–0.5	6	13	60	24	kg + 115	(95–145)	kg + 0.48
	0.5–1.0	9	20	71	28	kg + 105	(80–135)	kg + 0.44
Children	1–3	13	29	90	35	1300	(900–1800)	5.5
	4–6	20	44	112	44	1700	(1300–2300)	7.1
	7–10	28	62	132	52	2400	(1650–3300)	10.1
Males	11–14	45	99	157	62	2700	(2000–3700)	11.3
	15–18	66	145	176	69	2800	(2100–3900)	11.8
	19–22	70	154	177	70	2900	(2500–3300)	12.2
	23–50	70	154	178	70	2700	(2300–3100)	11.3
	51–75	70	154	178	70	2400	(2000–2800)	10.1
	76+	70	154	178	70	2050	(1650–2450)	8.6
Females	11–14	46	101	157	62	2200	(1500–3000)	9.2
	15–18	55	120	163	64	2100	(1200–3000)	8.8
	19–22	55	120	163	64	2100	(1700–2500)	8.8
	23–50	55	120	163	64	2000	(1600–2400)	8.4
	51–75	55	120	163	64	1800	(1400–2200)	7.6
	76+	55	120	163	64	1600	(1200–2000)	6.7
Pregnancy						+300		
Lactation						+500		

[a] The data in this table have been assembled from the observed median heights and weights of children, together with desirable weights for adults for the mean heights of men (70 in.) and women (64 in.) between the ages of 18 and 34 years as surveyed in the U.S. population (HEW/NCHS data).

The energy allowances for the young adults are for men and women doing light work. The allowances for the two older age groups represent mean energy needs over these age spans, allowing for a 2-percent decrease in basal (resting) metabolic rate per decade and a reduction in activity of 200 kcal/day for men and women between 51 and 75 years, 500 kcal for men over 75 years, and 400 kcal for women over 75 years. The customary range of daily energy output is shown in parentheses for adults and is based on a variation in energy needs of ±400 kcal at any one age, emphasizing the wide range of energy intakes appropriate for any group of people.

Energy allowances for children through age 18 are based on median energy intakes of children of these ages followed in longitudinal growth studies. The values in parentheses are 10th and 90th percentiles of energy intake, to indicate the range of energy consumption among children of these ages.

[b] Megajoules.

WHO/FAO RECOMMENDATIONS
RECOMMENDED INTAKES OF NUTRIENTS

Age	Body weight	Energy (1)		Protein (1, 2)	Vitamin A (3, 4)	Vitamin D (5, 6)	Thiamine (3)	Ribo-flavin (3)	Niacin (3)	Folic acid (5)	Vitamin B12 (5)	Ascorbic acid (5)	Calcium (7)	Iron (5, 8)
	kilo-grams	kilo-calories	mega-joules	grams	micro-grams	micro-grams	milli-grams	milli-grams	milli-grams	micro-grams	micro-grams	milli-grams	grams	milli-grams
Children														
<1	7.3	820	3.4	14	300	10.0	0.3	0.5	5.4	60	0.3	20	0.5–0.6	5–10
1–3	13.4	1360	5.7	16	250	10.0	0.5	0.8	9.0	100	0.9	20	0.4–0.5	5–10
4–6	20.2	1830	7.6	20	300	10.0	0.7	1.1	12.1	100	1.5	20	0.4–0.5	5–10
7–9	28.1	2190	9.2	25	400	2.5	0.9	1.3	14.5	100	1.5	20	0.4–0.5	5–10
Male adolescents														
10–12	36.9	2600	10.9	30	575	2.5	1.0	1.6	17.2	100	2.0	20	0.6–0.7	5–10
13–15	51.3	2900	12.1	37	725	2.5	1.2	1.7	19.1	200	2.0	30	0.6–0.7	9–18
16–19	62.9	3070	12.8	38	750	2.5	1.2	1.8	20.3	200	2.0	30	0.5–0.6	5–9
Female adolescents														
10–12	38.0	2350	9.8	29	575	2.5	0.9	1.4	15.5	100	2.0	20	0.6–0.7	5–10
13–15	49.9	2490	10.4	31	725	2.5	1.0	1.5	16.4	200	2.0	30	0.6–0.7	12–24
16–19	54.4	2310	9.7	30	750	2.5	0.9	1.4	15.2	200	2.0	30	0.5–0.6	14–28
Adult man (moderately active)	65.0	3000	12.6	37	750	2.5	1.2	1.8	19.8	200	2.0	30	0.4–0.5	5–9
Adult woman (moderately active)	55.0	2200	9.2	29	750	2.5	0.9	1.3	14.5	200	2.0	30	0.4–0.5	14–28
Pregnancy (later half)		+350	+1.5	38	750	10.0	+0.1	+0.2	+2.3	400	3.0	50	1.0–1.2	(9)
Lactation (first 6 months)		+550	+2.3	46	1200	10.0	+0.2	+0.4	+3.7	300	2.5	50	1.0–1.2	(9)

[1] Energy and Protein Requirements. Report of a Joint FAO/WHO Expert Group. FAO, Rome, 1972. — [2] As egg or milk protein. — [3] Requirements of Vitamin A, Thiamine, Riboflavin and Niacin. Report of a Joint FAO/WHO Expert Group, FAO, Rome, 1965. — [4] As retinol. — [5] Requirements of Ascorbic Acid, Vitamin D, Vitamin B12, Folate and Iron. Report of a Joint FAO/WHO Expert Group, FAO, Rome, 1970. — [6] As cholecalciferol. — [7] Calcium Requirements. Report of a FAO/WHO Expert Group, FAO, Rome, 1961. — [8] On each line the lower value applies when over 25 percent of the calories in the diet come from animal foods, and the higher value when animal foods represent less than 10 percent of calories. — [9] For women whose iron intake throughout life has been at the level recommended in this table, the daily intake of iron during pregnancy and lactation should be the same as that recommended for nonpregnant, nonlactating women of childbearing age. For women whose iron status is not satisfactory at the beginning of pregnancy, the requirement is increased, and in the extreme situation of women with no iron stores, the requirement can probably not be met without supplementation.

FOR VEGANS:
A SUMMARY OF GUIDELINES

HEALTHY ADULTS

Vegans should take care that their calorie needs are met, since a plant-based diet is generally not calorically dense. Good concentrated-calorie but healthful foods are legumes like beans, lentils, and peas, various nuts and seeds, and grains like rice, wheat, and barley (and their products).

Since protein is less digestible in plant foods, a vegan should figure his or her protein RDA at a slightly higher rate than for lacto-ovos. A vegan's weight in kilograms (pounds divided by 2.2) equals the RDA in grams.

A varied diet based on whole foods will provide enough protein if it provides enough calories. Eat whole grains, legumes, nuts, and seeds for the bulk of your protein, supplemented with dark green, leafy vegetables.

Vegans generally get generous amounts of most vitamins and minerals although they should take the same care as others regarding iron and zinc. Vitamin B_{12} need bears some examination, since nonanimal sources are sometimes hard to find. Bacterially fermented vegetable foods may contain abundant vitamin B_{12}. These include tempeh and kombu. Commercial soy milk and nutritional yeast may be fortified with the vitamin in production. Commercial supplements are *not* animal products, being made from extracts of bacteria cultures.

Vegans' intake of riboflavin may also be marginal since good vegetable sources are few and far between. The best are nutritional yeast, greens, grains, mushrooms, nuts, and beans.

Vegans don't consume the single best source of calcium for lacto-ovos, milk and milk products, so they must get it from other foods. Good plant sources include molasses, sesame, and greens. Hard water can also make a significant contribution to total intake. Vegans' need for calcium is probably much lower than the RDA of 800 mg; in fact, it is probably closer to the WHO recommendation of 400 to 500 mg. This should be easy to get from a plant diet if reasonable care is taken.

The primary vegan source of vitamin D is sunlight's action on cholesterol in the skin. Vegans who don't get much sun may run a slight risk of vitamin D deficiency, since they don't have the backup of the vitamin D present in dairy products. Obviously, they must either get more sun or take a supplement.

Vegans can meet almost all of their nutritional needs solely from easily available foods by eating a varied diet chosen from the food groups elaborated in this Appendix. The few nutrients that may be short in this diet, mainly vitamin B_{12} and iron, can be supplied by foods especially rich in those particular nutrients or by supplementation.

PREGNANT WOMEN

Pregnant women must eat an extremely well-balanced and complete diet, because they are building new tissue—the baby's growing body plus the placenta and an increased blood volume. This is the only time when more protein is actually better. Vegan mothers should get between 90 and 100 grams of protein a day. Soy products such as fortified soy milk, soy flour, and tofu are very helpful, and they can be added to a variety of foods, including casseroles and baked goods.

It is wise for pregnant vegans to eat from several food groups at the same meal and include grain products at every meal. A full complement of amino acids should always be present, since the pregnant vegan is in positive nitrogen balance.

Pregnant vegans need the same nutrients as other pregnant women and should consider supplementing iron and zinc. In addition, they should be especially careful of the nutrients that may be at risk in a normal vegan's diet—calcium, vitamins B_{12} and D, and riboflavin. Since vegans normally get high doses of folic acid, they may not need as great a supplement of this vitamin as other pregnant women.

CHILDREN

Vegan children can be just as healthy as lacto-ovo or omnivore children. As infants they should breast- or formula-feed for at least the first year to provide a firm nutritional foundation.

Since they are growing, their need for fully complemented protein is great. Growing vegan children should eat from several food groups at each meal, and include grains and soy foods to round out the diet.

Including foods from several food groups at each meal also insures that the other nutrient needs are met—those for vitamins, minerals, and energy.

Take extra care that vegan children get all the vitamin B_{12}, riboflavin, vitamin D, and zinc they need, as well as the iron, fluoride, and calcium all children need.

FOOD GROUP GUIDE

Whole Grain Products

Barley

Bread: whole wheat, rye, pumpernickel, triticale, corn, pita, French,
Italian

Breadsticks, rolls, and biscuits

Buckwheat berries and flour

Bulgur

Cereals: cooked oatmeal, whole wheat;
prepared granola, shredded wheat,
Grape Nuts

Corn: cracked, meal, and flour

Crackers: whole wheat, rye, rice

Kasha

Matzoh

Millet

Muffins

Oats

Pancakes and crepes

Pasta and noodles

Popcorn

Rice: whole grain, bran, and polishings

Rye berries and flour

Sorghum grain

Soybean flour

Sprouted grain berries

Tortillas

Triticale

Wheat: whole grain, cracked, rolled,
flour, bran, germ, meal

Wild rice

Legumes

Aduki beans

Bayo beans

Bean flakes

Bean sprouts

Black beans

Brown beans

Calico beans

Cannelini or white beans

Cowpeas (blackeyed peas)

Fava beans

Garbanzos or chick peas

Great Northern beans

Hyacinth beans

Kidney beans

Lentils

Miso

Mung beans

Navy or pea beans

Peanuts and peanut butter

Peas (dried)

Pigeonpeas

Pinto beans

Red beans

Red Mexican beans

Soybeans

Soy flour

Soy grits

Soy milk

Split peas

Tofu

Nuts and Seeds

Almonds

Brazil nuts

Cashews

Chestnuts

Coconut

Filberts

Macadamia nuts

Pecans

Pine nuts (pignolias)

Piñon nuts

Pistachio nuts

Poppyseed

Pumpkin seeds

Sesame seeds, hulled or unhulled

Squash seeds

Sunflower seeds

Walnuts

Vegetables

Amaranth
Artichokes
Asparagus
Bamboo shoots
Beets
Beet greens
Belgian endive
Broccoli
Brussels sprouts
Cabbage: common, Chinese, red, Savoy, bok choy
Carrots
Cauliflower
Celery
Chili peppers
Chives
Collards
Corn
Cucumbers
Escarole
Garlic
Garden cress
Ginger root
Green beans
Horseradish
Jerusalem artichokes
Kale
Kohlrabi
Lambsquarters
Leeks
Lettuce
Lima beans
Mushrooms
Mustard greens
New Zealand spinach
Okra
Onions
Parsley
Parsnips
Peas, common and edible-podded
Pokeweed shoots (must be cooked)
Potatoes
Pumpkin
Radishes
Rutabagas
Salsify
Scallions
Shallots
Sorrel
Spinach
Sprouts: mung, lentil, soy, alfalfa, wheat, other grains, other seeds
Summer squash: scallop, yellow, zucchini
Sweet peppers, red and green
Sweet potatoes
Swiss chard
Tomatoes, green, ripe, and canned
Tomato juice, paste, and purée
Turnips
Turnip greens
Vegetable juice cocktail
Water chestnuts
Watercress
Wax beans
Winter squash: acorn, butternut, Hubbard
Yams

Fruits (fresh, dried, or juice)

Apples
Apricots
Avocados
Bananas
Blackberries
Blueberries
Boysenberries
Cherries, sweet and sour
Cranberries
Currants
Dates
Dewberries
Figs
Gooseberries
Grapefruit
Grapes
Guava
Kumquats
Lemons
Limes

Loganberries
Loquats
Lychees
Mangoes
Muskmelons: cantaloupes, casabas, honeydews
Nectarines
Oranges
Papaws
Papayas
Peaches
Pears
Persimmons

Pineapples
Plantain
Plums
Pomegranates
Prunes
Raisins
Raspberries
Rhubarb
Strawberries
Tangelos
Tangerines
Watermelon
Youngberries

Dairy Products

Buttermilk
Cheeses:
    Bleu
    Brick
    Camembert
    Cheddar
    Cottage
    Fontina
    Gouda
    Jarlsberg
    Limburger
    Mozzarella

    Muenster
    Parmesan
    Ricotta
    Romano
    Swiss
    Tilsit
Eggs
Kefir
Milk: cow's, goat's, whole, part-skim, skim, dried
Whey, fresh or dried
Yogurt, whole, part-skim, or skim

MAIL ORDER SOURCES

Below are listed a few food suppliers who sell to individuals through the mail. Prices are usually quite reasonable, since they don't share the overhead costs of natural food or specialty stores (such as rent or mortgage on a retail store building). Many are not purely vegetarian, but they carry many good, natural, vegetarian foods.

Many of the companies will appreciate return postage and a self-addressed envelope accompanying your inquiry. Since parcel post and United Parcel Service charges increase by distance, it's a good idea to start with those closest to you.

For a more complete listing of food sources, get *Organic Directory* (Rodale Press, Emmaus, PA) or *Mail Order Food Guide,* by Anne Tilson and Carol Hersh Weiss (Simon and Schuster, New York).

General

Barth's of Long Island
270 West Merrick Rd.
Valley Stream, NY 11582

Deer Valley Farm
R. D. 1
Guilford, NY 13780

David Hodas
Pleasant Plains Natural and Organic
    Foods
P. O. Box 190
Toms River, NJ 08753

Erewhon Trading Co., Inc.
8454 Steller Dr.
Culver City, CA 93306
or
33 Farnsworth St.
Boston, MA 02210

Pavo's
119 N. Fourth St.
Minneapolis, MN 55401

Shiloh Farms
Sulphur Springs, AR 72768

Walnut Acres
Penns Creek, PA 17862

Grains, Beans, and Flour

Arrowhead Mills
P. O. Box 866
Hereford, TX 79045

El Molino Mills
P. O. Box 2025
Alhambra, CA 91803

Fearn Soya Foods (soy products)
4520 James Pl.
Melrose Park, IL 60160

Birkett Mills
Penn Yan, NY 14527

Chico-San, Inc. (brown rice products)
P. O. Box 1004
Chico, CA 95926

Leon R. Horsted Whole Grain Foods
Route 2
Waunakee, WI 53597

The Jolly Farmer
East Lempster, NH 03605

The Nauvoo Milling Co.
Nauvoo, IL 62354

Wesley K. Wilson
Wilson Milling
P. O. Box 481
La Crosse, KS 67548

Letoba Farms
Route 3, Box 180
Lyons, KS 07554

Fruits, Nuts, and Vegetables

All Organics, Inc. (mangoes and avocados)
15870 Southwest 216th St.
Miami, FL 33170

Cartwright Groves (citrus)
P. O. Box 372
Carrizo Springs, TX 78834

Covalda Date Co. (figs, dates, grapes)
P. O. Box 908
Coachella, CA 92236

Ira D. Ebersole (mangoes, limes, avocados)
25295 Southwest 194th Ave.
Homestead, FL 33030

Jaffe Brothers Natural Foods (dried and fresh fruit, nuts)
P. O. Box 636
Valley Center, CA 92082

Kaste's Morningside Orchards (apples)
Galesville, WI 54630

Lee's Fruit Co. (citrus)
P. O. Box 450
Leesburg, FL 32748

Timber Crest Farms (dried fruits)
4791 Dry Creek Rd.
Healdsburg, CA 95448

Valley Cove Ranch (citrus)
P. O. Box 603
Springville, CA 93265

Vita-Green Farms (fresh vegetables, fresh and dried fruits, nuts)
P. O. Box 878
Vista, CA 92083

Cheese

Crowley Cheese Factory (Colby)
Healdville, VT 05147

Diamond Dairy Goat Farm (goat cheese)
P. O. Box 133
North Prarie, WI 53153

The Don Edwardses (Cheddar and maple syrup)
Box 123, Townshend Road
Grafton, VT 05146

Christian Hansen's Laboratory (vegetable rennet for cheesemaking)
9015 W. Maple St.
Milwaukee, WI 53214

John Harman's Country Store (Cheddar)
Sugar Hill, NH 03585

Kutter's Cheese Factory (rennetless Cheddar and other cheeses)
857 Main Rd., Route 5
Corfu, NY 14036

Nauvoo Cheese Co. (blue-veined cheese)
Nauvoo, IL 62354

Nichols Garden Nursery (Cheddar)
1190 N. Pacific Hwy.
Albany, OR 97321

Sugarbush Farm (Cheddar)
Woodstock, VT 05091

Vegetarian Vitamin Supplements

Royal Laboratories, Inc.
633 Pearson Rd.
Paradise, CA 95969

Nonfood Products

These suppliers' products are not tested on animals nor do they contain any animal products.

Beauty Without Cruelty (cosmetics)
Distribution Center
2577 S. Superior St.
Milwaukee, WI 53207

Nermin's Dry Goods (nonanimal clothing and accessories)
R. D. #1, Box 53A
Barto, PA 19504

SUGGESTED READING

Vegetarianism

The Vegetarian Alternative—A Guide to a Healthful and Humane Diet, by Vic Sussman, 1978, Rodale Press, Emmaus, PA. Excellent all-around book on the issues involving vegetarianism.

Laurel's Kitchen—A Handbook for Vegetarian Cookery and Nutrition, by Laurel Robertson, Carol Flinders, and Bronwen Godfrey, 1976, Nilgiri Press, Petaluma, CA. Wonderful cookbook and nutrition advice. Time-in-the-kitchen oriented.

Diet for a Small Planet, by Frances Moore Lappé, revised 1975, Ballantine Books (Random House), New York. Revolutionized the concept of complementarity. Good background—not necessary to live by.

The Vegetarian Handbook—A Guide to Vegetarian Nutrition, by Roger Doyle, 1979, Crown Publishers, New York. Interesting assessment of the current literature and opinions.

General Nutrition

Some of these books are obviously geared to meat-eaters and take a somewhat conservative approach. We don't agree with everything therein; however, they are generally informative and helpful.

Realities of Nutrition, by Ronald M. Deutsch, 1976, Bull Publishing Company, Palo Alto, CA. Explained simply, logically, and completely.

Nutrition: Concepts and Controversies, by Eva May Hamilton and Eleanor Whitney, 1979, West Publishing Company, St. Paul, MN. An exhaustive, intelligent, concerned approach to the nutritional issues. Well organized.

Eating Your Way Through Life—A No-nonsense Guide to Good Nutrition for All Ages and All Eating Styles, by Judith J. Wurtman, 1979, Raven Press, New York. An approach to nutrition in daily life.

Problems with Meat, by John A. Scharffenberg, 1979, Woodbridge Press, Santa Barbara, CA. Self-explanatory, logically presented.

No-nonsense Nutrition for Your Baby's First Year, by Jo-Ann Heslin, Annette B. Natow, and Barbara C. Raven, 1978, CBI Publishing Company, Boston. Not for vegans.

As You Eat, So Your Baby Grows, by Nikki Goldbeck, 1978, Ceres Press, Woodstock, NY. A handy little book on nutrition during pregnancy.

Recommended Dietary Allowances, by the Committee on Dietary Allowances, the Food and Nutrition Board, National Research Council, ninth revision 1980, National Academy of Sciences, Washington. A complete explanation of the reasoning behind these influential numbers.

Composition of Foods . . . Raw, Processed, Prepared, by Bernice K. Watt and Annabel L. Merrill, revised 1963, U. S. Department of Agriculture, Washington (Agriculture Handbook No. 8).

Nutritive Value of American Foods in Common Units, by Catherine F. Adams, 1975, U. S. Department of Agriculture, Washington, (Agriculture Handbook No. 456).

Handbook on Human Nutritional Requirements, by R. Passmore, B. M. Nicol, and M. Narayana Rao, 1974, World Health Organization, Geneva, Switzerland. This joint effort of WHO and the Food and Agriculture Organization of the United Nations gives an international perspective on nutrient needs. Interesting comparison to the RDAs.

Shopping

The Supermarket Handbook—Access to Whole Foods, by Nikki and David Goldbeck, revised 1976, Signet Books (New American Library), New York. A great book on how to shop, including lists of exemplary brands in every food category.

Eater's Digest—The Consumer's Factbook of Food Additives, by Michael F. Jacobson, revised 1976, Anchor Press (Doubleday), Garden City, NY. The facts on food additives.

International Vegetarian Health Food Handbook, 1979–80 (published every two years), edited by Bronwen Humphreys and Derek McEwen, 1979, The Vegetarian Society of the United Kingdom, Altrincham, Cheshire, England. A listing of vegetarian societies, restaurants, products, worldwide.

Cookbooks

Tassajara Cooking, by Edward Espe Brown, 1973, Shambhala Publications, Berkeley, CA. A wonderful guide to confidence in the kitchen.

The Vegetarian Epicure, by Anna Thomas, 1972, Alfred A. Knopf, New York (hardcover), Vintage Books, division of Random House, New York (paperback), and *The Vegetarian Epicure Book Two,* by Anna Thomas, 1978, Alfred A. Knopf, New York. Delicious but very rich.

Laurel's Kitchen—A Handbook for Vegetarian Cookery and Nutrition, by Laurel Robertson, Carol Flinders, and Bronwen Godfrey, 1976, Nilgiri Press, Petaluma, CA. Good, down-to-earth, everyday recipes.

A Passion for Vegetables, by Vera Gewanter, 1980, the Viking Press, New York. Any book with a separate section on garlic sauces meets with our approval.

The Deaf Smith Country Cookbook—Natural Foods for Family Kitchens, by Marjorie Winn Ford, Susan Hillyard, and Mary Faulk Koock, 1973, Collier Books, New York. Interesting, original recipes.

The Vegetarian Feast, by Martha Rose Shulman, 1979, Harper & Row, New York. Delicious caterer-tested recipes.

Good Food Without Meat, by Ann Seranne, 1973, William Morrow, New York. Good basic recipes. Some very high in fat.

Cooking What Comes Naturally—A Natural Foods Cookbook Featuring a Month's Worth of Natural-Vegetarian Menus, by Nikki Goldbeck, 1972, Doubleday & Company, New York.

Bean Cuisine—A Culinary Guide for the Ecogourmet, by Beverly White, 1977, Beacon Press, Boston. A multitude of simple, bean-based vegetarian meals.

The Complete Vegetarian Cookbook, by Karen Brooks, 1974, Rodale Press, Emmaus, PA, re-released 1976, Pocket Books, New York.

The New York Times Natural Foods Cookbook, by Jean Hewitt, 1971, Avon
   Books, New York. Not completely vegetarian, but enough to be worth it.
Recipes for a Small Planet, by Ellen Buchman Ewald, 1973, Ballantine Books,
   New York. Interesting, creative recipes. Ignore the accounting.
International Vegetarian Cookery, by Sonya Richmond, 1965, Arco Publishing
   Company, New York.
The Vegan Kitchen, by Freya Dinshah, North American Vegetarian Society,
   Malaga, NJ.
The Oats, Peas, Beans, and Barley Cookbook, by Edyth Young Cottrell, Wood-
   bridge Press, Santa Barbara, CA. Vegan recipes.
Florence Lin's Chinese Vegetarian Cookbook, by Florence Lin, 1976, Hawthorne
   Books, New York.
Flavors of India, by Shanta Nimbark Sacharoff, 1972, 101 Productions, San
   Francisco. All vegetarian recipes.
The Complete Book of Pasta—An Italian Cookbook, by Jack Denton Scott, 1968,
   William Morrow & Company, paperback edition 1970, Bantam Books, New
   York. Not all vegetarian, but many good vegetarian examples of the versatil-
   ity of pasta.
The Book of Tofu, by William Shurtleff and Akiko Aoyagi, 1975, Autumn Press,
   Brookline, MA. Instructions for tofu-making, plus hundreds of recipes.
The All Kids' Natural Foods Cookbook, Tom Morton and the All Kids Daycare
   Center, revised 1978, Unigraphics, East Lansing, MI. Good, fun food to cook
   with your kids.

ORGANIZATIONS AND NEWSLETTERS

Vegetarian Information Service
P. O. Box 5888
Washington, DC 20014
    Nonprofit organization, press releases and packets.

North American Vegetarian Society
P. O. Box 72
Dolgeville, NY 13329
    Vegetarian Voice, $6.00 a year.

Center for Science in the Public Interest
1755 S St. NW
Washington, DC 20009
    Nutrition Action, $10.00 for one year, $18.00 for two. Many other publications.

Syndicated Vegetarian News Service
Vegetarian Society of D.C.
1455 Harvard St. NW
Washington, DC 20009
    Weekly news transcripts on vegetarian issues, $1.00.

Beauty Without Cruelty
Dr. Ethel Thurston
175 West 12th St.
New York, NY 10011
    Membership information, literature on cruelty-free products.

Vegetarian Action
835 Carroll St.
Brooklyn, NY 11215

American Vegan Society
P. O. Box H
Malaga, NJ 08328

Vegetarian Times
41 East 42nd St., Suite 921
New York, NY 10017
    One year, $12.00; two years, $22.00; three years, $30.00.

CONVERSION TABLES

WEIGHT

1 pound = 16 ounces = 454 grams = 0.454 kilograms
1 kilogram = 1000 grams = 2.2 pounds = 35.2 ounces
1 ounce = 28.375 grams
1 gram = 0.035 ounces = 0.0022 pounds
1 kilogram = 1000 grams = 1,000,000 milligrams = 1,000,000,000 micrograms

VOLUME

1 quart = 32 fluid ounces = 946 milliliters = 0.946 liters
1 liter = 1000 milliliters = 1.06 quarts = 33.83 ounces
1 milliliter = 0.034 ounces = 0.068 tablespoons = 0.203 teaspoons
1 quart = 2 pints = 4 cups = 32 fluid ounces = 64 tablespoons = 192 teaspoons
1 pint = 473 milliliters
1 cup = 236.5 milliliters
1 fluid ounce = 29.56 milliliters
1 tablespoon = 14.78 milliliters
1 teaspoon = 4.93 milliliters

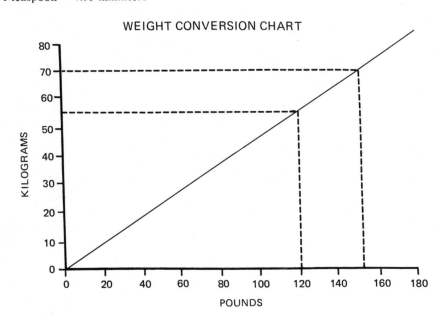

WEIGHT CONVERSION CHART

BIBLIOGRAPHY

Bibliography

GENERAL

Committee on Dietary Allowances, Food and Nutrition Board, National Research Council. *Recommended Dietary Allowances*. 9th ed. Washington: National Academy of Sciences, 1980.

Deutsch, Ronald M. *Realities of Nutrition*. Palo Alto: Bull Publishing Company, 1976.

Goodhart, Robert S., and Shils, Maurice E. (eds.). *Modern Nutrition in Health and Disease*. 5th ed. Philadelphia: Lea & Febiger, 1973.

Hamilton, Eva May, and Whitney, Eleanor. *Nutrition: Concepts and Controversies*. St. Paul: West Publishing Company, 1979.

Mitchell, Helen S., Rynbergen, Henderika J., Anderson, Linnea, and Dibble, Marjorie V. *Nutrition in Health and Disease*. 16th ed. Philadelphia: J. B. Lippincott Company, 1976.

Nutrition Foundation. *Present Knowledge in Nutrition*. 4th ed. Washington: The Nutrition Foundation, Inc., 1976.

Passmore, R., Nicol, B. M., and Narayana Rao, M. *Handbook on Human Nutritional Requirements*. Geneva: World Health Organization, 1974.

Williams, Sue. *Mowry's Basic Nutrition and Diet Therapy*. St. Louis: The C. V. Mosby Company, 1975.

American Dietetic Association. "Position Paper on food and nutrition misinformation on selected topics." *Journal of the American Dietetic Association* 66 (March 1975), pp. 277–280.

American Dietetic Association. "Position Paper on the vegetarian approach to eating." *Journal of the American Dietetic Association* 77 (July 1980), pp. 61–69.

Committee on Nutrition Misinformation, Food and Nutrition Board, National Research Council. "Vegetarian Diets." *Journal of the American Dietetic Association* 65 (August 1974), pp. 121-122.

Fleshman, Ruth P. "Eating rituals and realities." *Nursing Clinics of North America* 8 (March 1973), pp. 91-104.

Hardinge, Mervyn G., and Stare, Fredrick J. "Nutritional studies of vegetarians." *Journal of Clinical Nutrition* 2 (March 1954), pp. 73-82.

311

Hardinge, Mervyn G., and Crooks, Hulda. "Non-flesh dietaries. I. Historical background." *Journal of the American Dietetic Association* 43 (December 1963), pp. 545-549. "II. Scientific literature." *Journal of the American Dietetic Association* 43 (December 1963), pp. 550-558. "III. Adequate and inadequate." *Journal of the American Dietetic Association* 45 (December 1964), pp. 537-542.

Register, U. D., and Sonnenberg, L. M. "The vegetarian diet." *Journal of the American Dietetic Association* 62 (March 1973). pp. 253-261.

Sonnenberg, Lydia, and Hardinge, Mervyn G. "Vegetarian diets in health and disease." *Ross Timesaver* 1 (November 1974), pp. 1-5.

United States Department of Agriculture and United States Department of Health and Human Needs. "Nutrition and Your Health—Dietary Guidelines for Americans." Washington: U. S. Departments of Agriculture and Health and Human Needs, 1980.

Williams, Eleanor R. "Making vegetarian diets nutritious." *American Journal of Nursing* 75 (December 1975), pp. 2168-2173.

CHAPTER 2
CARBOHYDRATE

Brewster, Letitia, and Jacobson, Michael F. *The Changing American Diet.* Washington: Center for Science in the Public Interest, 1978.

Stillman, Irwin M., and Baker, Samm S. *The Doctor's Quick Weight Loss Diet.* Englewood Cliffs, N.J.: Prentice-Hall, Inc., 1967.

Brody, Jane E. "Alcohol offers some benefits to health as well as drawbacks." *The New York Times,* 3 October 1979.

Huang, Charles T. L., Gopalakrishna, G. S., and Nichols, Buford L. "Fiber, intestinal sterols, and colon cancer." *The American Journal of Clinical Nutrition* 31 (March 1978), pp. 516-526.

Institute of Food Technologists' Expert Panel on Food Safety and Nutrition. *Sugars and Nutritive Sweeteners in Processed Foods* Chicago: Institute of Food Technologists, 1979.

Institute of Food Technologists' Expert Panel on Food Safety and Nutrition and the Committee on Public Information. *Dietary Fiber.* Chicago: Institute of Food Technologists, 1979.

CHAPTER 3
FAT

Castelli, William (Director, Framingham Heart Study, National Heart, Lung, and Blood Institute). Telephone conversation, 11 August 1980.

Consumer Liaison Panel to the Food and Nutrition Board, National Academy of Sciences. "Consumer Nutrition Panel Breaks Ties in Protest over National Academy of Sciences Report—Heart Disease Expert Refutes Report's Conclusions" (press release). Washington: Consumer Liaison Panel to the Food and Nutrition Board, National Academy of Sciences, 11 June 1980.

Food and Nutrition Board, National Academy of Sciences. *Toward Healthful Diets.* Washington: National Academy of Sciences, 1980.

Levy, Robert I., Rifkind, Basil M., Dennis, Barbara H., and Ernst, Nancy D. *Nutrition, Lipids, and Coronary Heart Disease—A Global View.* Nutrition in Health and Disease Series, vol. 1. New York: Raven Press Publications, 1979.

Glueck, Charles J., and Connor, William E. "Diet-coronary heart disease relationships reconnoitered." *The American Journal of Clinical Nutrition* 31 (May 1978), pp. 727-737.

Hausman, Patricia. "Unscrambling the Egg 'Controversy.' " *Nutrition Action,* December 1978, pp. 3-6.

Hausman, Patricia. "Are Small Changes Small Change?" *Nutrition Action,* December 1978, p. 5.

Hausman, Patricia. "Exposing Hidden Fat." *Nutrition Action,* June 1979, pp. 3-7.

Hausman, Patricia. Telephone interviews, 29 October 1979, 8 January 1980, 11 February 1980, 6 August 1980.

Rifkind, Basil M. (Chief, Lipid Metabolism Branch, Division of Heart and Vascular Diseases, National Institutes of Health). Private letter, 26 September 1979.

Rifkind, Basil M. and Levy, Robert I. "Does Hypolipidemic Therapy Prevent Coronary Heart Disease?" *Cardiovascular Drug Therapy,* undated offprint, 8 pp.

Sanders, T. A. B., Ellis, Frey R., Path, F. R. C., and Dickerson, J. W. T. "Studies of vegans: the fatty acid composition of plasma choline phosphoglycerides, erythrocytes, adipose tissue, and breast milk, and some indicators of susceptibility to ischemic heart disease in vegans and omnivore controls." *The American Journal of Clinical Nutrition,* 31 (May 1978), pp. 805-813.

Simons, L. A., Gibson, J. Corey, Paino, C., Hosking, M., Bullock, J., and Trim, J. "The influence of a wide range of absorbed cholesterol on plasma cholesterol levels in man." *The American Journal of Clinical Nutrition* 31 (August 1978), pp. 1334-1339.

Troll, Walter, Belman, Sidney, Wiesner, Rakoma, and Shellabarger, Claire J. "Protease Action in Carcinogenesis." New York University Medical Center and Brookhaven National Laboratory, 1979.

CHAPTER 4
PROTEIN

Brewster, Letitia, and Jacobson, Michael F. *The Changing American Diet.* Washington: Center for Science in the Public Interest, 1978.

Lappe, Frances M. *Diet for a Small Planet.* Rev. ed. New York: Random House, Ballantine Books, 1975.

Scharffenberg, John A. *Problems with Meat.* Santa Barbara: Woodbridge Press Publishing Company, 1979.

Calloway, Doris. Telephone interview, 8 November 1979.

Nasset, E. S. "Role of the digestive tract in the utilization of protein and amino acids." *Journal of the American Medical Association* 164, pp. 172-177.

Nasset, E. S. "Amino acid homeostasis in the gut lumen and its nutritional significance." *World Review of Nutrition and Dietetics* 14, pp. 134-153.

Nasset, E. S., Schwartz, P., and Weiss, H. V. "The digestion of protein *in vivo.*" *Journal of Nutrition* 56, pp. 83-94.

Register, U. D., Inano, Mitsuko, Thurston, C. E., Vyhmeister, Irma B., Dysinger, P. W., Blankenship, J. W., and Horning, M. C. "Nitrogen-balance studies in human subjects on various diets." *American Journal of Clinical Nutrition* 20 (July 1967), pp. 753-759.

Williams, Eleanor. Telephone interview, 14 February 1980.

CHAPTER 5
VITAMINS AND MINERALS

Williams, Roger J. *Nutrition in a Nutshell.* Doubleday & Company, Dolphin Books, 1962.

Armstrong, Bruce K., Davis, Richard E., Nicol, Darryl J., van Merwyk, Anthony J., and Larwood, Carol J. "Hematological, vitamin B_{12}, and folate studies on Seventh Day Adventist vegetarians." *American Journal of Clinical Nutrition* 27 (July 1974), pp. 712-718.

Brody, Jane E. "Some trace elements in our diets are nutrients essential to health." *The New York Times,* 10 January 1979.

Brody, Jane E. "ABC of Vitamins Is Far from Simple." *The New York Times,* 30 May 1979.

Carmel, Ralph. "Nutritional vitamin B_{12} deficiency—possible contributory role of subtle vitamin-B_{12} malabsorption." *Annals of Internal Medicine* 88 (May 1978), pp. 647-649.

Gleeson, M. H., and Graves, P. S. "Complications of dietary deficiency of vitamin B_{12} in young Caucasians." *Postgraduate Medical Journal* 50 (July 1974), pp. 462-464.

Higginbottom, Marilyn C., Sweetman, Lawrence, and Nyhan, William L. "A syndrome of methylmalonic aciduria, homocystinuria, megaloblastic anemia and neurological abnormalities in a vitamin B_{12}-deficient breast-fed infant of a strict vegetarian." *New England Journal of Medicine* 299 (August 1978), pp. 317-323.

Hirwe, Rashmi, Jathar, V. S., Desai, Shanta, and Satoskar, R. S. "Vitamin B_{12} and potential fertility in male lactovegetarians." *Journal of Biosocial Science* 8 (1976), pp. 221-227.

Weisburger, John H., Marquardt, H., Mower, H. F., Hirota, N., Mori, H., and Williams, G. "Inhibition of Carcinogenesis: Vitamin C and the Prevention of Gastric Cancer." *Preventive Medicine* 9 (May 1980), pp. 352-361.

CHAPTER 7
PREGNANCY

Goldbeck, Nikki. *As You Eat, So Your Baby Grows.* Woodstock, N.Y.: Ceres Press, 1978.

Slattery, Jill S., Pearson, Gayle A., and Torre, Carolyn T. *Maternal and Child Nutrition: Assessment and Counseling.* New York: Appleton-Century-Crofts, 1979.

Wurtman, Judith J. *Eating Your Way Through Life*. New York: Raven Press, 1979.

Brody, Jane E. "Feeding the Unborn: Some Diet Wisdom for Mothers-to-Be." The *New York Times*, 28 November 1979.

Hasan, Judith W. "Of Pregnancy and Nutrition." *The New York Times*, 21 October 1979.

Thomas, J., and Ellis, F. R. "The health of vegans during pregnancy." *Abstracts of Communications* 36 (1977), p. 46A.

Williams, Eleanor R. "Vegetarian diets in pregnancy." *Birth and the Family Journal* 3, pp. 83–86.

CHAPTER 8
BABIES AND CHILDREN

Dinshah, Freya. *Feeding Vegan Babies*. Malaga, N. J.: American Vegan Society, Ahimsa Booklet Number 9, 1975.

Goldbeck, Nikki, and Goldbeck, David. *The Supermarket Handbook—Access to Whole Foods*. Rev. ed. New York: New American Library, Signet Books, 1976.

Heslin, Jo-Ann, Natow, Annette B., and Raven, Barbara C. *No-nonsense Nutrition for Your Baby's First Year*. Boston: CBI Publishing Company, 1978.

Howard, Frances, and Howard, Friedenstern. *Parents Handbook of Breastfeeding and Plant Foods*. Hitchin, Hertsfordshire, England, 1975.

Slattery, Jill S.; Pearson, Gayle A.; and Torre, Carolyn T. *Maternal and Child Nutrition: Assessment and Counseling*. New York: Appleton-Century-Crofts, 1979.

Wurtman, Judith J. *Eating Your Way Through Life*. New York: Raven Press, 1979.

Brody, Jane E. "New Studies Explain Protective Benefits of Mother's Milk." *The New York Times*, 4 December 1979.

Dwyer, Johanna T., Palombo, Ruth, Thorne, Halorie, Valadian, Isabelle, and Reed, Robert B. "Preschoolers on alternate life-style diets." *Journal of the American Dietetic Association* 72 (March 1978), pp. 264-270.

"Exotic diets and the infant." *British Medical Journal*, 1 April 1978.

Henig, Robin M. "The Case for Mother's Milk." *The New York Times Magazine*, 8 July, 1979.

Potterton, David. "Growing up a vegetarian." *Nursing Times*, 30 March 1978, pp. viii-xi.

Shull, Margaret W., Reed, Robert B., Valadian, Isabelle, Palombo, Ruth, Thorne, Halorie, and Dwyer, Johanna T. "Velocities of growth in vegetarian preschool children." *Pediatrics* 60 (October 1977), pp. 410-417.

"Vegetarian Diet." *Journal of the American Medical Association* 228 (April 1974), p. 460 (three letters to the editor).

Vyhmeister, Irma B., Register, U. D. and Sonnenberg, Lydia M. "Safe vegetarian diets for children." *Pediatric Clinics of North America* 24 (February 1977), pp. 203-210.

"Warning on Breast Milk." *The New York Times*, 27 November 1979.

CHAPTER 9
ATHLETES

Bogert, L. J., et al. *Nutrition and Physical Fitness.* 9th ed. Philadelphia: W. B. Saunders Company, 1973.

Mirkin, Gabe, and Hoffman, Marshall. *The Sportsmedicine Book.* Boston: Little, Brown and Company, 1978.

Åstrand, Per-Olaf. "Something old and something new . . . very new." *Nutrition Today,* June 1968, pp. 9-11.

Brody, Jane E. "Fact vs. Fantasy in the Athlete's Diet." *The New York Times,* 22 August 1979.

Fisher, Irving. "The influence of flesh eating on endurance." *Yale Medical Journal* 13 (March 1907), pp. 205-221.

CHAPTER 10
A WEIGHT-LOSS DIET

Ahrens, Richard A. *Nutrition for Health.* Basic Concepts in Health Science Series, edited by Herbert L. Jones. Belmont, CA: Wadsworth Publishing Company, 1970.

Wurtman, Judith J. *Eating Your Way Through Life.* New York: Raven Press, 1979.

CHAPTER 11
IS VEGETARIANISM HEALTHIER?

Brewster, Letitia, and Jacobson, Michael F. *The Changing American Diet.* Washington: Center for Science in the Public Interest, 1978.

Hur, Robin. *Food Reform: Our Desperate Need.* Austin: Heidelberg Publishers, 1975.

Jacobson, Michael F. *Eater's Digest—The Consumer's Factbook of Food Additives.* Rev. ed. Garden City. N. Y.: Doubleday & Company, 1976.

Scharffenberg, John A. *Problems with Meat.* Santa Barbara: Woodbridge Press, 1976.

United States Department of Health, Education, and Welfare; Public Health Service: National Institutes of Health. *Everything Doesn't Cause Cancer.* Washington: National Cancer Institute, NIH Publication No. 79-2039, 1979.

United States Senate, Select Committee on Nutrition and Human Needs. *Dietary Goals for the United States.* 2nd ed. Washington: U. S. Government Printing Office, 1977.

National Live Stock and Meat Board. *Meat and Your Heart—Heart Disease: A Matter of Diet, or Life Style?* Chicago: National Live Stock and Meat Board, 1977.

National Live Stock and Meat Board. *Meat and the Vegetarian Concept—The Case for Meat in the Human Diet: A Review of the Evidence.* Chicago: National Live Stock and Meat Board, 1976.

Adventist Health Study. "Summary of results of Adventist mortality study—

1958-65." Loma Linda, CA: School of Health, Loma Linda University, undated. (Two-page pamphlet.)

Burkitt, Denis P. "Epidemiology of cancer of the colon and rectum." *Cancer* 28 (July 1971), pp. 3-13.

Commoner, Barry, Vithayathil, Anthony J., Dolara, Piero, Nair, Subhadra, Madyastha, Prema, and Cuca, Gregory C. "Formation of mutagens in beef and beef extract during cooking." *Science* 201 (8 September 1978), 913-916.

Drasar, B. S., and Irving, D. "Environmental factors and cancer of the colon and breast." *British Journal of Cancer* 27 (1973), p. 167.

"Drugged Cows—Antibiotics are feed for thought." *Time*, 10 September 1979, p. 49.

Ellis, Frey R., Holesh, Schura, and Ellis, John W. "Incidence of osteoporosis in vegetarians and omnivores." *American Journal of Clinical Nutrition* 25 (June 1972), pp. 555-558.

Finegold, Sydney M., Sutter, Vera L., Sugihara, Paul T., Elder, Harvey A., Lehmann, Shirley M., and Phillips, Roland L. "Fecal microbial flora in Seventh Day Adventist populations and control subjects." *American Journal of Clinical Nutrition* 30 (November 1977), pp. 1781-1792.

Goldberg, Michael J., Smith, Jeffrey W., and Nichols, Ronald L. "Comparison of the fecal microflora of Seventh-Day Adventists with individuals consuming a general diet. Implications concerning colonic carcinoma." *Annals of Surgery* 186 (July 1977), pp. 97-100.

Haenszel, W. M., and Kurihara, M. "Studies of Japanese migrants: I. mortality from cancer and other diseases among Japanese in the U. S." *Journal of the National Cancer Institute* 40, p. 43.

Jakobsson, Erik. "The Nitrite Debate" (letter to the editor). *Science* 201 (8 September 1978), p. 930.

Lijinsky, W., and Shubik, P. "Benzo(α)pyrene and other polynuclear hydrocarbons in charcoal broiled meat." *Science* 145, p. 53.

National Cancer Institute. "Conference on Nutrition in the Causation of Cancer proceedings." *Cancer Research* 35 (November 1975), p. 11(2).

National Cancer Institute. "Symposium on the Role of Dietary Fiber in Health proceedings." *American Journal of Clinical Nutrition, Supplement* 31 (October 1978), p. 10.

Phillips, Roland L., Lemon, Frank R., Beeson, W. Lawrence, and Kuzma, Jan W. "Coronary heart disease mortality among Seventh-Day Adventists with differing dietary habits: a preliminary report." *American Journal of Clinical Nutrition* 31 (October 1978), pp. S191-S198.

Reddy, Bandaru W., Weisburger, John H., and Wynder, Ernst L. "Effects of high risk and low risk diets for colon carcinogenesis on fecal microflora and steroids in man." *Journal of Nutrition* 105 (1975), pp. 878-884.

Reddy, Bandaru S., and Wynder, Ernst L. "Large bowel carcinogenesis: fecal constituents of populations with disease incidence rates of colon cancer." *Journal of the National Cancer Institute* 50 (1973), p. 1437.

Walker, Alexander R. P. "Colon cancer and diet, with special reference to intakes of fat and fiber." *American Journal of Clinical Nutrition* 29 (December 1976), pp. 1417-1426.

Weisburger, John H., Marquardt, Hildegard, Mower, Howard F., Hirota, Norio,

Mori, Hideki, and Williams, Gary. "Inhibition of Carcinogenesis: Vitamin C and the Prevention of Gastric Cancer." *Preventive Medicine* 9 (May 1980), pp. 352-361.

Wynder, Ernst L., and Shigematsu, T. "Environmental factors of cancer of the colon and rectum." *Cancer* 20 (1967), p. 1520.

CHAPTER 12
SHOPPING AND STORING

Goldbeck, Nikki, and Goldbeck, David. *The Supermarket Handbook—Access to Whole Foods*. Rev ed. New York: New American Library, Signet Books, 1976.

Seelig, R. A. *Selection and Care of Fresh Fruits and Vegetables—A Consumer's Guide*. Alexandria, Va.: United Fresh Fruit Association, 1977. (Not copyrighted.)

United States. *Code of Federal Regulations*. Title 21—food and drugs—part 1 and part 101. Washington: U. S. Department of Health, Education, and Welfare, Public Health Service, Food and Drug Administration, 1980.

Brody, Jane E. "The Push for More Complete Food Labels." *The New York Times*, 21 December 1979.

Brody, Jane E. "Making Some Sense of Nutrition Labels." *The New York Times*, 2 January, 1980.

King, Seth S. "U. S. Seeking Clearer and More Precise Food Labels." *The New York Times*, 20 December 1979.

Newberry, R. E. (Assistant to the Director, Division of Regulatory Guidance, Bureau of Foods, Food and Drug Administration). Letter, 10 October 1979.

Salat, Barbara. "Natural Foods Labels, Loopholes and Lies." *Well-Being*, 44 (1979), pp. 10-14.

Sheraton, Mimi. "Vegetable Oils: Looking for What's Best." *The New York Times*, 22 August 1979.

CHAPTER 13
BRANCHING OUT FROM YOUR OWN RECIPES

Brown, Edward. *Tassajara Cooking*. Berkeley, Ca.: Shambhala, A Zen Center Book, 1973. For the inspiration.

CHAPTER 14
EATING OUT—AND OTHER MATTERS

Humphreys, Bronwen, and McEwen, Derek. *International Vegetarian Health Food Handbook, 1979-80*. Published every two years. Altrincham, Cheshire, England: The Vegetarian Society of the United Kingdom, 1979.

Morey, S. *Vegetarianism: Diets for Dogs and Cats*. Altrincham, Chesire, England: The Vegetarian Society of the United Kingdom, 1977.

Index

Vitamin B$_{12}$, 3, 79, 80, 93–96, 294; differences between vegetarian and omnivore diets, 213–214, 216; interrelationships, 114; pregnancy and, 147, 148–149; role of, RDA, sources, and comment, 119; vegans and, 94, 213–214; *See also* Cobalamin

Vitamin C, 80, 85–89, 90; deficiency, 86; nitrosamines and, 86–87; other nutrients and, 114–115; pregnancy and, 149–150; role of, RDA, sources, and comment, 118; sources of, 87; *See also* Ascorbic acid

Vitamin D, 33, 34, 80, 82–83, 101, 294–295; breastfeeding and, 161; milk and, 83; pregnancy and, 146–147; role of, RDA, sources, and comment, 118; sources for, 83; sunlight and, 83; *See also* Cholecalciferol

Vitamin E, 33, 34, 80, 83–85; interrelationships, 114; role of, RDA, sources, and comment, 118; sources of, 83–84; *See also* Tocopherol

Vitamin K, 33, 34, 80, 85; role of, RDA, sources, and comment, 118

Vitaminlike substances, 98

Vitamins, 55, 78–98; athlete's needs for, 182–184; categories of, 80; fat soluble, 80–85; guidelines, 122; interrelationships, 113–115; meaning of, 78–79; water soluble, 85–98; *See also* Minerals

Vitamin supplements, *see* Supplements

Voit, Carl von, 54

Water: athlete's need for, 174–177; flurodation of, 112

Water Diet, 28

Watermelons, season for, choosing, and storing, 260

Water-soluble vitamins, 85–98; recommended daily nutrient intake, 290; *See also* individual vitamins

Weaning, 161–163

Weight-loss diet, 189–206; activity level, 193–194; Basal Metabolic Rate (BMR) formula, 192–193; breakfast (every day), 198; decreasing calories, 194–195; dinner (recipes), 199–203; by expending calories, 191–192; guidelines, 206; lunch (every day), 198) medical problem and, 191; overweight question, 190; pinch test, 190–191; psychology of gaining and losing, 204–206; rules for, 196–198; 1200 calorie-a-day, 195–203

Wilson, Dr. Edward O., 5

Winter squash, season for, choosing, and storing, 259

World Health Organization, 42, 90, 100

World War II, 54

Xylose, 15

Yogurt, selecting and storing, 247–248

Zinc, 101, 107–108, 294; best sources of, 108; differences between vegetarian and omnivore diets, 214; interrelationships, 115; role of, RDA, sources, and comment, 120